Elaine Linderman   July 2015

Megan Galbally · Martien Snellen ·
Andrew Lewis

Editors

Psychopharmacology and Pregnancy

Treatment Efficacy, Risks, and Guidelines

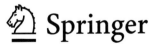 Springer

Editors
Megan Galbally
Martien Snellen
Perinatal Mental Health
Mercy Hospital for Women
Heidelberg, Australia

Andrew Lewis
School of Psychology
Deakin University
Victoria, Australia

ISBN 978-3-642-54561-0   ISBN 978-3-642-54562-7 (eBook)
DOI 10.1007/978-3-642-54562-7
Springer Heidelberg New York Dordrecht London

Library of Congress Control Number: 2014941111

Printed on acid-free paper

Springer is part of Springer Science+Business Media (www.springer.com)

Psychopharmacology and Pregnancy

Contents

Introduction: Pharmacological Treatments of Mental Disorders in Pregnancy

Megan Galbally, Andrew J. Lewis, and Martien Snellen

Abstract

This book provides an overview of the latest research and clinical practice recommendations for the use of psychopharmacology in pregnancy. Authors include leading researchers and clinicians in this field from across the globe with a focus on how the latest research findings can be translated into clinical care.

Keywords

Psychopharmacology • Pregnancy • Maternal mental illness

This book brings together experts from around the globe in the area of pharmacological treatment of mental disorders in pregnancy. In addition to chapters which focus on the treatment of specific mental disorders this book has included chapters which focus on the broader and highly relevant issues, such as informed consent, that face clinicians and researchers in examining treatment for perinatal mental illness. As the implications of maternal mental illness for maternal and fetal well-being become apparent, perinatal mental illness has become a focus for those working in mental health, obstetric and maternity care, pediatrics, and primary health care.

There is much room for optimism in the field of perinatal mental health. There is now a substantial improvement in the awareness and detection of mental disorder over pregnancy. The public awareness of postnatal depression in particular has grown substantially in the light of increasing media awareness, high profile members of the public discussing their experiences, and mental health promotional

M. Galbally (✉) • M. Snellen
Perinatal Mental Health, Mercy Hospital for Women, 163 Studley Rd, Heidelberg 3084, VIC, Australia
e-mail: mgalbally@mercy.com.au

A.J. Lewis
Faculty of Health, School of Psychology, Deakin University, Burwood, Australia

M. Galbally et al. (eds.), *Psychopharmacology and Pregnancy*,
DOI 10.1007/978-3-642-54562-7_1, © Springer-Verlag Berlin Heidelberg 2014

activities. There are also significant advances in population screening for high prevalence disorders such as depression and anxiety in pregnancy and in the postpartum. Traditional and religiously inspired views about mother's mental health over pregnancy have been replaced with scientific accounts of the no less miraculous processes of fetal development, and the profound interplay between maternal and fetal biology is increasingly a focus of research.

And yet there remain significant challenges in the psychiatric field, particularly in terms of the provision of adequate services to all members of the public and across both developed and developing countries. Also in terms of the availability of effective interventions targeted to those who are likely to benefit the most.

Alongside the increasing awareness of maternal mental health conditions over pregnancy, there have been increases in antidepressant prescription rates in countries such as Canada, the USA, and Denmark (Andrade et al. 2008; Cooper et al. 2007; Oberlander et al. 2006; Jimenez-Solem et al. 2013), although studies also suggest that many women precipitously cease antidepressants upon becoming pregnant due to concerns about fetal well-being with one study showing up to 60 % ceased upon becoming pregnant (Ververs et al. 2006). A study of those women who abruptly discontinued their antidepressants found 70 % had adverse effects and 30 % became suicidal (Einarson 2005). A study specifically of relapse of depression in pregnancy found of those who continued to take their antidepressant medication only 26 % relapsed compared to 68 % who discontinued their treatment (Cohen et al. 2006).

While much of the focus of perinatal mental health research and clinical care is concerned with high prevalence disorders such as depression and anxiety. A focus on low prevalence disorders, such as schizophrenia and bipolar disorder, is emerging as evidence for high-risk pregnancies associated with both these conditions and the treatments used emerges. Antipsychotic medications, particularly the second generation, have increased in rates of prescription in the general population including women during the fertile period (Alexander et al. 2011). The increasing rate of use is attributed to a broadening of indications and common uses for these medications and hence understanding the risks and benefits of treatment in pregnancy is now relevant to conditions beyond bipolar disorder and schizophrenia.

Understanding the research basis upon which risks and benefits of antidepressant treatment are assessed is vital to accurately convey and translate the latest findings to women in this ever-growing field of literature. This book has therefore sought not just to provide comprehensive chapters on managing women in pregnancy with psychopharmacological agents but provide some of the essential background tools to allow ongoing appraisal of the literature. This includes the ethical and legal obligations around informed consent which in pregnancy takes on the added dimension of fetal and child well-being which is covered in this chapter. Understanding the principles of research methodology specifically to exposure research in pregnancy is essential to any appraisal of research findings and this is discussed in Chap. 2. The biological basis upon which concerns arise for exposure to psychotropic medication during fetal development and equally relevant an understanding of maternal mental illness as an exposure in its own right form Chaps. 3 and 4.

The remainder of the book systematically covers specific mental illnesses in pregnancy with a review of the current literature of risks and benefits of pharmacological treatment. This has deliberately been structured under the disorder rather than the treatment to keep a strong clinical focus and ensure relevance to day-to-day clinical care in pregnancy.

Each of these chapters is focused on a specific disorder and covers the natural history of the condition across the perinatal period. In addition, the chapters examine the evidence for the efficacy of drug treatments for that specific disorder in the perinatal period. This includes a discussion of the issue of study quality and replication as well as gaps in the evidence base. Special attention is paid to the potential dangers of different treatment options for both mother and fetus, covering risks of malformation, pregnancy and obstetric risks, neonatal risks, and possible long-term consequences.

The final chapters cover Complementary and Alternative treatments and ECT in pregnancy. Both are important areas of clinical care which can be indicated or requested treatments for mental illness in pregnant women.

This book is designed for a range of professionals and interested member of the public. The consideration of clinical risk *vs.* benefit of pharmacological treatment is also highlighted in each chapter. The emphasis throughout is on a collaborative model of care between treating clinicians and women and their families to seek the best outcomes in pregnancy. We have sought to ensure this book has wide relevance with an international focus and hence we have solicited papers from a wide range of clinicians and researchers across from around the globe.

The wide range of research covered in this book indicates the importance of perinatal mental health with implications for maternal, child, and wider family well-being. This book serves as a resource of current findings in this important area of health care but also serves as a lens to view future research in perinatal mental health.

References

Alexander GC, Gallagher SA, Mascola A, Moloney RM, Stafford RS. Increasing off-label use of antipsychotic medications in the United States, 1995–2008. Pharmacoepidemiol Drug Saf. 2011;20(2):177–84. doi:10.1002/pds.2082.

Andrade SE, Raebel MA, Brown J, Lane K, Livingston J, Boudreau D, et al. Use of antidepressant medications during pregnancy: a multisite study. Am J Obstet Gynecol. 2008;198(2):194.e1–5. doi:10.1016/j.ajog.2007.07.036. S0002-9378(07)00915-5.

Cohen LS, Altshuler LL, Harlow BL, Nonacs R, Newport DJ, Viguera AC, et al. Relapse of major depression during pregnancy in women who maintain or discontinue antidepressant treatment. JAMA. 2006;295(5):499–507. doi:10.1001/jama.295.5.499. 295/5/499.

Cooper WO, Willy ME, Pont SJ, Ray WA. Increasing use of antidepressants in pregnancy. Am J Obstet Gynecol. 2007;196(6):544.e1–5. doi:10.1016/j.ajog.2007.01.033. S0002-9378(07) 00144-5.

Einarson A. Abrupt discontinuation of psychotropic drugs following confirmation of pregnancy: a risky practice. J Obstet Gynaecol Can. 2005;27(11):1019–22.

Jimenez-Solem E, Andersen JT, Petersen M, Broedbaek K, Andersen NL, Torp-Pedersen C, et al. Prevalence of antidepressant use during pregnancy in Denmark, a Nation-Wide Cohort Study. PLoS One. 2013;8(4):e63034.

Oberlander TF, Warburton W, Misri S, Aghajanian J, Hertzman C. Neonatal outcomes after prenatal exposure to selective serotonin reuptake inhibitor antidepressants and maternal depression using population-based linked health data. Arch Gen Psychiatry. 2006;63 (8):898–906. doi:10.1001/archpsyc.63.8.898. 63/8/898.

Ververs T, Kaasenbrood H, Visser G, Schobben F, de Jong-van den Berg L, Egberts T. Prevalence and patterns of antidepressant drug use during pregnancy. Eur J Clin Pharmacol. 2006;62 (10):863–70. doi:10.1007/s00228-006-0177-0.

The Process of Obtaining Informed Consent When Prescribing Psychopharmacology in Pregnancy

2

Martien Snellen, Geoff Thompson, and Neill Murdoch

Abstract

As with most things, in order to understand a modern concept it is useful to have knowledge as to its historical evolution. To comprehend fully the ethical and legal principle of informed consent in the context of the provision of psychopharmacological treatment in pregnancy this is essential. It is a story of transformation that began with the Beneficence model that is characterised by maximum physician discretion, and ends with the Autonomy model that emphasises increased patient involvement.

Keywords

Informed consent • Psychopharmacology • Pregnancy • Guidelines

As with most things, in order to understand a modern concept it is useful to have knowledge as to its historical evolution. To comprehend fully the ethical and legal principle of informed consent in the context of the provision of psychopharmacological treatment in pregnancy this is essential. It is a story of transformation that began with the Beneficence model that is characterised by maximum physician discretion, and ends with the Autonomy model that emphasises increased patient involvement.

The current approach to decision-making in medicine is governed by the informed consent doctrine that aims to philosophically and legally preserve a patient's right to self-determination. It was once considered ill-advised to include

M. Snellen (✉)
Mercy Hospital for Women, Heidelberg, Australia
e-mail: msnellen@iprimus.com.au

G. Thompson
Private practitioner, Melbourne, Australia

N. Murdoch
Victorian Bar, Melbourne, Australia

M. Galbally et al. (eds.), *Psychopharmacology and Pregnancy*,
DOI 10.1007/978-3-642-54562-7_2, © Springer-Verlag Berlin Heidelberg 2014

patients in treatment decision-making: now it is mandatory. The history of the concept of informed consent is also the history of the nature of the doctor–patient relationship and discloses a shift in the focus of control from one to the other.

The evolution of the modern doctrine of informed consent began with the idea that the medical profession should determine what information regarding the risks of any proposed treatment is sufficient. The irony here was that the law had started to recognise that doctors were obliged to inform their patients as to the relevant risks, but left the question of whether that obligation had been complied with in the sole hands of the medical profession itself. Thus, the decision as to what course to follow might have been the patient's, but that decision could only be made on the basis of the information that a doctor thought reasonable to provide in accordance with contemporary medical standards. This situation continues in the UK (Bolam v Friern Hospital Management Committee 1957; Sidaway v Board of Governors of Bethlehem Royal Hospital 1985) and elsewhere, including many states in the USA (Wear 1998; Faden and Beauchamp 1986). In other places, including a number of other states in the USA (Canterbury v Spence 1972), Canada (Reibl v Hughes 1980), South Africa (Castell v De Greef 1994) and Australia (Rogers v Whitaker 1992), the courts determined what amount of imparted information should be considered sufficient by reference to a notional standard of a reasonable person in the position of the particular patient. Further, in some jurisdictions like Australia, a subjective element has been added as an alternative so that it is the particular patient who determines sufficiency, at least to the extent that the doctor knows or ought to know of that person's views.

2.1   Beneficence

Until the middle of the last century the prevailing doctrine that informed medical practice was that of Beneficence which emerged from the Hippocratic tradition and its requirement for doctors to have an ethical obligation to act, to the best of their judgment, for the medical benefit of their patients, whilst at the same time doing no harm. In this tradition doctors were encouraged to exercise authority over obedient patients, albeit in a benign and paternalistic way. It was very much a situation where doctor knew best and patients, if they wanted to continue to be treated, acted accordingly. Essentially, at a time where therapies were often of limited benefit and the reliance on the placebo effect was great, it was considered that benevolent deception was a moral and justifiable act. Should the withholding of information be deemed by the doctor to be potentially beneficial for the patient it was considered clearly justifiable. As the word itself conveys, beneficence was the practice of one person doing good for, or acting for the benefit of, another. The "other" in this sense, being the patient, had a purely passive role and barely participated in the decision-making process. What was sought was consent for treatment that was implied by the very act of consulting a doctor.

During the Enlightenment, under the tutorage of such men as Benjamin Rush in America and John Gregory in Scotland, it was advocated that doctors have a duty to be truthful in their disclosures to patients. They introduced a sentiment that improved medical outcomes would emerge from greater patient understanding; however, they did not consider that doctors should deviate from their requirement that patients act exactly as they suggested. It was, in fact, the patients' ability to share in their doctor's wisdom that was thought to contribute to overall medical prognosis and thus to be beneficial. Thomas Percival's *Medical Ethics* (1803) continued to support this tradition (Percival 1803) and it was not until 1980 that the American Medical Association amended their code of conduct to remove much of this ethic.

2.2   Autonomy

The term informed consent was first used in a legal context by a Californian court in 1957 (Salgo v Leland Stanford Junior University Board of Trustees 1957) and it was not until the 1970s that the informed consent doctrine was broadly developed by bioethicists and lawmakers and widely applied within medical practice (Dolgin 2010). The driving force behind this transformation was the emergence of the right to self-determination in the context of litigation in the USA addressing a constitutional right to privacy (Griswold v Connecticut 1965). The right to self-determination was equated to personal autonomy, itself a concept familiar to the common law where it reflects the "central tenet" that a person is legally responsible for their choices, as a corollary of which that person is entitled to make those choices free from unjustifiable interference from others (McHugh 1999) The development in the law of express notions of self-determination and autonomy in informed consent was associated with the promotion of these ideas in moral theory and, most relevantly, clinical practice (Faden and Beauchamp 1986).

It was determined that patients have the right to protect their bodily integrity, which entitles them to evaluate the different risks and dangers associated with each medical decision prior to giving consent (Beauchamp and Childress 2009). Associated rights include the rights to receive information, to consent to or refuse treatment and to have confidentiality and privacy maintained. At the same time the obligation of beneficence has been maintained.

It has been asserted that the initial imperative to seek consent for medical treatment emerged in the early twentieth century as a response to lawsuits rather than a moral imperative to respect patient autonomy (Will 2011). In the second half of the century the bioethics movement gained momentum in its endeavour to address the imbalance of knowledge within the doctor–patient relationship. In a seminal American case the right to self-determination was expanded when a judge considered that "true consent to what happens to one's self is the informed exercise of a choice, and that entails an opportunity to evaluate knowledgeably the options available" (Canterbury v Spence 1972). The Autonomy model is founded on the assumption that a patient will be able to make an informed decision consistent with their subjective sense of well-being so long as they are given adequate information.

In most cases the doctor's ethical duty to act in the patient's best interests and, above all, to do no harm will coincide with both the legal duty to exercise reasonable care and skill in the management of that patient's condition and with the patient's right to determine what course that management should take. However, there will be some cases where these principles conflict. What is still not universally accepted by the medical profession is the notion that the patient's right to autonomy overrides the doctor's view of what is best for the patient. To respect patient autonomy is to accept that the patient has the right to make bad decisions. In these circumstances the doctor's ethical and legal obligations are discharged in most jurisdictions by providing the patient with all relevant information as to the patient's options, including the risks and benefits of each, advising the patient as to what the doctor considers to be the best course to follow, thereby giving the patient the benefit of the doctor's expertise and experience and then allowing the patient to decide what to do.

Informed consent is now considered to be given when a patient agrees to a proposed treatment based on their participation in a risk: benefit analysis. For this to occur a patient acting autonomously must be competent to understand and decide for themselves, be free of any third party coercion and be provided with all of the relevant facts needed to make a decision. The informed consent principle is still one that exists in evolution with the medical and legal professions, and bioethicists and philosophers exerting influence on the fine-tuning. This is so despite the relative lack of change in the law over the last two decades in most of the common law world.

In the area of perinatal psychiatry there is a potential for the unborn child to come to harm secondary to any proposed treatment. A mother will, in effect, be consenting on its behalf. This raises difficult questions. Plainly, the unborn (or yet to be conceived) foetus is not an autonomous being. It cannot make any determination for itself and is wholly dependent on its mother. In many legal systems it has no legal status at all until it is born alive. In others, legislatures have intervened to create legal personality in the foetus, usually for the purposes of the law in relation to abortion.

It is well accepted that, once born, a person may sue a third party for injuries caused in utero. For the doctor considering the prescription of medication to a woman considering pregnancy this confirms the need for the interests of the unborn to be given due weight. There will be circumstances where the interests of the mother and her foetus will not coincide: where the mother's mental illness requires treatment without which her life may be in danger but where that treatment will endanger the health of the foetus. Informed consent in such a case will be of the greatest importance, for the psychiatrist treating the mother will have to do so while owing duties both to her and the unborn child.

2.3 What Is "Informed Consent"?

Much has been written about what is meant by the expression "informed consent" and we do not propose to add greatly to it. It has come to be used as a term of art, although plainly it means different things to different people. We regard it as a useful shorthand expression for a complex and critically important clinical tool with important legal ramifications. However, the law has disparaged the phrase as "somewhat amorphous" (Rogers v Whitaker 1992) and "apt to mislead" (Rogers v Whitaker 1980). In the legal context this may be so, as the phrase does not reflect the fundamental precepts of the law of negligence, in which so many of the cases have arisen that require there to be a duty to take reasonable care, a breach of that duty and damage as a result.

Even in the clinical context the phrase has its limitations, as it must cover situations where, by way of example, there is no consent but refusal. The fact is that the phrase is too well established in different disciplines now to be avoided. As with any other such convenient expression, it must be used with care.

We use it to refer to the process whereby a clinician secures the authorisation of their patient to follow a particular course of medical management, having disclosed to the patient the important features and risks of that course, together with the features and risks of any alternative course open to the patient so that the patient's decision can be regarded as relevantly informed. The requirements of this broad definition are a different matter and it to them we now turn.

2.4 Requirements of the Law and of Ethical Practice

The relevant legal requirements are principally derived from the law of negligence. That is to say, the relevant requirements did not arise from any ethical obligation or clinical practice but from the content of the duty owed by the medical practitioner to a patient where a breach of that duty causes injury.

It is the medical practitioner's duty to communicate to a patient who is considering a medical intervention the material risks of the proposed intervention. The High Court of Australia (Rogers v Whitaker 1980) has held that a risk inherent in the proposed treatment is material if, in the circumstances of a particular case, either:

1. A reasonable person in the patient's position, if warned of the risk, would be likely to attach significance to it (the objective limb); or
2. if the medical practitioner is or should reasonably be aware that the particular patient, if warned of the risk, would be likely to attach significance to it (the subjective limb).

They later added that it is in every case, barring emergency or necessity, the choice of the patient whether to undergo particular medical treatment and that the choice is meaningless unless it is made on the basis of relevant information and advice.

As to the materiality of the risks which may be entailed in the proposed treatment, Australian law requires that the doctor must consider reasonably foreseeable risks, being those which are not farfetched or fanciful, even though they may be extremely unlikely to occur; the precise and particular character of an injury or the precise sequence of events leading to an injury need not be foreseeable. It is sufficient if the kind or type of injury was foreseeable (Rosenberg v Percival 2001). In considering the materiality of a risk, however, some reference must be made to particular rather than general risks if accurate information is to be conveyed concerning the severity of the potential injury or the likelihood of its occurrence.

The situation, which pertains in Australia, is to be contrasted with the law in the UK. There, the House of Lords have determined that a doctor is not negligent if he acts in accordance with a practice accepted at the time as proper by a responsible body of medical opinion even though other doctors adopt a different practice. In short, the law imposes the duty of care, but the standard of care is a matter of medical judgment (Sidaway v Board of Governors of Bethlehem Royal Hospital 1985). This is the so-called Bolam principle (Bolam v Friern Hospital Management Committee 1957). The only requirement imposed on the body of professional opinion supportive of the doctor's position is that it be, variously, respectable, responsible or reasonable in the sense of not being illogical (Bolitho v City and Hackney Health Authority 1998).

The contrast between the two approaches is clear: in the former, the question of what information must be conveyed is determined by reference to the patient and their perspective. In the latter, the question is determined by reference to a body of responsible professional opinion.

It has been the complaint of the medical profession that while the law has imposed a set of mandatory requirements it has made no attempt to inform as to how compliance with those requirements can be achieved.

A different perspective is indicated. Informed consent should not be seen as onerous compliance with minimum legal requirements but as means of ensuring good communication with patients which is positively beneficial in its own right, through increasing patient understanding, managing expectations, improving compliance and fostering a sense of empowerment and control. This perspective requires consideration of what the doctor is engaged in and trying to achieve.

2.5   Principles of Informed Consent

The bioethicists Beauchamp and Childress (2009) suggest that there are seven key elements that constitute the principle of informed consent: threshold elements (competence and voluntariness), transformation elements (disclosure, recommendation and understanding) and consent elements (decision and authorisation). These will be considered with specific reference to the prescribing of psychopharmacological medicines during pregnancy.

2.6 Competence

In general, a patient is considered to be competent if they can understand a treatment option, deliberate regarding its risks and benefits, form a decision based on this deliberation and communicate their decision adequately. Whilst competence may be easy to define, incompetence is not. A patient may be competent in that they meet these criteria but may be a minor according to the law of the land and incompetent for that reason. Similarly, a person committed for involuntary treatment may lawfully be so treated even though they express an unwillingness to be treated. There is great variation across legal jurisdictions as to what age a person must be before they are allowed to make certain autonomous decisions and the extent of mental and psychological disturbance of capacity required before a third party or surrogate is able to make decisions on their behalf. As a general principle all adults are presumed competent to consent and all children are presumed to be incompetent. In practice, the process of obtaining informed consent may not differ where the patient is incompetent but not lacking the capacity to understand, deliberate, decide and communicate. Their involvement in discussions and agreement to what is proposed should be obtained.

Competence can be seen in absolute terms: it either exists or it does not. Capacity in the competent is to be distinguished: it exists on a spectrum between the highly educated, materially well off, physically and mentally unimpaired mature adult to the illiterate, poor, physically unwell, depressed, brain injured person suffering chronic pain and under the influence of medication or other substances. Capacity in this way overlaps to a large extent with the voluntary nature of the process.

2.7 Voluntariness

Voluntariness is a key element of the greater principle of autonomy. It refers to the idea that a person acts voluntarily if they will an action in the absence of external constraints and coercions. However, in many jurisdictions surrogate decision makers are authorised to treat patients when they are deemed to lack the competence to make decisions on their own behalf that are conducive to their best health outcome. The involuntary treatment of psychosis and depressive suicidality sit as prime examples.

Coercion may involve the making of a threat that will, if carried out, be to the perceived detriment of the patient. A doctor who informs a patient that they will commit them to involuntary treatment unless they take their medication is acting in a coercive way, even though their goal is in the patient's interests. The same result may be achieved in another more acceptable way, if the doctor were to explain to the patient that the patient needs to continue to take their medication lest they become so unwell that they require hospitalisation.

Perceptions are important in considering how a doctor's disclosure of information is to be regarded. There is an imbalance of knowledge and authority between doctor and patient, not least in a mental health setting. This imbalance may create a perception in the patient that they have no real choice but to comply with the doctor's suggested course of action. If the patient's will is in fact overborne the authorisation given by the patient to the doctor is not valid.

Others may inappropriately influence a patient, including family members. Partners and spouses of pregnant women are relevant here. Care must be taken to see that it is the patient who makes the relevant decision, and that the patient takes it freely, rather than at the behest of or to please someone else. Mostly, putative fathers of unborn children do not have legal rights in relation to those children although they may have, with the agreement of the patient, an important supportive role to play in obtaining informed consent.

2.8   Disclosure and Recommendation

Disclosure refers to the provision by a doctor to a patient of relevant information regarding the condition from which the patient suffers, any investigations required, its prognosis, the possibilities for management, a recommended course of management together with information as to the material risks and benefits of a proposed course and such alternative courses of management which might be open (which may include doing nothing).

Disclosure is about communication between doctor and patient. It is made in furtherance of the patient's autonomy, which is achieved by increasing the patient's understanding of their situation. Like all forms of communication, disclosure has to be tailored to the circumstances in order to be effective.

As a matter of general principle, the following must be considered in relation to disclosure of risks:
1. the nature of the risk (what it is)
2. the magnitude of the risk (how big it is)
3. the probability the risk might materialise (how likely it is)
4. the imminence of risk materialisation (when it will happen)

As a result of legal proceedings within courtrooms across the globe three basic standards of disclosure have emerged: the proper professional practice standard, the reasonable person standard and the subjective standard.

The first two of these standards have been discussed above. The third, which requires the informational needs and concerns of each patient, no matter how idiosyncratic, to be ascertained and addressed by their doctor in order for the informed consent process to be properly completed, is not legally required practice everywhere. The difficulties of complying with such a standard are obvious. What the patient regards as relevant is deemed to be so regardless of the doctor's views as to its importance. It may objectively be unimportant. With subjectivity comes the dilemma as to how can a doctor know what is important to any particular patient? Good practice, and to some extent legal requirement, indicates an investigation into what the particular patient is worried about. Legal requirement, in Australia, renders necessary a simple question of the patient, at an appropriate stage in the process, as to what their concerns are.

Many cases present an obvious path to follow: some less so. Some involve insoluble dilemmas—notably in this area where a medication necessary to treat a maternal mental illness creates an adverse risk to the foetus of such magnitude and probability that either the mother takes a chance by not taking the medication (to her own detriment and thereby that of the foetus), or by taking the medication (to the risk of the foetus's well-being and thereby the mother later on) or there is no pregnancy. Where the decision involves these considerations the ethical implications for the advising doctor are great.

Disclosure is not exclusively a matter of substance. It cannot be achieved solely by dissemination of written information. Where, when and how it occurs, the type of language used and the patient's underlying cultural beliefs all affect the effectiveness of the doctor's attempts to communicate.

When it comes to the prescription of psychopharmacological medicines during pregnancy both doctors and patients are inevitably required to tolerate many uncertainties. The knowledge base regarding the full implications for both mother and child are incomplete at best. However, decisions need to be made and actions taken in order to relieve the suffering of the mentally ill. As data accumulates recommendations and standard practice may change. What can be considered reasonable practice at one particular point in time can be considered to be ill-advised at another.

One issue that causes a struggle at the interface between medicine and the law relates to the degree of certainty regarding research. A difference exists between what is established and what is speculated. As we will see in the next chapter methodological issues frequently make it difficult to advise regarding risk with any certainty. The courts and patients alike frequently find it difficult to distinguish between evidence-based risk and reports that suggest an association between exposure and outcome.

Unfortunately this has often resulted in the "knee jerk" response to cease all prescribing of psychotropic medications in the perinatal setting. If it becomes a choice between the doctor being held to account or the illness itself being held to account for any adverse outcome many doctors feel that it is legally safer to expose the patient to the latter risk. All in all there have been far fewer lawsuits filed as a consequence of non-treatment than there have been for negative outcomes associated with treatment. Such defensive medicine can but only lead to a lowering of health-care standards. Thus balancing the risk of foetal exposure with the risk of untreated psychiatric disorder places the clinician "between a teratologic rock and a clinical hard place" (Cohen et al. 1989).

2.9   Understanding

The concept of understanding is a vexed issue. It cannot be presumed that the provision of medical information results in any particular patient appreciating the full nature and implications of any proposed treatment. Studies have consistently revealed that following any medical consultation only around 20–60 % of the disclosed information is actually retained by the patient, the greater the amount of information presented the lower the proportion correctly recalled, and almost half of the information that is recalled is incorrect (Kessels 2003).

It is the doctor's obligation to ensure that his or her patient has understood the information that has been disclosed. This may be done by discussing the information with the patient, asking that the information be repeated in summary by the patient and asking questions of the patient as to what they think is likely to happen to them (and their baby) and why. Again, the language used is critical.

In order to enhance a patient's right to exercise autonomy they need to be given the best opportunity possible to understand the information that is given to them. Being provided with written material and time before a decision is made to adopt any particular treatment certainly increases the chances that a patient is able to offer informed consent. We advise that whenever possible the prescribing of psychopharmacological treatment in the perinatal context be separated in time from the consultation that offers opinion and recommendations, that patients are encouraged to explore with their doctor any uncertainties or lack of understanding and that this always occurs in a setting conducive to good communication.

2.10 Decision and Authorisation

Once again, it needs to be stated that for informed consent to be obtained any decision made by a patient to accept treatment needs to be free of coercion, undue persuasion, manipulation by misinformation or otherwise and maleficence. The principle of autonomy requires that a patient is able to not only give consent to any proposed treatment, but they are also allowed to withhold such consent either temporarily or permanently, or to change their position, and to do any of these things without incurring the wrath of their doctor or to find the therapeutic relationship ended.

Once a joint decision is made to embark on any particular treatment this action needs to be authorised. For this to be achieved the patient must unequivocally inform the doctor as to their decision—as to what course of management is to be followed. How this is to be evidenced is a matter of no clinical importance but may be forensically significant. In surgery this action has been enshrined in the signing of a consent form, a practice that has come to be synonymous (wrongly) with obtaining informed consent. In psychiatry consent forms are not much used outside of the context of Electroconvulsive Therapy, although there is no particular reason why this is so. When it comes to the prescribing and administration of medicines in psychiatry the patient's authorisation is given orally in the course of a consultation with their doctor.

We have described the obtaining of informed consent as a process for good reason. It should not be seen as a one-off event to be attended to in the course of a single consultation. We envisage that the necessary steps—consultation, investigation, diagnosis, disclosure, recommendation, discussion, understanding, consideration, further discussion if need be, followed by decision, authorisation and communication—may take place over a number of consultations each taking some time.

2.11   What to Make of It All?

Doctors frequently find themselves in the uncomfortable position of having to treat a woman with mental illness who is either pregnant or planning to become pregnant. The issue is further complicated by the fact that more than half of the pregnancies in this population group are unplanned and exposure to psychotropic medications may have already occurred during the formative first trimester before they become aware of the fact of pregnancy. As a further complication the statute of limitations in many jurisdictions allows for the filing of civil lawsuits for medical malpractice related to pregnancy and birth for many years after exposure to any prescribed medication and any proposed injury. The net result is that fewer doctors may be willing to treat women with mental illness during the reproductive years, thus rendering more vulnerable an already vulnerable patient population (Einarson and Koren 2007). In the absence of established clinical guidelines for the prescribing of psychotropic medications during pregnancy each doctor and patient is forced to run a medico-legal gauntlet.

It needs to be remembered that the baseline risk for malformation in the general population is 2–4 %. When a birth defect or negative pregnancy outcome occurs it cannot be automatically assumed that any prescribed medication was the causative agent. As will be discussed in other chapters untreated mental illness in itself has been shown to adversely affect many pregnancy- and birth-related outcomes.

In order to provide optimal patient care and reduce overall medico-legal risk we wish to propose the following:

Guidelines for obtaining informed consent for psychopharmacological treatment in pregnancy

1. Establish the diagnosis through standard practice: interview, examination and investigation, explaining each step to the patient. Inform the patient of the diagnosis once reached, explaining the nature of the illness and its natural course if untreated. Should doubt remain, or disagreement exist between the offered opinion and the patient's conceptualization of their problems, seek a second opinion from a suitable colleague.
2. Ascertain whether the proposed treatment can be considered to be standard practice and openly disclose any proposed actions that exist outside of established clinical guidelines.
3. Propose suggested treatment whilst at the same time elaborating upon alternative treatment options. Explain that it is the patient who must decide what course to follow but that it is for the doctor to give advice as to what to do. Explain the nature of the proposed treatment and compare it to the alternatives—including the option, if it is one, of doing nothing.

4. Establish that a patient is competent to agree to any proposed treatment and that they are able to give this consent voluntarily. Any external influences should be assessed and influences that might interfere with the patient's independent judgment addressed; if the patient is not competent, or cannot decide voluntarily, consideration should be given to the requirements of local mental health legislation before proceeding with any form of involuntary treatment.
5. Given that the implications of any therapeutic action could expose an unborn child to particular risks the baby's father should be involved in the decision-making process whenever possible.
6. Perform a risk:benefit analysis of your proposed treatment giving consideration to the risks for the mother as well as the risks to the foetus, and the risks to either of non-treatment. Identify and disclose all material risks, both proven and speculative, giving particular consideration to what is of significance to your particular patient and to what she wishes to know. Disclose that presently no database regarding the safety of any psychopharmacological treatment is established to the point of certainty.
7. Material risks need to be considered in the following domains:
   – Risk to mother
   – Risk of teratogenicity
   – Risk of obstetric complications
   – Risk to the newborn
   – Risk of negative long-term neurodevelopmental or other health outcome
   – Risk of non-treatment
8. Establish that your patient's understanding of your risk: benefit analysis is adequate (i.e. substantial) and answer any specific question asked as fully and accurately as possible.
9. Seek a decision and authorization of your proposed treatment from the patient and preferentially also their partner.
10. Document all of the above with rigorous precision, ensuring that the record of the informed consent process is capable of being understood by anyone reading it years later. The details of the process of obtaining informed consent should be recorded in clinical records and as a written communication and distributed to the patient, the referring doctor and the engaged obstetrician and paediatrician.

References

Beauchamp TL, Childress JF. Principles of biomedical ethics. 6th ed. New York, NY: Oxford University Press; 2009.
Bolam v Friern Hospital Management Committee. 1 WLR 582. 1957.
Bolitho v City and Hackney Health Authority. AC 232. 1998
Canterbury v Spence. 464 F. 2d. 772. 1972.
Castell v De Greef. (4) SA 408 (C). 1994.
Cohen LS, Heller VL, Rosenbaum JE. Treatment guidelines for psychotropic drug use in pregnancy. Psychosomatics. 1989;30(1):25–33.

Dolgin JL. The legal development of the informed consent doctrine: past and present. Camb Q
    Healthc Ethics. 2010;19:97–109.
Einarson A, Koren G. Prescribing antidepressants to pregnant women: what is a family physician
    to do? Can Fam Physician. 2007;53(9):1412–4.
Faden RR, Beauchamp TL. A history and theory of informed consent. New York, NY: Oxford
    University Press; 1986.
Griswold v Connecticut. 381 U.S. 479. 1965.
Kessels RPC. Patients' memory for medical information. J R Soc Med. 2003;96(5):219–22.
McHugh J, in Perre v Apand Pty Ltd. 198 CLR 180 at 223-4. 1999.
Percival T. Medical ethics; or a code of institutes and precepts, adapted to the professional conduct
    of physicians and surgeons. Manchester: S. Russell; 1803.
Reibl v Hughes. 2 S.C.R. 880. 1980.
Rogers v Whitaker. 175 CLR 479. 1992.
Rogers v Whitaker, supra, at 490, citing Reibl v Hughes. 2 S.C.R. 880 at 892 (Supreme Court of
    Canada). 1980.
Rosenberg v Percival. HCA 18 at [64] per Gummow J. 2001.
Salgo v Leland Stanford Junior University Board of Trustees. 317 Pacific Reporter 2nd
    170 (California Court of Appeals 1957). 1957.
Sidaway v Board of Governors of Bethlehem Royal Hospital. AC 871. 1985.
Wear S. Informed consent: patient autonomy and clinician beneficence within health care.
    Washington, DC: Georgetown University Press; 1998.
Will JF. A brief historical and theoretical perspective on patient autonomy and medical decision
    making. Part II: the autonomy model. Chest. 2011;139(6):1491–7.

Critical Evaluation of the Literature: Understanding the Complexities of Observational Research

3

Adrienne Einarson

Abstract

Studying the safety of drugs used in pregnancy, especially psychotropics, is a complicated process with currently no ideal model for conducting studies. Because of the ethical issues surrounding pregnancy it is highly unlikely Randomized Controlled Trials (RCTs) will ever be conducted. Consequently, observational studies are used and all of the models have their limitations, such as small sample size, retrospective bias, inability to know exactly if the women took their medication in pregnancy, and other missing data. However, this does not mean that the data collected are not valuable and useful to provide evidence-based information. Psychopharmacology and pregnancy is a highly sensitive topic with healthcare providers, with the media being very interested and eager to report findings, especially if adverse effects are reported. Consequently, it is of great importance when evaluating these studies, to point out the limitations of each study and how it may affect the results. For best evidence, a combination of these different types of observational studies will assist women and their healthcare providers in making informed decisions as to whether or not to take a particular drug during pregnancy.

Keywords

Observational studies • Models • Examination • Knowledge

3.1   Introduction

Since the advent of evidence-based medicine, students in all medical disciplines are expected to learn the skills necessary to allow them to keep up to date with the continuous changes in the field and to practice state-of-the-art medicine. However,

A. Einarson (✉)
The Hospital for Sick Children, Toronto, ON, Canada M5G 1X8
e-mail: einarson@sickkids.ca

M. Galbally et al. (eds.), *Psychopharmacology and Pregnancy*,
DOI 10.1007/978-3-642-54562-7_3, © Springer-Verlag Berlin Heidelberg 2014

this is not as easy as it may appear, as critical evaluation of the literature is no simple task and most clinicians do not have the background in epidemiology and statistics to fully understand the complex nature of what they have read. Consequently, information on treatments, such as an antidepressant medication, may or may not be given appropriately to a patient, perhaps causing harm to the individual, which is definitely not the anticipated outcome (Einarson 2010).

It is possible that clinicians can critically evaluate the literature appropriately if they have enough basic knowledge to be able to know, for example, the difference between statistical significance and clinical relevance of the results. In fact, this is one of the most important pieces of information to understand, as significant (or positive) results are easier to get published, whether they have clinical importance or not (Easterbrook et al. 1991; Gluud 2006).

3.2 Types of Studies

Before critically evaluating the literature, the reader must have comprehensive knowledge regarding the different types of studies that are used in observational research, which is the methodology used in the published literature involving pregnant women. The randomized controlled trial (RCT) is considered the highest form of evidence, but it is not ethical to conduct such trials in pregnant women due to the unknown risk to the developing fetus. The following are different types of studies ranging from the lowest to the highest evidence in observational studies.

3.2.1 The Case Report

A case report is a signal generator, which may identify a potential problem and can prompt a more formal investigation. However, the main limitation of case reports is that they cannot determine causation, unless many other cases describe the same defect with the same exposure. The most classic example in pregnant women was the case report regarding thalidomide, where Dr W McBride reported in the Lancet that he had seen several cases of exposure to thalidomide which had resulted in polydactyly, syndactyly, and failure of development of long bones (abnormally short femora and radii). He then asked the question, "have any of your readers seen similar abnormalities after taking this drug?" (McBride 1961). We now know that there were many other case reports and the study of teratology began.

In those more than 40 years, only one other drug has caused major abnormalities in a large percentage of cases (50 %) to an infant exposed during pregnancy which is Accutane® (isotretinoin). However, because of the heightened awareness due to the thalidomide tragedy, it was known to be a teratogen in a much shorter time than thalidomide, due to the many case reports published in the literature, reporting on infants exposed in utero to the drug who exhibited the same pattern of malformations. Consequently, very quickly, guidelines were put in place to prevent women from taking this drug during pregnancy (Pochi et al. 1988).

3.2.2   Case Series

These are usually more than one case and could be hundreds, occasionally thousands as in some drug company pregnancy registries. They can be presented as cases of exposure or cases of outcome. However, the main limitation of these studies is that there is no comparison group to examine variables, which may affect outcomes. On the other hand, these reports can be useful if the drug is new on the market and there is no information at all regarding safety in pregnancy in the literature (Yaris et al. 2004).

3.2.3   Prospective Comparative Cohort Studies

Studies of this type are most commonly used when examining the safety of drug exposures in pregnancy and are considered a relatively high level of evidence, mainly because there is a comparison group. It is quite usual to match these women with respect to maternal demographics, such as smoking and alcohol consumption and produce a group that is as similar as possible in all demographics, apart from exposure to the drug being studied. For example, in Teratology Information Services studies, pregnancy outcomes of interest are collected and compared to one or two groups of other women who are either (1) exposed to different antidepressants (in an attempt to control for depression) or (2) neither depressed nor taking an antidepressant, called the non-teratogen group, consisting of women who called the service regarding an innocuous exposure. The outcomes of interest are then compared between groups, the primary one often being major malformations. These studies are relatively simple and require no comprehensive knowledge of statistics, as the results are usually reported as p values and Odds Ratios (ORs) with occasional logistic regression. These studies are conducted by the individual service or in collaboration with other services in the world. The main strength of these studies is a personal interview with the individual, which includes detailed history taking and whether she actually took the drug, the dose, and in which trimester of pregnancy. It is also a prospective approach, as when a woman is enrolled in the study when she is in early pregnancy, so the outcome is unknown, preventing recall bias.

The major limitation of these types of studies is the sample size. For example, examining 100 patients is small for statistical purposes as it only has an 80 % power to detect a fourfold increase in major malformations over the baseline rate, since major malformations occur in 1–3 % of all pregnancies, whether the women took any medications or not.

Approximately 800 cases in each group would be required to detect a twofold increase in risk of relatively common malformations, and with most of the study sample sizes around 200–250 cases, thousands more cases would be required to detect rare malformations. Other limitations include samples that are not randomly selected and women calling a teratogen information service generally have a higher socioeconomic status (SES) who may not reflect the general population (Chambers et al. 1996; Einarson et al. 2012a; Sivojelezova et al. 2005).

3.2.4 Case–Control Studies

These are retrospective studies where the outcome is known and the group with a given outcome (e.g., major malformation) is compared to another group who did not have that outcome with respect to the exposure of interest. This methodology is often used in teratology studies because far fewer cases are required to examine rare birth defects, compared to prospective comparative cohorts. The main limitation is the retrospective bias and the inability to match for all confounders. Some important studies have been published regarding use of antidepressants during pregnancy using this model which will be discussed later.

3.2.5 Meta-analysis

This can be a very useful method when studying drug use in pregnancy; as discussed previously, most observational pregnancy outcome studies have small sample sizes. Meta-analysis is a way of combining results across different studies, enlarging the sample size, so as to make a more definitive statement regarding safety/risk of the drug. Usually a minimum of at least two reviewers independently search for studies published in the literature on the drug of interest. A literature search is conducted by these two individuals, using all available databases. Both case–control and cohort studies can be accepted for analysis, as well as abstracts presented at scientific meetings, as long as the subjects were similar. The inclusion and exclusion process is then carried out by the two reviewers, who independently evaluate the articles for acceptance into the study. If necessary, a third reviewer may act as an adjudicator for any unresolved disputes. The reviewers then extract the data from the included studies into 2×2 tables and the data are analyzed. The first meta-analysis carried out using pregnancy outcome data and birth defects was conducted regarding Bendectin® (doxylamine/pyridoxine), a drug used for the treatment of nausea and vomiting of pregnancy (NVP). This study was prompted by several lawsuits against the company alleging that this drug was a teratogen. It was estimated that at one time 30 million women were exposed to this drug in the USA and 25 epidemiologic studies had been performed regarding its safety during pregnancy. Following the combination of all of these studies, with more than 17,000 women, there was no evidence of an increased risk for major malformations above the population based 1–3 % (Einarson et al. 1988).

3.3   Administrative Databases

Databases are not typically set up for pharmacoepidemiologic research as they are primarily developed for various administrative claims payments. For this reason, important data are often missing, especially for studies of drug use and pregnancy outcomes. However, they often contain data from large numbers of individuals with important information, so have been increasingly used in research, most frequently to conduct post-marketing surveillance. Many studies that have produced positive results are from prescription databases with samples compiled using data from prescriptions that have been filled by the patient. The main strength of this method is the very large sample sizes. However, there are several limitations, the main one being that it is only known if a person filled the prescription, not that the drug was actually taken (Källén et al. 2011). Due to the extremely large sample sizes, there can be a potential for false positives, as statistical significance is a function of sample size. That is, the larger the sample size, the higher is the probability of chance findings of statistically significant results that may have no clinical relevance. In addition, results are usually given as an Odds Ratio (OR) and the baseline rate is rarely documented. For example, it is not very meaningful if, after comparing the results of two groups, there is a statistically significant OR, and if the risk in both groups is below the baseline rate of what is expected in the population. In one publication, researchers examined the quality of 100 abstracts from published studies that had examined the safety of various drugs in pregnancy. In 94 % of the results, when a significant OR was reported, baseline rates were not documented (Einarson et al. 2006), and without knowing what rates are expected in the population, it is difficult to evaluate whether there really is an increased risk. For example, in a study reporting results from a prescription data base examining rates of spontaneous abortions (SA) comparing two groups of women, one group taking a nonsteroidal anti-inflammatory drug (NSAID) and one group not, it was documented that the OR was 2, which meant that women taking an NSAID had twice the risk of having an SA. However, there was no record of the actual rates of SA in the paper, and only after contacting the author, the actual rates of SA were identified in the unexposed group. Considering that rates of SA are believed to be approximately 10–15 % it was evident that in both groups, rates were considerably below what is expected in the population, so the clinical relevance of this study was definitely questionable (Nielsen et al. 2001). Recently, a study with women enrolled prospectively and outcomes verified with medical records did not find an increased risk for use of NSAIDs associated with an increased risk for SA (Edwards et al. 2012).

3.3.1   National Birth Registries

Some European countries operate government-supported registries where data from the mother and child pairs are entered after birth and are followed up prospectively. For example, many studies have been published with data from The Swedish Birth

Registry (Källén and Otterblad 2006). The Hungarian Case-Control Surveillance System of Congenital Abnormalities is another group in this category who have published many pregnancy outcome studies following exposure during pregnancy (Kazy et al. 2007).

When practicing evidence-based medicine, all of these methodologies loosely fit into the category Level 2 "Evidence obtained from well-designed cohort or case–control analytic studies, preferably from more than one center or research group" (Elstein 2004).

3.4   Evaluating Studies

Critical appraisal is not difficult if one knows what needs careful examination in each individual study. A relatively new guideline which has been introduced to help design, conduct, and report observational studies and is currently required by some high impact journals, is the STROBE statement which was developed to strengthen the reporting of observational studies in Epidemiology (von Elm et al. 2007). In journals in which this is a requirement, a questionnaire has to be completed and submitted to the journal together with the manuscript. Although this checklist is primarily for authors, it can be an extremely useful tool for the reader, as the authors are required to check items that should be included in the study which are compulsory. The STROBE checklist covers each section of the study and is available online at: http://www.strobe-statement.org/?id=available-checklists

3.5   Understanding the Results of the Statistical Analysis

Following a close examination of the study design using the STROBE guidelines, it is now time to examine how the statistical analysis was conducted and how it was reported. The analysis of studies can vary greatly and the results even more so, most often depending on the sample sizes. The larger the sample size, the easier it is to conduct more statistical tests to find significance, just because it can be done, which does not necessarily make the results of the particular study more important than a smaller one. A large sample size is considered to be able to produce more robust results; however, sometimes the sample size can be so large that even the smallest differences can become statistically significant with no clinical relevance. For example, women should not smoke cigarettes during pregnancy and many studies have been published reporting significant differences in birth weight in women who smoke. Smaller sample sizes such as the Motherisk studies with about 200 cases did not find any differences in birth weight (Einarson et al. 2001; Gallo et al. 2000); however, huge sample sizes with thousands of women did find statistical differences, albeit with often less than 100-g difference in birth weight between the smokers and nonsmokers (Conter et al. 1995). When considering a full-term infant is born weighing on average 3,500 g, one wonders if this really has any real clinical relevance. However, in this example, because women are advised to stop smoking in pregnancy and rightfully so, much is made of this clinically insignificant result, because hopefully, if a women believes she is harming her baby, this will give her more incentive to quit.

3.5.1 Statistical Tests

An Odds Ratio (OR) is a measure of association between an exposure and an outcome. The OR represents the odds that an outcome will occur given a particular exposure, compared to the odds of the outcome occurring in the absence of that exposure. Odds ratios are most commonly used in case–control studies; however, they can also be used in cohort study designs as well. The 95 % confidence interval (CI) is used to estimate the precision of the OR. A large CI indicates a low level of precision of the OR, whereas a small CI indicates a higher precision of the OR. It is important to note, however, that unlike the p value, the 95 % CI does not directly report a measure's statistical significance, but it does provide comparable information. In practice, the 95 % CI is often used as a proxy for the presence of statistical significance if it does not contain the null value (e.g., OR $= 1$).

Relative Risk (RR) is the risk of an adverse event (or of developing a disease) in an exposed group relative to a nonexposed group. It is used in cohort studies; however, the study must be large enough to accurately measure the outcome in the control group (i.e., the baseline risk). As with the OR, a RR of 2 means that the probability of the outcome is twice as high in the exposed as in the nonexposed group.

Logistic Regression (LR) is used when one wants to produce odds ratios while controlling for the possible influence of other factors. For example, one could examine whether smoking status during pregnancy was related to the development of depression while controlling for maternal age, body mass index, and previous episodes of depression. The outcome variable must have two categories. Observational cohorts, such as Motherisk studies, rarely do LR as the women are already matched on these variables, which is an alternate approach to control for these variables (Einarson et al. 2012a; Sivojelezova et al. 2005).

Understanding these basic statistical tests is a good foundation to be able to evaluate most studies examining safety/risk of drugs in pregnancy.

3.6 Evaluation of the Abstract

It is likely, for a variety of reasons, that many clinicians read only the abstract of a paper in a scientific journal. Therefore, it is very important that abstracts contain as much information about the study as possible, especially the results and conclusions. Most journals have reduced the number of words in their abstracts from 300–350 to 200–250 maximum and some do not include an introduction, simply an objective, the study design, results, and conclusions. In a previously discussed study (Einarson et al. 2006), details frequently absent were baseline risk

(94 %), drug dose (91 %), nonsignificant p-values (72 %), significant p-values (57 %), confounders (69 %), and risk difference (48 %). Two examples of why one should not read only the abstract and were misunderstood are as follows: the first study (case control) was one where the authors examined whether taking an antidepressant in pregnancy was associated with an increased risk of Persistent Pulmonary Hypertension in the Newborn (PPHN). 14 infants with PPHN who had been exposed to an SSRI as compared with 6 control infants revealed an OR 6.1 (95 % confidence interval, 2.2–16.8), which appears to be a really large risk. However, in the conclusion of the main text, these results were clearly put into perspective; "on the assumption that the relative risk of 6.1 is true and that the relationship is causal, the absolute risk for PPHN in their infants among women who use SSRIs in late pregnancy is relatively low (about 6–12 per 1,000), put in other terms, about 99 % of these women will deliver a baby unaffected by PPHN" (Chambers et al. 2006). This study caused a great deal of angst among both pregnant women and their healthcare providers, especially because it was published in the New England Journal of Medicine. The second (an observational cohort) was to determine the association of maternal psychotropic medication use during pregnancy with preterm delivery and other adverse perinatal outcomes using a cohort of 2,793 pregnant women. In the abstract, the authors reported that the maternal use of benzodiazepines during pregnancy was associated with an increased risk of preterm delivery (adjusted odds ratio, 6.79; 95 % confidence interval, 4.01–11.5) and an increased risk of low birth weight, low Apgar score, higher neonatal intensive care unit admissions, and respiratory distress syndrome. The authors' conclusion was that benzodiazepine use in pregnancy was associated highly with preterm delivery and other adverse perinatal outcomes. However, when reading the complete paper, their conclusions simply did not match the results for varying reasons. The reporting in the abstract suggested that the entire cohort were psychotropic medication users; in the text the sample size of psychotropic medication users was 10.7 % (300/2,793) of their cohort. They reported that benzodiazepines are highly associated with an increased risk of preterm delivery, despite the fact that the sample size was only $N = 85$. In addition, decreasing the sample size further, hydroxyzine, an antihistamine, was listed as a psychotropic drug ($n = 107$), so the real sample of psychotropic drug exposures was only ($N = 193$), or 6.9 % of 2,793 women. Consequently, this sample size was too small to make a definitive conclusion, as the authors had stated in the conclusion (Calderon-Margalit et al. 2009). That paper was also published in a highly respected obstetrics and gynecology journal, which behooves readers to not allow the high impact of the journal to affect their critical examination of the manuscript.

3.7   Questioning the Validity of the Results

When evaluating the literature, one should always examine if the results appear to be valid, based on the authors' conclusions. In one example, the authors reported an increase risk for major malformation (RR 1.84) in women taking antidepressants.

The validity of these results was questionable for the following reasons: (1) there was no pattern of specific defects, (2) there was no separation of major versus minor malformations, (3) as this was a prescription events monitoring study, it was not known whether the medications were actually taken, and (4) psychiatrically ill patients frequently use other psychotropic medications, alcohol, and illicit drugs and these potential confounders were not addressed (Wogelius et al. 2006). In another study, the authors conducted a large number of tests, but made no adjustment for multiple testing, without acknowledging that their results could all be random error. They also attempted to identify depressed untreated pregnant women, but provided no solid evidence that they actually succeeded in doing so. They also found two very trivial differences in birth weights (30 g difference between groups) and stated they had found an increased risk for low birth weight (Oberlander et al. 2006). In another study (meta-analysis) the authors pooled the results of 12 studies that examined poor neonatal adaptation syndrome PNAS. There was a significant association between exposure to antidepressants during pregnancy and overall occurrence of poor neonatal adaptation syndrome PNAS (OR $= 5.07$; 95 % CI, 3.25–7.90; $p < 0.0001$). It is well known that that infants can suffer from PNAS (up to 30 %) information derived from different published reports as stated by the authors. However, in neither the abstract or main text, there was no baseline frequency of occurrence, so the reader still has no idea of how often this syndrome actually occurs (Grigoriadis et al. 2013). Finally, in another study (meta-analysis) the authors concluded that the summary estimate indicated an increased prevalence of combined cardiac defects with first trimester paroxetine use. However, the authors opted to exclude the Motherisk study $n = 1,174$ cases for trivial reasons that reported no increased risk for cardiovascular defects, which likely would have lowered the OR (Einarson and Koren 2010; Wurst et al. 2010).

3.8   Selective Bias in Reviews of the Literature

Bias is inherent in all research, whether or not the researchers are even aware and good research is conducted so as to control for any obvious bias in the data. Recently, a review was published regarding the use of antidepressants in pregnancy and the authors' conclusion was "Antidepressant use during pregnancy is associated with increased risks of miscarriage, birth defects, preterm birth, newborn behavioral syndrome, persistent pulmonary hypertension of the newborn and possible longer term neurobehavioral effects. There is no evidence of improved pregnancy outcomes with antidepressant use." Unfortunately for readers, the authors selected only papers that reported adverse outcomes following exposure to antidepressants and did not include any that found no association with adverse outcomes. This was not a systematic review, there were no ORs stated in the abstract, and it is the most blatant example of selection bias (Domar et al. 2013). In this case, the authors had no basis for their conclusions because they did not examine all of the literature and their conclusions should be disregarded. Again, this study was published in a respected journal and received a great deal of media attention, which again caused a great deal of anxiety for pregnant women taking antidepressant and their healthcare providers.

In contrast, with no apparent bias a national pregnancy registry recently published a study in which 10,511 infants of women who had used SSRI drugs but no other central nervous system-active drug, 1,000 infants born of women who had used benzodiazepines and no other CNS-active drug, and 406 infants whose mothers had used both SSRI and benzodiazepines but no other CNS-active drug were compared to a nonexposed group. Their conclusions were as follows: none of the three groups showed a higher risk for any relatively severe malformation or any cardiac defect when comparison was made with the general population risk (adjusted RR for the combination of SSRI and benzodiazepines and a relatively severe malformation = 1.17; 95 % CI, 0.70–1.73). Similar results were obtained for the combination of SSRI with other sedative/hypnotic drugs. Conclusions: "The previously stated increased risk associated with the combined use of these drug categories, notably for a cardiac defect, could not be replicated" (Reis and Källén 2013). Therefore, all available studies should be examined before making a conclusion.

3.9   Does Research Design Affect Results?

To date, there have been more than 30,000 pregnancy outcomes of infants exposed to antidepressants during pregnancy, published in studies where the researchers used different methodologies and reported different conclusions although odds ratios were rarely >2.

A study (meta-analysis) was conducted to examine the possibility that the seemingly conflicting results may be different because of the variety of models that were used.

Designs that were compared included prospective cohort, retrospective cohort, and case–control studies. Rates of major malformations and cardiac malformations were combined by study type using random effects meta-analytic models. Overall ORs for major malformations ranged from 1.03 to 1.24 and 0.81 to 1.32 for cardiac malformations. The authors discovered that diverse observational models with differing strengths and weaknesses produced remarkably similar nonsignificant results. Perceived conflicting results may be due to subsequent dissemination of results with attention given to small statistically differences with negligible clinical relevance. The authors concluded that a combination of methods is appropriate to produce evidence-based information on the safety of drugs during pregnancy, provided the study design is rigorous and the limitations are stated clearly (Einarson et al. 2012b).

Conclusion

Understanding simple statistics and evaluating published studies are critical, as all study designs have limitations and authors do not always fully disclose details. It should not be assumed that high impact journals, renowned authors, and prestigious institutions automatically publish high-quality research. Application of results requires careful interpretation, most importantly, to consider when confronted with marginally increased ORs to examine whether the results have any real clinical significance.

This process is extremely important in the Knowledge Transfer Translation (KT) process. This is observational research, and consequently, there are some deficiencies in study design and analysis among all of the studies. However, this does not mean that the information provided from the results of these studies is not valuable, as long as the methodology and analyses are critically evaluated. It is unlikely that in the near future, pregnant women will be included in randomized controlled trials, so this reinforces the need to improve the rigor of the available study methods.

The apparent conflicting evidence regarding the results of the antidepressant studies are not conflicting after all, as it appears likely due to the way selected results were interpreted and disseminated. Finally and of great importance, improved knowledge transfer and translation will ensure that pregnant women with mental health disorders and their healthcare providers receive the most accurate evidence-based information, for decision making regarding the use of psychotropic drugs during pregnancy.

References

Calderon-Margalit R, Qiu C, Ornoy A, Siscovick DS, Williams MA. Risk of preterm delivery and other adverse perinatal outcomes in relation to maternal use of psychotropic medications during pregnancy. Am J Obstet Gynecol. 2009;201(6):579.

Chambers CD, Johnson KA, Dick LM, Felix RJ, Jones KL. Birth outcomes in pregnant women taking fluoxetine. N Engl J Med. 1996;335(14):1010–5.

Chambers CD, Hernandez-Diaz S, Van Marter LJ, Werler MM, Louik C, Jones KL, et al. Selective serotonin-reuptake inhibitors and risk of persistent pulmonary hypertension of the newborn. N Engl J Med. 2006;354(6):579–87.

Conter V, Cortinovis I, Rogari P, Riva L. Weight growth in infants born to mothers who smoked during pregnancy. BMJ. 1995;310(6982):768.

Domar AD, Moragianni VA, Ryley DA, Urato AC. The risks of selective serotonin reuptake inhibitor use in infertile women: a review of the impact on fertility, pregnancy, neonatal health and beyond. Hum Reprod. 2013;28(1):160–71.

Easterbrook PJ, Berlin JA, Gopalan R, Matthews DR. Publication bias in clinical research. Lancet. 1991;337(8746):867–72.

Edwards DRV, Aldridge T, Baird DD, Funk MJ, Savitz DA, Hartmann KE. Periconceptional over-the-counter nonsteroidal anti-inflammatory drug exposure and risk for spontaneous abortion. Obstet Gynecol. 2012;120(1):113–22.

Einarson A. Antidepressants and pregnancy: complexities of producing evidence-based information. CMAJ. 2010;182(10):1017–8.

Einarson A, Koren G. First trimester exposure to paroxetine and prevalence of cardiac defects: meta-analysis of the literature: unfortunately incomplete. Birth Defects Res A Clin Mol Teratol. 2010;88(7):588.

Einarson TR, Leeder JS, Koren G. A method for meta-analysis of epidemiological studies. Drug Intell Clin Pharm. 1988;22(10):813–24.

Einarson A, Fatoye B, Sarkar M, Lavigne SV, Brochu J, Chambers C, et al. Pregnancy outcome following gestational exposure to venlafaxine: a multicenter prospective controlled study. Am J Psychiatry. 2001;158(10):1728–30.

Einarson TR, Lee C, Smith R, Manley J, Perstin J, Loniewska M, et al. Quality and content of abstracts in papers reporting about drug exposures during pregnancy. Birth Defects Res A Clin Mol Teratol. 2006;76(8):621–8.

Einarson A, Smart K, Vial T, Diav-Citrin O, Yates L, Stephens S, et al. Rates of major malformations in infants following exposure to duloxetine during pregnancy: a preliminary report. J Clin Psychiatry. 2012a;73(11):1471.

Einarson TR, Kennedy D, Einarson A. Do findings differ across research design? The case of antidepressant use in pregnancy and malformations. J Popul Ther Clin Pharmacol. 2012b;19 (2):e334–48.

Elstein AS. On the origins and development of evidence-based medicine and medical decision making. Inflamm Res. 2004;53(S2):S184–9.

Gallo M, Sarkar M, Au W, Pietrzak K, Comas B, Smith M, et al. Pregnancy outcome following gestational exposure to echinacea: a prospective controlled study. Arch Intern Med. 2000;160 (20):3141.

Gluud LL. Bias in clinical intervention research. Am J Epidemiol. 2006;163(6):493–501.

Grigoriadis S, Vonderporten EH, Mamisashvili L, Eady A, Tomlinson G, Dennis CL, et al. The effect of prenatal antidepressant exposure on neonatal adaptation: a systematic review and meta-analysis. J Clin Psychiatry. 2013;74(4):e309–20.

Källén BA, Otterblad OP. Use of oral decongestants during pregnancy and delivery outcome. Am J Obstet Gynecol. 2006;194(2):480–5.

Källén B, Nilsson E, Olausson PO. Antidepressant use during pregnancy: comparison of data obtained from a prescription register and from antenatal care records. Eur J Clin Pharmacol. 2011;67(8):839–45.

Kazy Z, Puhó EH, Czeizel AE. Effect of doxycycline treatment during pregnancy for birth outcomes. Reprod Toxicol. 2007;24(3):279–80.

McBride WG. Letters to the editor: thalidomide and congenital abnormalities. Lancet. 1961;278 (7216):1358.

Nielsen GL, Sørensen HT, Larsen H, Pedersen L. Risk of adverse birth outcome and miscarriage in pregnant users of non-steroidal anti-inflammatory drugs: population based observational study and case-control study. BMJ. 2001;322(7281):266–70.

Oberlander TF, Warburton W, Misri S, Aghajanian J, Hertzman C. Neonatal outcomes after prenatal exposure to selective serotonin reuptake inhibitor antidepressants and maternal depression using population-based linked health data. Arch Gen Psychiatry. 2006;63 (8):898–906.

Pochi PE, Ceilley RI, Coskey RJ, Drake LA, Jansen GT, Rodman OG, et al. Guidelines for prescribing isotretinoin (Accutane) in the treatment of female acne patients of childbearing potential. Acne Subgroup, Task Force on Standards of Care. J Am Acad Dermatol. 1988;19 (5):920.

Reis M, Källén B. Combined use of selective serotonin reuptake inhibitors and sedatives/hypnotics during pregnancy: risk of relatively severe congenital malformations or cardiac defects. A register study. BMJ Open. 2013;3(2):e002166.

Sivojelezova A, Shuhaiber S, Sarkissian L, Einarson A, Koren G. Citalopram use in pregnancy: prospective comparative evaluation of pregnancy and fetal outcome. Am J Obstet Gynecol. 2005;193(6):2004–9.

von Elm E, Altman DG, Egger M, Pocock SJ, Gøtzsche PC, Vandenbroucke JP, et al. The strengthening the reporting of observational studies in epidemiology (STROBE) statement: guidelines for reporting observational studies. Lancet. 2007;370(9596):1453–7.

Wogelius P, Nørgaard M, Gislum M, Pedersen L, Munk E, Mortensen PB, et al. Maternal use of selective serotonin reuptake inhibitors and risk of congenital malformations. Epidemiology. 2006;17(6):701–4.

Wurst KE, Poole C, Ephross SA, Olshan AF. First trimester paroxetine use and the prevalence of congenital, specifically cardiac, defects: a meta-analysis of epidemiological studies. Birth Defects Res A Clin Mol Teratol. 2010;88(3):159–70.

Yaris F, Kadioglu M, Kesim M, Ulku C, Yaris E, Kalyoncu NI, et al. Newer antidepressants in pregnancy: prospective outcome of a case series. Reprod Toxicol. 2004;19(2):235–8.

Maternal and Fetal Factors That Influence Prenatal Exposure to Selective Serotonin Reuptake Inhibitor Antidepressants

4

Alison K. Shea, Tuan-Anh Thi Nguyen, Ursula Brain, Dan Rurak, and Tim F. Oberlander

Abstract

Prenatal serotonin reuptake inhibitor (SRI) exposure is common and neonatal outcomes vary greatly, often leading to confusion about whether to use or even continue antenatal use of these antidepressants. Importantly, some but not all infants are affected, which raises questions about how maternal drug metabolism contributes to fetal drug exposure. To address this question, this chapter reviews the role of key maternal, fetal, and placental pharmacokinetic, metabolic, and genetic factors that affect the extent of fetal drug exposure. Considering the role of these factors may further our understanding of variables that might assist in optimizing maternal psychopharmacotherapy during pregnancy and neonatal outcomes.

Keywords

Antidepressants • Pharmacodynamics • Pregnancy • Depression • Fetus

4.1 Introduction/Background

Up to one-third of neonates exhibit neonatal neurobehavioral disturbances following prenatal exposure to a serotonin reuptake inhibitor (SRI) antidepressant (Moses-Kolko et al. 2005). While this has been assumed to be an effect of an acute drug exposure, these behavioral disturbances may not be related to maternal

A.K. Shea
Department of Obstetrics and Gynecology, University of Toronto, Toronto, ON, Canada

T.-A.T. Nguyen • U. Brain • D. Rurak
Department of Pediatrics, Child & Family Research Institute, University of British Colombia, Vancouver, BC, Canada

T.F. Oberlander (✉)
Child & Family Research Institute, 950 West 28th Avenue, Vancouver, BC, Canada V5Z 4H4
e-mail: toberlander@cw.bc.ca

M. Galbally et al. (eds.), *Psychopharmacology and Pregnancy*,
DOI 10.1007/978-3-642-54562-7_4, © Springer-Verlag Berlin Heidelberg 2014

drug dose, length of gestational exposure, or timing of gestational exposure (Oberlander et al. 2009). These considerations subsequently raise critical questions about what factors affect fetal drug exposure and predict these neonatal outcomes. Determining why some infants and not others are affected by perinatal SRI use remains challenging. Central to addressing this question is our ability to consider the impact of physiological factors of the pregnancy itself and SRI-related pharmacological factors that influence maternal drug metabolism and by extension, fetal exposure. Neonatal outcomes following in utero SRI exposure depend largely on the degree of fetal drug exposure. As such, understanding factors that affect fetal drug pharmacology may offer important clues to any associated developmental risks. Importantly, SRI treatment occurs in the context of antenatal maternal mood disturbances which themselves have a critical impact on fetal and neonatal health (Hanley and Oberlander 2012). However, this chapter will focus on reviewing the key maternal, placental, fetal metabolic, and genetic factors that influence SRI pharmacology and fetal drug exposure. Both selective serotonin reuptake inhibitors (SSRIs, e.g., citalopram, escitalopram, fluoxetine, fluvoxamine, paroxetine, sertraline) and serotonin norepinephrine reuptake inhibitors (SNRIs, e.g., desvenlafaxine, duloxetine, venlafaxine) are increasingly used to manage antenatal mood disturbances (Cooper et al. 2007) and will be referred to as SRIs (serotonin reuptake inhibitors). This chapter is offered as a review to highlight key maternal and fetal variables that account for the variations in maternal perinatal SRI pharmacology, fetal drug exposure, and neonatal outcomes that should serve as a guide to the clinician regarding the benefits and risks associated with SRI use in this setting.

4.2   Fetal Drug Exposure During Pregnancy

The management and treatment of antenatal mood disturbances present an important public health concern. Each year, 15–20 % of women experience mood and anxiety disorders (e.g., major depression, generalized anxiety disorder) during their pregnancy (Cooper et al. 2007). Approximately one-third of these women will be treated with a serotonin reuptake inhibitor (SRI) antidepressant (Oberlander et al. 2006). Importantly, up to 50 % of women discontinue their medication within the first 60 days of their pregnancy (Vesga-Lopez et al. 2008; Oberlander et al. 2006; Bennett et al. 2004; Warburton et al. 2010). This highlights the need to recognize and manage perinatal mood disturbances and to establish evidence to guide SRI medication use in conjunction with non-pharmacological treatments that may be less effective (Yonkers et al. 2009). Discontinuation of pharmacological treatment leads to increased risk for relapse in these patients (Cohen et al. 2006). It is critical to understand the pharmacological and physiological effects when weighing the risks and benefits of SRI medication use in pregnant women—particularly in relation to maternal mental health and infant neurodevelopment (Yonkers et al. 2009).

Soon after the advent of SRI pharmacological treatment in 1988, reports of use during pregnancy cited a shortening of gestational age, lower birth weights, and neonatal neurobehavioral disturbances (irritability, weak or absent cry, increased motor activity) suggesting a neonatal "withdrawal" condition (Moses-Kolko et al. 2005). While shortening gestational age at birth (Kallen and Olausson 2008) might explain some of these findings, the severity of behavioral disturbances has been linked to increased maternal and cord SRI drug levels (Oberlander et al. 2004) as well as with altered neonatal monoamine neurotransmitter levels (Laine et al. 2004), suggesting a direct role for pharmacological factors. During gestation, disrupted fetal nonrapid eye movement sleep (Zeskind and Stephens 2004; Mulder et al. 2011) and reduced cerebral blood flow indices and fetal heart rate variability (Rurak et al. 2011) have been associated with SRI exposure, which suggests that neurobehavioral changes may be present even before the prenatal period ends. Importantly, not all neonates are affected (Moses-Kolko et al. 2005), suggesting that genetic variations may moderate such associations (Oberlander et al. 2008; Davidson et al. 2009). The heterogeneity of outcomes following SRI exposure raises critical questions about fetal and maternal factors that affect the extent of drug metabolism and fetal drug exposure.

4.3 Fetal and Neonatal Effects of SRIs Exposure: Preclinical Evidence

Findings from animal studies suggest that prenatal SRI exposure alters fetal behaviors and physiology well before the gestational exposure ends. For example, sheep fetuses exposed to SRI medication in utero showed an alteration in behavioral state (i.e., increased quiet sleep, decreased REM sleep, and fetal breathing movements) and increased ACTH and cortisol surges (Morrison et al. 2002, 2004).

In newborn lambs exposed to 12 days of fluoxetine in late pregnancy, increased newborn activity during the first 2 weeks after birth has also been observed (Nguyen 2013).

Importantly, findings from this sheep model showed no changes in cardiovascular, metabolic, endocrine, and behavior in the newborn lambs (~4 days old) with acute fluoxetine IV injection. In addition, there were low and undetectable plasma fluoxetine and norfluoxetine concentrations in the postnatal lambs exposed to fluoxetine in utero, who exhibited hyperactivity for 2 weeks after birth. This may suggest that acute toxicity may not be the mechanism underlying poor neonatal adaptation in human infants exposed to these drugs (Nguyen 2013).

The effects of SRIs exposure on brain development have also been studied using a mouse model. Prenatal fluoxetine exposure for 14 days leads to a decreased cell count in the nucleus accumbens and in the raphe nucleus, a key brain region responsible for reward response systems (Forcelli and Heinrichs 2008). Using rodent models akin to the human third trimester, early postnatal SRI exposure reduced novelty exploration, increased immobility, sleep abnormalities, reduced sexual activity and anhedonia (Lee 2009; Ansorge et al. 2004; Maciag et al. 2006; Popa et al. 2008). These effects are associated with alterations in brain structure, including neuronal structure in the somatosensory cortex (Lee 2009), a decreased synthesis of tryptophan hydroxylase (a key rate-limiting enzyme for serotonin synthesis) in the dorsal raphe, and decreased serotonin transporter expression in the cortex (Maciag et al. 2006). However, not all outcomes associated with early SRI exposure using mouse models reflect developmental disturbances. Increased locomotor activity and increased spatial task ability have been observed in mice exposed to citalopram from postnatal days 8–21, respectively (Maciag et al. 2006).

4.4   Drug Metabolism and Genetic Variations

All SRIs are metabolized by phase 1 and 2 hepatic pathways, with only 0–12 % of the drugs being excreted as intact compounds (Hiemke and Hartter 2000; DeVane 1999) (Table 4.1). Phase 1 reactions, which are dependent on hepatic cytochrome P450 enzymes (CYP), typically, CYPs 1A2, 2C9, 2C19, 2D6, and 3A4, are involved in the metabolism of SSRIs and the SNRI, venlafaxine (Table 4.1) (Fogelman et al. 1999). Genetic variations have been identified for each enzyme and some variants are associated with reduced or no catalytic activity (Martinez et al. 1999). For CYP 2D6 and 2C19, there are alleles with no catalytic activity, whereas for CYP 2C9, there are two alleles with significantly reduced catalytic activity and for CYP 3A4 there are many alleles with varying degrees of activity loss (Martinez et al. 1999). While metabolic capacity varies with genetic and pharmacological factors, a linear relationship has been demonstrated between maternal and fetal fluoxetine levels, suggesting that fetal exposure depends on maternal concentrations (Kim et al. 2006).

For example, the gene for the CYP2D6 enzyme has more than 80 genetic variants characterized to date (http://cypalleles.ki.se). However, not all are active and some variants encode an inactive protein or no enzyme product, reflecting an autosomal recessive polymorphism. When two nonfunctional alleles occur, the carrier is referred to as a "poor metabolizer" (PM), versus those heterozygous for the defect allele, "intermediate metabolizers" (IMs). Those carrying two functional alleles are classified as "extensive metabolizers" (EMs), while those with >2 functional copies are "ultrarapid metabolizers" (UMs), which may require higher than average doses of medication. Approximately 5–10 % of the Caucasian population is classified as PM, which is relevant to treatment during pregnancy as it leads to higher plasma concentrations of SRIs, particularly since most SRIs depend on the CYP 2D6 enzyme (Bradford 2002). Differences in SRI metabolism accompanying such allelic variants have been demonstrated by several studies (Bijl et al. 2008; Tsai et al. 2010). For the SRIs that depend on multiple CYP enzymes for metabolism, such as fluoxetine, citalopram, and sertraline, the individual genetic variation of one enzyme appears to be less critical. Alternately, desvenlafaxine metabolism and measured serum levels are not dependent on 2D6 variability (Preskorn et al. 2008).

Table 4.1 The cytochrome P450 enzymes utilized during SRI metabolism (Shea et al. 2012)

SRI	CYP1A2	CYP2C9	CYP2C19	CYP2D6	CYP3A4
Citalopram	−	−	+	+	+
Desvenlafaxine	−	−	−	−	+
Duloxetine	+	−	−	+	−
Escitalopram	−	−	−	+	+
Fluoxetine	−	+	+	+	−
Paroxetine	−	−	−	+	+
Sertraline	−	+	+	+	+
Venlafaxine	−	−	−	+	+

4.5 Maternal Adaptations to Pregnancy and Their Impact on SSRI/SNRI Disposition

Pregnancy itself alters key drug metabolic enzyme activities, leading to changes in SRIs disposition. Increased maternal blood volume, decreased plasma protein concentrations, increased cardiac output and renal function (GFR), and decreased intestinal mobility all potentially alter drug disposition and SRI dosing (Anderson 2005; Jeong 2010) during pregnancy. This may be reflected in decreased plasma concentrations of fluoxetine, citalopram, and sertraline during pregnancy (Wadelius et al. 1997). While the decrease in maternal antidepressant concentrations reduces fetal drug exposure, it often leads to the need to increase the maternal drug dose to maintain maternal euthymia (Anderson 2005).

Induced CYP2D6 activity during pregnancy has been linked to increased SRI levels (Wadelius et al. 1997). Comparing CYP2D6 activity in late pregnancy with 7–11 weeks postpartum, Wadelius et al. (1997) reported that CYP2D6 activity increased progressively during pregnancy and in the third trimester was ~48 % higher than in the postpartum period. Similarly, Anderson (2005) reported that CYP3A4 increased 35–38 % during all stages of pregnancy, whereas CYP1A2 activity decreased progressively across gestation. Further, increased CYP2C9 and increased uridine diphosphate glucuronosyltransferase activities and decreased CYP2C19 activity have been reported during pregnancy (Jeong 2010). Of note, declining sertraline levels have been reported by Freeman et al. (2008) from the second to the third trimester for most but not all women, reflecting individual variations in enzyme activity. Another prospective investigation found decreasing paroxetine levels from 16 to 40 weeks gestation in ultrarapid and extensive metabolizers of 2D6 (Ververs et al. 2009), while drug levels in the intermediate and poor metabolizers increased with gestational age. In the same study, maternal depression scores also increased as pregnancy progressed in the extensive metabolizers, suggesting a gene x environment (pregnancy) effect (Ververs et al. 2009). Given the differences in CYP metabolic capacities and CYP inhibitory potencies of the drug themselves, further study of links between an individual antidepressant used in pregnancy and CYP genotypes is needed to characterize the alterations in the disposition of these drugs during pregnancy.

4.6   Interactions with SRIs

SRIs influence their metabolism by inducing and inhibiting the action of CYP enzymes (Tables 4.2 and 4.3). The use of other drugs that are substrates for the same CYPs may lead to competitive inhibition when co-administered with SRIs. Notably, CYP2D6 is inhibited by some, but not all SRIs (Preskorn et al. 2006; Pelkonen et al. 2008). Fluoxetine inhibits 2D6 after only 8 days of treatment (Alfaro et al. 1999). Further, antidepressant–drug interactions have been extensively investigated and impacts of the antidepressants on the pharmacokinetics of a large number of drugs have been identified. It has been argued that, on the basis of the existing in vitro, in vivo, and epidemiologic evidence, antidepressant–drug interactions are rarely clinically significant (DeVane et al. 2006). However, an increased risk for poor neonatal adaptation in neonates with higher levels of paroxetine following combined prenatal exposure to paroxetine and clonaze-pam—both CYP3A4 substrates—might illustrate the impact of a fetal drug–drug interaction (Oberlander et al. 2004).

Given multiple medical conditions may also be present when the pregnancy begins (e.g., gastroesophageal reflux, chronic hypertension, heart disease) or arise during pregnancy (e.g., preeclampsia, preterm rupture of membranes, preterm labor, cholestasis of pregnancy), the potential for antidepressant–drug interactions is substantial. Drugs used to treat these conditions are administered during pregnancy, and many of them are substrates for the CYPs that are inhibited by fluoxetine, paroxetine, and fluvoxamine (Oberlander et al. 2004), and affecting these enzymes may potentially increase fetal SRI exposure (Garnett 2001) (see http://medicine.iupui.edu/clinpharm/DDIs/clinicalTable.aspx).

Pregnancy-related increased gastroesophageal reflux is often treated with proton-pump inhibitors (PPIs), such as pantoprazole or the H2 antagonist cimetidine, which inhibit P450 enzymes (Li et al. 2004; Martinez et al. 1999). Dexamethasone, used to advance fetal lung maturation in threatened preterm labor, inhibits CYP2C9, but induces CYP3A4 (Zhou et al. 2009; Pascussi et al. 2001). When preterm rupture of membranes occurs, erythromycin (an inhibitor of 3A4) is often used to prolong the pregnancy and decrease maternal and neonatal morbidity (Yudin et al. 2009). Nifedipine, a 2C9 inhibitor, is used extensively to treat high blood pressure during pregnancy and is used also as a tocolytic agent in threatened preterm labor (Magee et al. 2011). Psychotropic medications, such as quetiapine, inhibit several SRI-metabolizing enzymes (Arranz and de Leon 2007). Interactions may also unexpectedly occur among commonly prescribed as well as OTC medications during pregnancy. Yeast infections are treated with fluconazole and miconazole, which inhibit key P450 enzymes involved in SRI metabolism (Niwa et al. 2005). These interactions may increase maternal plasma SRI levels, may affect fetal plasma concentrations, and thus increase the risk of drug-elicited

Table 4.2 List of cytochrome P450 enzyme inhibitors and inducers, relevant for SRI metabolism (Shea et al. 2012)

	CYP1A2	CYP2C9	CYP2C19	CYP2D6	CYP3A4
Inhibitors	Cimetidine	PPIs	Fluoxetine	Bupropion	Grape fruit juice
	Olanzapine	Fluconazole	PPIs	Duloxetine	Fluoxetine
	Clozapine	Metronidazole	Amitriptyline	Fluoxetine	Cimetidine
		Miconazole	Cimetidine	Paroxetine	Quetiapine
		Valproic acid nifedipine	Miconazole	Sertraline	Risperidone
			Fluconazole	Methadone	Aripiprazole
				Haldol	Clarithromycin
				Valproic acid	Erythromycin
				Celecoxib	Fluconazole
				Cimetidine	Miconazole
				Risperidone	
				Aripiprazole	
Inducers	Smoking	Dexamethasone	St. John's Wort		Dexamethasone
	Vegetables[a]	St. John's Wort			St. John's Wort
	Grilled meat				

PPI proton-pump inhibitor
[a]Cruciferous vegetables only

Table 4.3 Cytochrome P450 (CYP) isozymes involved in the metabolism of SRIs and the CYPs that they inhibit

Antidepressant	CYPs involved in metabolism	CYPs inhibited[g]
Fluoxetine	2C9, 2C19, 2D6[a]	CYPs 2D6 (strong), 2C9 (moderate), 2C19 (weak to moderate), 3A4 (weak)
Paroxetine	2D6, 3A4[b]	2D6 (strong), 1A2 (weak), 2C9 (weak), 2C19 (weak, 3A4 (weak)
Fluvoxamine	1A2, 2D6[c]	1A2 (strong), 2C9 (moderate), 2C19 (strong) 2D6 (weak), 3A4 (moderate)
Sertraline	2B6, 2C9, 2C19, 2D6, 3A4[d]	1A2 (weak) 2D6 (weak to moderate), 2C9 (weak), 2C19 (weak), 3A4 (weak)
Citalopram	2C19, 3A4[e]	CYPs 2D6 (weak to moderate), 2C9 (weak), 2C19 weak), 3A4 (weak
Venlafaxine	2C9 , 2C19, 2D6, 3A4[f]	CYP2D6 (weak)

[a]Ring et al. (2001); [b]Tang and Helmeste (2008); [c]DeVane (1999); [d]Obach et al. (2005); [e]Kobayashi et al. (1997); [f]Fogelman et al. (1999); [g]Spina et al. (2008)

adverse effects with consequences for fetal cardiovascular, neurologic, endocrine, or metabolic function.

Lifestyle-related factors may also influence SRI-metabolizing enzymes. For example, cigarette smoking and intake of cruciferous vegetables (such as broccoli) and grilled meat induce CYP1A2, which also metabolizes duloxetine (Lampe et al. 2000; Kall and Clausen 1995). Serum levels of duloxetine were found to be significantly lower among smokers possibly due to CYP1A2 induction by the polycylic hydrocarbons found in cigarettes (Fric et al. 2008). See Table 4.2 for a summary of CYP enzyme inducers and inhibitors, relevant to pregnancy.

Together, an awareness of key pharmacological and environmental factors could decrease (via induction of enzymes, EM, UM) or increase (enzyme inhibition, PM) drug levels in the mother and her fetus. Individualized therapeutic drug monitoring has been suggested by DeVane et al. (2006). Although it may offer a way to optimize pharmacotherapy and reduce side effects for women and their fetuses, it also raises questions about the ethics, cost, and complexity of care inherent to genotyping. At the very least, understanding the metabolic implications of multiple co-administered drugs, OTC mediations, and environmental influences, as well as prescribing SRIs that utilize more than one enzyme, increases the likelihood that metabolism will be less affected by drug–drug interactions or enzyme genetic variability.

4.7   Placental Contributions to Fetal SRI Exposure

While the role the placenta plays in determining fetal SRI exposure remains unclear, fetal levels are comparable to maternal levels (Kim et al. 2006). Maternal–fetal exchange of drugs occurs via the chorioallantoic placenta, which in humans is of the villous hemochorial type (Carter and Enders 2004). As with other epithelial structures, the extent of placental transfer of a molecule depends in large part upon its physicochemical properties, with placental permeability being inversely related to molecular size, polarity, and charge and directly related to lipophilicity (Faber and Thornburg 1983). All SRIs are lipophilic (Wishart et al. 2006), leading to high placental permeability and extensive maternal to fetal SRI transfer in humans (Kim et al. 2006; Rampono et al. 2009), although the fetal/maternal concentrations vary substantially. Associations between cord SRI levels and risk for neonatal behavioral disturbances remain inconsistent (Rampono et al. 2009; Oberlander et al. 2004; Laine et al. 2004), suggesting that other factors such as fetal metabolism, variations in drug potency that influence the inhibition of serotonin reuptake, or the presence of psychoactive metabolites may also be important predictors of neonatal outcomes.

4.8   Fetal Contributions to SRI Metabolism

For lipophilic drugs, two factors are important in determining fetal to maternal concentration ratios and hence the extent of fetal drug exposure. First, maternal and fetal differences in plasma protein drug binding are a key determinant of drug availability (Hill and Abramson 1988) and this is particularly important for SRIs that are highly protein bound (Hiemke and Hartter 2000; DeVane 1999). Second is the magnitude of drug clearance in the fetus, which is important in a setting with chronic drug dosing that results in steady-state plasma drug concentrations, as is

Table 4.4 Summary of ontogenesis of the hepatic CYPs involved in the metabolism of SRIs in the human

	Fetus		New born	Infants	Children	Adults
Genes and proteins	<20 weeks	>20 weeks	<1 month	<1 year	<12 years	>12 years
CYP2C9	−	+				+++
CYP2C9	−/+	+	++	+++	+++/++++	++++
CYP2C19	−	−/+				+++
CYP2C19	−	−/+	+	+	++	+++
CYP2D6	+	+	++	+++	+++	+++
CYP2D6	−/+	+	++	+++	+++	++++
CYP3A4	+	+				++++
CYP3A4	−	+	++	+++	+++/++++	++++
CYP3A7	++++	+++				+
CYP3A7	++++	++++/+++	++/++++	++	+/−	−

Data from Hines et al. 2002

+++++ very high expression, ++++ high expression, +++ moderate expression, ++ low expression; + very low expression; − no or negligible expression

typical for SRI drug therapy. Further, fetal drug clearance can be divided into placental (i.e., fetal to maternal drug transfer) and non-placental clearance, including hepatic drug metabolism and renal drug excretion (Szeto et al. 1982). The main route of non-placental clearance of drugs appears to be via metabolism in the liver (Kumar et al. 1997). Renal drug excretion does not serve as a route of drug elimination in the fetus. Fetal urine is excreted into the amniotic cavity, and from there can be returned to the fetus via fetal swallowing of amniotic fluid and reuptake by the intra-membranous pathway into the vasculature in the fetal membranes overlying the placenta (Brace 1997; Rurak et al. 1991), then metabolized in the fetal liver, or transferred back to the mother across the placenta when fetal/maternal drug concentration ratios permit.

Fetal drug metabolic capacity is limited by the low expression of phase I and II enzymes in the liver. With the exception of the high expression of CYP3A7, which is involved in the metabolism of endogenous steroids and declines progressively after birth, the expression of most of CYPs is low or absent in the fetus, with more or less progressive increases after birth (Hines and McCarver 2002; McCarver and Hines 2002). This is summarized in Table 4.4, which gives the CYP enzyme mRNA and protein levels in the human fetus, newborn, child, and adult (Hines and McCarver 2002; McCarver and Hines 2002). It is likely that the differences in the fetal/maternal drug ratios (Table 4.3) reflect the degree of CYP expression in the fetus and the extent of inhibition of these CYPs by the various SSRIs and SNRIs.

4.9   Considerations for Perinatal Mental Health Clinicians

Prenatal SRI exposure is common and neonatal outcomes vary greatly. Identification of the factors that contribute to both positive (e.g., maternal remission of depression, neonatal health) and negative outcomes (e.g., continued maternal depression and anxiety, neonatal SRI syndrome) in maternal–infant pairs must be prioritized as critical research topics to improve the benefits to both mother and her infant following SRI use in pregnancy. By considering the role of key maternal, fetal, and placental pharmacokinetic, metabolic, and genetic factors that affect the extent of fetal drug exposure we may develop evidence to guide optimal treatment with SRIs in pregnancy. Knowledge to inform pharmacologic care for pregnant women and their offspring is a critical investment in the health of the next generation. Overall, a key clinical approach should recognize the role of both fetal and maternal factors that influence pharmacological efficacy, a history of previous SRI treatment and related effects that might offer clues to pharmacological and genetic barriers to drug efficacy, the influence of environmental exposure that might influence drug effects (i.e., reduce drug–drug interactions), and efforts to minimize drug exposure where possible. The value of therapeutic drug monitoring and pharmacogenetic CYP testing for SRIs is unclear, given the limited evidence for clear drug concentration–effect relationships with the reported adverse fetal and neonatal consequences of antenatal drug exposure.

In providing antenatal care that requires SRI antidepressants, one needs to recognize risk characteristics that are inherent to an individual mother (and her child), in contrast to seeing them as just part of a population of prenatally treated mothers and their exposed children. There is a need to effectively diagnose and address antenatal maternal mental health considering all treatment options (cognitive/behavioral therapy, social support, diet, housing, etc.), remembering that medications may just be one of many options available. Recognizing interrelated risks of both antenatal maternal mood disorders and SRI exposure is critical for developing empirical, evidence-based approaches that identify the best fit between a pharmacological agent, non-pharmacological therapy, and maternal and neonatal factors so as to balance risks and benefits for both mothers and their children. Given increased risks associated with both untreated maternal depression and in utero SRI exposure, the clinical application of these findings may be challenging. This is not a setting where neonatal outcomes can be easily attributed to one causal factor— either maternal depression or SRI antidepressants. Rather, for most infants, the health risk is the result of an interplay between psychological, pharmacological, genetic, and social factors related to both the mother and the child. SRIs are prescribed with the expectation of treating the underlying maternal mood disorders to improve both maternal and infant health; however, such pharmacologic treatment during pregnancy does not guarantee remission of the underlying maternal mental illness. Identifying mothers who are likely to benefit from SRI treatment is a pressing issue. Clinicians may guide their management approaches by identifying patients who have a previous history of remission of depression/or anxiety with an SRI; however, this is not possible in all situations. Algorithms are available to guide clinical decision making regarding treatment for maternal mental illness for mothers who are planning to conceive and for those who are already pregnant (Yonkers et al. 2009). The decision to initiate SRI treatment during pregnancy rests with the mother and her physician carefully weighing the risks and benefits, understanding that the implications—both for better and worse—may last far longer than the pregnancy. Risks to infant health do not end in the newborn period and are not confined to neonatal behavior or heart and lung development. Given ongoing life with a depressed mother, our challenge is to find ways to "stack the deck" in favor of optimal neonatal health in the context of family well-being, extending well into childhood. Recognition of multiple and ongoing "environmental pathogens" requires ongoing surveillance and timely interventions that reduce risk exposures and maximize the benefits of treatment.

Acknowledgment We are grateful to Ursula Brain for her editorial assistance in the preparation of this chapter. TFO is the R. Howard Webster Professor in Early Child Development (UBC, College of Interdisciplinary Studies). DR was supported by an Investigatorship Award from the Child & Family Research Institute. None of the authors have conflicts of interest, including financial interests that are relevant to the study reported in this chapter.

References

Alfaro CL, Lam YW, Simpson J, Ereshefsky L. CYP2D6 status of extensive metabolizers after multiple-dose fluoxetine, fluvoxamine, paroxetine, or sertraline. J Clin Psychopharmacol. 1999;19:155–63.

Anderson GD. Pregnancy-induced changes in pharmacokinetics: a mechanistic-based approach. Clin Pharmacokinet. 2005;44:989–1008.

Ansorge MS, Zhou M, Lira A, Hen R, Gingrich JA. Early-life blockade of the 5-HT transporter alters emotional behavior in adult mice. Science. 2004;306:879–81.

Arranz MJ, de Leon J. Pharmacogenetics and pharmacogenomics of schizophrenia: a review of last decade of research. Mol Psychiatry. 2007;12:707–47.

Bennett HA, Einarson A, Taddio A, Koren G, Einarson TR. Prevalence of depression during pregnancy: systematic review. Obstet Gynecol. 2004;103:698–709.

Bijl MJ, Visser LE, Hofman A, Vulto AG, van Gelder GT, Stricker BH, et al. Influence of the CYP2D6*4 polymorphism on dose, switching and discontinuation of antidepressants. Br J Clin Pharmacol. 2008;65:558–64.

Brace RA. Physiology of amniotic fluid volume regulation. Clin Obstet Gynecol. 1997;40:280–9.

Bradford LD. CYP2D6 allele frequency in European Caucasians, Asians, Africans and their descendants. Pharmacogenomics. 2002;3:229–43.

Carter AM, Enders AC. Comparative aspects of trophoblast development and placentation. Reprod Biol Endocrinol. 2004;2:46.

Cohen LS, Altshuler LL, Harlow BL, Nonacs R, Newport DJ, Viguera AC, et al. Relapse of major depression during pregnancy in women who maintain or discontinue antidepressant treatment. JAMA. 2006;295:499–507.

Cooper WO, Willy ME, Pont SJ, Ray WA. Increasing use of antidepressants in pregnancy. Am J Obstet Gynecol. 2007;196:544–5.

Davidson S, Prokonov D, Taler M, Maayan R, Harell D, Gil-Ad I, et al. Effect of exposure to selective serotonin reuptake inhibitors in utero on fetal growth: potential role for the IGF-I and HPA axes. Pediatr Res. 2009;65:236–41.

DeVane CL. Metabolism and pharmacokinetics of selective serotonin reuptake inhibitors. Cell Mol Neurobiol. 1999;19:443–66.

DeVane CL, Stowe ZN, Donovan JL, Newport DJ, Pennell PB, Ritchie JC, et al. Therapeutic drug monitoring of psychoactive drugs during pregnancy in the genomic era: challenges and opportunities. J Psychopharmacol. 2006;20:54–9.

Faber JJ, Thornburg KL. Placental physiology. New York, NY: Raven Press; 1983.

Fogelman SM, Schmider J, Venkatakrishnan K, von Moltke LL, Harmatz JS, Shader RI, et al. O- and N-demethylation of venlafaxine in vitro by human liver microsomes and by microsomes from cDNA-transfected cells: effect of metabolic inhibitors and SSRI antidepressants. Neuropsychopharmacology. 1999;20:480–90.

Forcelli PA, Heinrichs SC. Preclinical study: teratogenic effects of maternal antidepressant exposure on neural substrates of drug-seeking behavior in offspring. Addict Biol. 2008;13:52–62.

Freeman MP, Nolan Jr PE, Davis MF, Anthony M, Fried K, Fankhauser M, et al. Pharmacokinetics of sertraline across pregnancy and postpartum. J Clin Psychopharmacol. 2008;28:646–53.

Fric M, Pfuhlmann B, Laux G, Riederer P, Distler G, Artmann S, et al. The influence of smoking on the serum level of duloxetine. Pharmacopsychiatry. 2008;41:151–5.

Garnett WR. Clinical implications of drug interactions with coxibs. Pharmacotherapy. 2001;21:1223–32.

Hanley GE, Oberlander TF. Neurodevelopmental outcomes following prenatal exposure to serotonin reuptake inhibitor antidepressants: a "social teratogen" or moderator of developmental risk? Birth Defects Res A Clin Mol Teratol. 2012;94:651–9.

Hiemke C, Hartter S. Pharmacokinetics of selective serotonin reuptake inhibitors. Pharmacol Ther. 2000;85:11–28.

Hill MD, Abramson FP. The significance of plasma protein binding on the fetal/maternal distribution of drugs at steady-state. Clin Pharmacokinet. 1988;14:156–70.

Hines RN, McCarver DG. The ontogeny of human drug-metabolizing enzymes: phase I oxidative enzymes. J Pharmacol Exp Ther. 2002;300:355–60.

Jeong H. Altered drug metabolism during pregnancy: hormonal regulation of drug-metabolizing enzymes. Expert Opin Drug Metab Toxicol. 2010;6:689–99.

Kall MA, Clausen J. Dietary effect on mixed function P450 1A2 activity assayed by estimation of caffeine metabolism in man. Hum Exp Toxicol. 1995;14:801–7.

Kallen B, Olausson PO. Maternal use of selective serotonin re-uptake inhibitors and persistent pulmonary hypertension of the newborn. Pharmacoepidemiol Drug Saf. 2008;17:801–6.

Kim J, Riggs KW, Misri S, Kent N, Oberlander TF, Grunau RE, et al. Stereoselective disposition of fluoxetine and norfluoxetine during pregnancy and breast-feeding. Br J Clin Pharmacol. 2006;61:155–63.

Kobayashi K, Chiba K, Yagi T, Shimada N, Taniguchi T, Horie T, et al. Identification of cytochrome P450 isoforms involved in citalopram N-demethylation by human liver microsomes. J Pharmacol Exp Ther. 1997;280:927–33.

Kumar S, Tonn GR, Kwan E, Hall C, Riggs KW, Axelson JE, et al. Estimation of transplacental and nonplacental diphenhydramine clearances in the fetal lamb: the impact of fetal first-pass hepatic drug uptake. J Pharmacol Exp Ther. 1997;282:617–32.

Laine K, Kytola J, Bertilsson L. Severe adverse effects in a newborn with two defective CYP2D6 alleles after exposure to paroxetine during late pregnancy. Ther Drug Monit. 2004;26:685–7.

Lampe JW, King IB, Li S, Grate MT, Barale KV, Chen C, et al. Brassica vegetables increase and apiaceous vegetables decrease cytochrome P450 1A2 activity in humans: changes in caffeine metabolite ratios in response to controlled vegetable diets. Carcinogenesis. 2000;21:1157–62.

Lee LJ. Neonatal fluoxetine exposure affects the neuronal structure in the somatosensory cortex and somatosensory-related behaviors in adolescent rats. Neurotox Res. 2009;15:212–23.

Li XQ, Andersson TB, Ahlstrom M, Weidolf L. Comparison of inhibitory effects of the proton pump-inhibiting drugs omeprazole, esomeprazole, lansoprazole, pantoprazole, and rabeprazole on human cytochrome P450 activities. Drug Metab Dispos. 2004;32:821–7.

Maciag D, Simpson KL, Coppinger D, Lu Y, Wang Y, Lin RC, et al. Neonatal antidepressant exposure has lasting effects on behavior and serotonin circuitry. Neuropsychopharmacology. 2006;31:47–57.

Magee LA, Abalos E, von Dadelszen P, Sibai B, Easterling T, Walkinshaw S. How to manage hypertension in pregnancy effectively. Br J Clin Pharmacol. 2011;72:394–401.

Martinez C, Albet C, Agundez JA, Herrero E, Carrillo JA, Marquez M, et al. Comparative in vitro and in vivo inhibition of cytochrome P450 CYP1A2, CYP2D6, and CYP3A by H2-receptor antagonists. Clin Pharmacol Ther. 1999;65:369–76.

McCarver DG, Hines RN. The ontogeny of human drug-metabolizing enzymes: phase II conjugation enzymes and regulatory mechanisms. J Pharmacol Exp Ther. 2002;300:361–6.

Morrison JL, Chien C, Riggs KW, Gruber N, Rurak D. Effect of maternal fluoxetine administration on uterine blood flow, fetal blood gas status, and growth. Pediatr Res. 2002;51:433–42.

Morrison JL, Riggs KW, Chien C, Gruber N, McMillen IC, Rurak DW. Chronic maternal fluoxetine infusion in pregnant sheep: effects on the maternal and fetal hypothalamic-pituitary-adrenal axes. Pediatr Res. 2004;56:40–6.

Moses-Kolko EL, Bogen D, Perel J, Bregar A, Uhl K, Levin B, et al. Neonatal signs after late in utero exposure to serotonin reuptake inhibitors: literature review and implications for clinical applications. JAMA. 2005;293:2372–83.

Mulder EJ, Ververs FF, de Heus R, Visser GH. Selective serotonin reuptake inhibitors affect neurobehavioral development in the human fetus. Neuropsychopharmacology. 2011;36:1961–71.

Nguyen TA. Cardiovascular, metabolic, endocrine and behavioral aspects of development in postnatal lambs in relation to age, sex, lamb number and acute fluoxetine administration. Thesis, University of British Columbia. 2013.

Niwa T, Inoue-Yamamoto S, Shiraga T, Takagi A. Effect of antifungal drugs on cytochrome P450 (CYP) 1A2, CYP2D6, and CYP2E1 activities in human liver microsomes. Biol Pharm Bull. 2005;28:1813–6.

Obach RS, Cox LM, Tremaine LM. Sertraline is metabolized by multiple cytochrome P450 enzymes, monoamine oxidases, and glucuronyl transferases in human: an in vitro study. Drug Metab Dispos. 2005;33:262–70.

Oberlander TF, Misri S, Fitzgerald CE, Kostaras X, Rurak D, Riggs W. Pharmacologic factors associated with transient neonatal symptoms following prenatal psychotropic medication exposure. J Clin Psychiatry. 2004;65:230–7.

Oberlander TF, Warburton W, Misri S, Aghajanian J, Hertzman C. Neonatal outcomes after prenatal exposure to selective serotonin reuptake inhibitor antidepressants and maternal depression using population-based linked health data. Arch Gen Psychiatry. 2006;63:898–906.

Oberlander TF, Weinberg J, Papsdorf M, Grunau R, Misri S, Devlin AM. Prenatal exposure to maternal depression, neonatal methylation of human glucocorticoid receptor gene (NR3C1) and infant cortisol stress responses. Epigenetics. 2008;3:97–106.

Oberlander TF, Gingrich JA, Ansorge MS. Sustained neurobehavioral effects of exposure to SSRI antidepressants during development: molecular to clinical evidence. Clin Pharmacol Ther. 2009;86:672–7.

Pascussi JM, Drocourt L, Gerbal-Chaloin S, Fabre JM, Maurel P, Vilarem MJ. Dual effect of dexamethasone on CYP3A4 gene expression in human hepatocytes. Sequential role of glucocorticoid receptor and pregnane X receptor. Eur J Biochem. 2001;268:6346–58.

Pelkonen O, Turpeinen M, Hakkola J, Honkakoski P, Hukkanen J, Raunio H. Inhibition and induction of human cytochrome P450 enzymes: current status. Arch Toxicol. 2008;82:667–715.

Popa D, Lena C, Alexandre C, Adrien J. Lasting syndrome of depression produced by reduction in serotonin uptake during postnatal development: evidence from sleep, stress, and behavior. J Neurosci. 2008;28:3546–54.

Preskorn SH, Borges S, Flockhart D. Clinically relevant pharmacology of neuropsychiatric drugs approved over the last three years: part I. J Psychiatr Pract. 2006;12:244–9.

Preskorn SH, Nichols AI, Paul J, Patroneva AL, Helzner EC, Guico-Pabia CJ. Effect of desvenlafaxine on the cytochrome P450 2D6 enzyme system. J Psychiatr Pract. 2008;14:368–78.

Rampono J, Simmer K, Ilett KF, Hackett LP, Doherty DA, Elliot R, et al. Placental transfer of SSRI and SNRI antidepressants and effects on the neonate. Pharmacopsychiatry. 2009;42:95–100.

Ring BJ, Eckstein JA, Gillespie JS, Binkley SN, VandenBranden M, Wrighton SA. Identification of the human cytochromes p450 responsible for in vitro formation of R- and S-norfluoxetine. J Pharmacol Exp Ther. 2001;297:1044–50.

Rurak DW, Wright MR, Axelson JE. Drug disposition and effects in the fetus. J Dev Physiol. 1991;15:33–44.

Rurak D, Lim K, Sanders A, Brain U, Riggs W, Oberlander TF. Third trimester fetal heart rate and Doppler middle cerebral artery blood flow velocity characteristics during prenatal selective serotonin reuptake inhibitor exposure. Pediatr Res. 2011;70:96–101.

Shea AK, Oberlander TF, Rurak D. Fetal serotonin reuptake inhibitor antidepressant exposure: maternal and fetal factors. Can J Psychiatry. 2012;57:523–9.

Spina E, Santoro V, D'Arrigo C. Clinically relevant pharmacokinetic drug interactions with second-generation antidepressants: an update. Clin Ther. 2008;30:1206–27.

Szeto HH, Umans JG, Rubinow SI. The contribution of transplacental clearances and fetal clearance to drug disposition in the ovine maternal-fetal unit. Drug Metab Dispos. 1982;10:382–6.

Tang SW, Helmeste D. Paroxetine. Expert Opin Pharmacother. 2008;9:787–94.

Tsai MH, Lin KM, Hsiao MC, Shen WW, Lu ML, Tang HS, et al. Genetic polymorphisms of cytochrome P450 enzymes influence metabolism of the antidepressant escitalopram and treatment response. Pharmacogenomics. 2010;11:537–46.

Ververs FF, Voorbij HA, Zwarts P, Belitser SV, Egberts TC, Visser GH, et al. Effect of cytochrome P450 2D6 genotype on maternal paroxetine plasma concentrations during pregnancy. Clin Pharmacokinet. 2009;48:677–83.

Vesga-Lopez O, Blanco C, Keyes K, Olfson M, Grant BF, Hasin DS. Psychiatric disorders in pregnant and postpartum women in the United States. Arch Gen Psychiatry. 2008;65:805–15.

Wadelius M, Darj E, Frenne G, Rane A. Induction of CYP2D6 in pregnancy. Clin Pharmacol Ther. 1997;62:400–7.

Warburton W, Hertzman C, Oberlander TF. A register study of the impact of stopping third trimester selective serotonin reuptake inhibitor exposure on neonatal health. Acta Psychiatr Scand. 2010;121(6):471–9.

Wishart DS, Knox C, Guo AC, Shrivastava S, Hassanali M, Stothard P, et al. DrugBank: a comprehensive resource for in silico drug discovery and exploration. Nucleic Acids Res. 2006;34:D668–72.

Yonkers KA, Wisner KL, Stewart DE, Oberlander TF, Dell DL, Stotland N, et al. The management of depression during pregnancy: a report from the American Psychiatric Association and the American College of Obstetricians and Gynecologists. Gen Hosp Psychiatry. 2009;31:403–13.

Yudin MH, van Schalkwyk J, Van Eyk N, Boucher M, Castillo E, Cormier B, et al. Antibiotic therapy in preterm premature rupture of the membranes. J Obstet Gynaecol Can. 2009;31:863–74.

Zeskind PS, Stephens LE. Maternal selective serotonin reuptake inhibitor use during pregnancy and newborn neurobehavior. Pediatrics. 2004;113:368–75.

Zhou SF, Zhou ZW, Yang LP, Cai JP. Substrates, inducers, inhibitors and structure-activity relationships of human Cytochrome P450 2C9 and implications in drug development. Curr Med Chem. 2009;16:3480–675.

Depression in Pregnancy and Child Development: Understanding the Mechanisms of Transmission

5

Andrew J. Lewis

Abstract

The impact of depression in pregnancy and in the early postpartum period on neonatal and early child development has been well documented. Perinatal depression predicts poorer cognitive function, behavioural development, and emotional regulation in offspring. However, the mechanism through which this occurs requires clarification. This chapter provides a commentary on existing research, particularly that emerging from fetal programming, to consider possible mechanisms for this transmission of risk. This body of literature suggests that the timing of depression across the perinatal period is significant, and should be separated into exposures across each trimester of pregnancy and across the postnatal period with the timing and dose of depressive symptoms being clearly distinguished. Other cofounding exposures are both psychosocial in nature such as anxiety and stress and also teratogenic such as smoking, nutritional deficiencies, and medication exposures. Such confounds need to be carefully considered when interpreting the depression literature. Putative mechanisms through which prenatal depression impacts child development include direct genetic inheritance, shared adverse environments, elevated maternal stress response, alteration in vascular and placental function, and inflammatory pathways. Postnatal pathways have been more substantially investigated and probably involve maternal sensitivity, lower stimulation, and ongoing environmental stressors. The cumulative effect of both prenatal and postnatal factors should be a greater focus of research design in this field. Prevention and intervention models to reduce the deleterious effects of maternal depression in the preconception, antenatal, and postnatal period can be informed by further research on these mechanisms of transmission.

A.J. Lewis (✉)
Faculty of Health, School of Psychology, Deakin University, Burwood, NSW, Australia
e-mail: andrew.lewis@deakin.edu.au

M. Galbally et al. (eds.), *Psychopharmacology and Pregnancy*,
DOI 10.1007/978-3-642-54562-7_5, © Springer-Verlag Berlin Heidelberg 2014

Keywords

Prevention • Maternal mental health • Perinatal depression • Fetal programming • Epigenetics • Developmental origins of health and disease (DOHaD)

Optimising child developmental outcomes requires a life-course model able to consider the complex unfolding of developmental processes that commence prior to the child's conception. The key developmental transitions are those leading up to conception, from pregnancy to birth, the period of lactation and early infancy, childhood, and then the pubertal transitions into the reproductive years of adult life. Conceptualising each transition provides a bio-developmental framework upon which all interventions, be they pharmacological, psychosocial, or lifestyle based, can be properly conceived, developed, and evaluated (Shonkoff 2010). Although it goes without saying that optimal early child development builds upon optimal fetal development, too much developmental research has considered birth to be a starting point to investigate development and too much psychiatric research has failed to consider the reproductive and child developmental consequences of adult psychiatric disorders.

At birth a neonate in a state of good health is able to thrive over the neonatal period by eliciting and receiving the benefit of high-quality parental investment. However, earlier developmental setbacks such as reduced gestation, low birth weight, deleterious pregnancy exposures, or complications during pregnancy or birth can negatively impact on the health and mental health of an individual across the life course. It follows that a child's development across such transitions cannot be considered apart from the mother's health, mental health, and well-being. An infant is more likely to experience optimal development in a context of good maternal health and mental health commencing in the preconception period and extending across her pregnancy.

Maternal mental health during pregnancy is not only a major psychosocial stressor, but increasingly understood to also be a major physiological stressor. The most prevalent issues are depression, anxiety, and stress exposure. Alongside obesity, nutrition, and metabolic disorders, compromised maternal mental health is increasingly recognised as one of the major complications of pregnancy. Efforts to optimise child development require researchers, clinicians, and policymakers to address such complications through interventions delivered at preconception, pregnancy, and postnatally. The high population prevalence of mood and anxiety disorders over pregnancy is of considerable public health concern given the impact on mothers themselves, their offspring, and child's experience of postnatal care. This chapter will focus on perinatal depression and, following a brief review of the findings on child and maternal outcomes, will consider in detail the putative biological mechanisms by which perinatal depression translates into poor outcomes for offspring.

5.1   Epidemiology of Perinatal Depression

Perinatal Depression is one of the most common complications of pregnancy affecting 7–13 % of pregnant women and 10–15 % of women in the 6 months following their child's birth (Bennett et al. 2009). There is a wide range of severity in depressive symptoms ranging from the so-called maternity blues, which is very common and typically transitory, through to postpartum psychosis which has a prevalence of less than 1 %. Depressive symptoms meet diagnostic criteria and require clinical intervention once they are characterised by persistently dysphoric mood and anhedonia as well as additional symptoms which can include sleep and appetite disturbance, fatigue, irritability, lack of concentration, and in some cases suicidal ideation and attempts. It is not uncommon that depressive disorders are also accompanied by feelings of lowered self-worth, hopelessness, social withdrawal, and an inability to cope. These symptoms are related to neurobiological changes that have mostly been investigated in terms of monoaminergic and glutamatergic systems or as dysregulations of the hypothalamic–pituitary–adrenal (HPA) axis and its interface with hippocampal activation. This neuroendocrine system involves corticotropin-releasing hormone (CRH), glucocorticoids, and brain-derived neurotrophic factor (BDNF). Clearly, other neural regions are involved and research has examined the nucleus accumbens and amygdala as brain regions involved in the regulation of motivation, eating, sleeping, energy level, circadian rhythm, and reward systems which are all known to be dysregulated in depression (Nestler et al. 2002). This complex group of depressive symptoms occurring within the context of the profound biological and psychosocial changes that accompany pregnancy suggests that our use of the term 'perinatal depression' is shorthand for a complex and highly disabling condition.

The prevalence of perinatal depression has also been well established: both antenatally and postnatally. Gaynes and colleagues systematically reviewed 28 papers reporting prevalence of perinatal depression and found that the combined point prevalence estimates ranged from 6.5 % to 12.9 %. Over the perinatal period from pregnancy up to 3 months postpartum the cumulative prevalence reached 19.2 % of women diagnosed with a major depressive episode with the majority occurring after delivery (Gaynes et al. 2005). Other studies have shown that the duration of the perinatal depressive episode is related to two key factors: the severity of symptoms and access to treatment (Dennis 2005). Antenatal mood disorders are also highly prevalent with a systematic review by Bennett reporting prevalence rates of depressive disorders in pregnancy as 7.4 %, 12.8 %, and 12.0 % across each trimester (Bennett et al. 2004). Leigh and Milgrom reported Australian data from the *Beyondblue* National Postnatal Depression Program showing a prevalence rate for depression at 28–32 weeks of pregnancy at 16.9 % and at 10–12 weeks postnatally at 11.2 % (Leigh and Milgrom 2008).

It is particularly important given this paper's focus on mechanisms to note that the continuity between antenatal depression and postnatal depression is high. Around 50 % of women with postnatal depressive symptoms have also experienced depression during their pregnancy (Gotlib et al. 1989). Using data from the Avon

Longitudinal Study of Parents and Children (ALSPAC) Heron reported that the majority of cases of postnatal depression and anxiety were preceded by antenatal depression and anxiety, respectively (Heron et al. 2004). This study found that women presenting with antenatal anxiety were more than three times more likely to present with postnatal depression at 8 weeks and 8 months. Leigh and Milgrom used a multivariate regression model which included a large number of demographic and historical factors, antenatal depression, anxiety and stressors, as well as personality variables to show that, in the final model, antenatal depression ($\beta = 0.47$), parenting stress ($\beta = 0.32$), and history of depression ($\beta = 0.15$) were the only significant predictors of postnatal depression after controlling for these other variables. The final regression model explained an impressive 66 % of the variance in postnatal depressive symptoms (Leigh and Milgrom 2008).

5.2   Offspring Outcomes Following Maternal Depression

Child outcomes following perinatal depression have been investigated in many studies. A significant body of research investigating perinatal depression has now examined outcomes including birth outcomes, child and adolescent mental and behavioural disorders, cognitive development including language development and attention capacity, and socio-emotional development in terms of temperament and attachment. These studies have been well reviewed in several recent papers (Schlotz and Phillips 2009; Talge et al. 2007; Swanson and Wadhwa 2008).

    In short, for prenatal exposure, maternal prenatal stress in various forms has been found to be associated with a number of mental health disorders. Some of this previous research has been based on ecological exposures such as disaster records or retrospective assessment of prenatal stress. Khashan et al. (2008) used two Danish national registries and found that maternal prenatal exposure to a family bereavement during the first trimester was related to an increased risk of schizophrenia. Similar studies have found associations between high pregnancy stress and risk of psychosis (Spauwen et al. 2004), storm or hurricane exposure and autism (Kinney et al. 2008), and earthquake exposure predicting depressive symptoms in offspring (Watson et al. 1999). A number of large prospective cohort studies have more convincingly measured maternal anxiety and depressive symptoms experienced in pregnancy and also show that these predict child mental health outcomes. Loomans et al. (2011) found that maternal state anxiety measured at 16 weeks gestation was significantly associated with an increased likelihood of inattention/hyperactivity problems for boys but not for girls. O'Connor et al. (2002, 2003) reported that prenatal maternal anxiety measured at 32 weeks predicted inattention/hyperactivity symptoms also in boys at 4 and 6.5 years. Clavarino et al. (2010) also found that high prenatal maternal anxiety was associated with attention problems at 5, but that these remitted by 14 years, while anxiety problems persisted from 5 to 14 years. Robinson et al. (2008) found that major life stressors were associated with small increases in behavioural problems at ages 2 and 5 and emotional problems at age 5. These are a small selection of the studies with larger samples, which consistently show an impact of maternal mental health in pregnancy on child behavioural, attention, and emotional outcomes.

In terms of postnatal depression, infants of depressed mothers show more negative affect and lower sensitivity (Dawson et al. 1992) and offspring may experience inadequate physical and verbal stimulation (Field 1998). These effects of postnatal depression have been shown to extend to adolescents who continue to display increased waking cortisol levels (Murray et al. 2010). It is well established that postnatal depression reduces the sensitivity of mother when interacting with the child and this results in poorer stress regulation and insecure attachments. A meta-analysis of seven studies found that the infants of depressed mothers were less likely to have a secure attachment and more likely to display avoidant and disorganised attachment (Martins and Gaffan 2000). Essentially, the putative mechanism here is the negative effects of *postnatal* maternal caregiving in the context of maternal depression.

The literature on temperament outcomes for infants and in early childhood is particularly interesting since it suggests important mechanistic pathways to what has previously been considered a highly genetically heritable trait of emotional regulation. Field reports in her systematic review that raised cortisol levels in pregnancy have been associated with increased fussiness and negative behaviour in previous studies and maternal reports of infant negative reactivity (Field 2011; Davis et al. 2007). Recent studies have found that maternal life stressors over pregnancy predict infant cortisol levels, reactive temperament (Lewis and Olsson 2011), and higher resting cortisol throughout the day in adolescence (Van Den Bergh et al. 2008).

There are important caveats to consider when interpreting this literature. Our own study of antidepressant use in Australia using the population Longitudinal Study of Australian Children (LSAC) showed that not only was antidepressant use associated with higher levels of depression, but was also associated with higher rates of multiple exposures such as smoking, other medication use, and health difficulties (Lewis et al. 2012). There is also high comorbidity between maternal obesity and mental health symptoms in pregnancy.

5.3   Mechanisms of Transmission

Broadly, there are three potential mechanisms whereby maternal perinatal depression could be transmitted to negative offspring outcomes. In summary, these are a model based purely on genetic heritability, secondly, the influence of shared environmental factors which contribute equally to maternal perinatal depression and impact on child development, and thirdly, there is the idea that maternal depression, in a variety of possible mechanisms, programmes fetal and early infant development in a manner which leads to poor outcomes for the child.

In terms of a genetic model, it is widely accepted that genetic factors play an important part in the risk for depression. Epidemiologic studies using behavioural genetic approaches generally suggest that 30–40 % of the risk for depression is heritable (Sullivan et al. 2000). However, the isolation of which specific mechanisms of heritability are responsible encounters several issues. The first is the pervasive 'missing heritability' problem which plagues studies of association that are based on candidate genes which typically account for a small fraction of the heritability estimates (Manolio et al. 2009). One example which has been prominent in the literature is a repeat length polymorphism in the serotonin transporter promoter region (*SLC6A4*) which codes for a protein that transports synaptic serotonin and is the target of SSRIs. However, the effect of this genetic variant is small and tends to be stronger for depression-associated personality or behavioural traits such as neuroticism or suicidality (Costas et al. 2010). Polymorphisms in *MAOA* and *COMT* have also been found to be associated with perinatal depression onset in the context of stressful events (Doornbos et al. 2009). Using data from the Cardiovascular Risk in Young Finns birth cohort followed since 1980 Jokela examined the serotonin receptor 2A gene and found that a polymorphism appears to moderate the relationship between mother's self-reported maternal nurturance of the child and the development of depressive symptoms in adulthood (Jokela et al. 2007). Perhaps a more profound limitation in the genetic heritability model concerns the rapidly shifting concept of heritability itself, which is moving beyond gene-based models in the light of germ line heritability conferred with epigenetic heritability (Lewis 2012).

While such findings are suggestive, there remains difficulty isolating specific candidate genes for depression that is probably due to there being many genes involved which produce such a complex phenotype, each gene only contributing a small effect. It is also important to recognise that a purely genetic model is itself biologically implausible given that genes operate within a complex biological system which provides the context of their biological action (Meaney 2010). There may also be a number of different genetic pathways that confer risk and there are complex interactions over time between genes, epigenetic effects, and environmental factors.

Recent evidence concerning common genetic variants for a range of mental health disorders adds an intriguing possibility that across disorders such as schizophrenia, depression, and bipolar disorder common genetic variants confer a genetic risk disposition which becomes shaped into different disorders by subsequent developmental, environmental, or stochastic factors. A recent meta-analysis examined whether variants in methylenetetrahydrofolate reductase (*MTHFR*), a gene involved in processing folic acid, contribute to shared genetic vulnerability to a combined group of psychiatric disorders (schizophrenia, bipolar disorder, and unipolar depressive disorder) and found a 26 % increased association with one polymorphism (Peerbooms et al. 2011).

Here we have said nothing of the possible genetic links between perinatal depression and non-mental health outcomes in children such as cognitive and psychosocial outcomes via pleiotropic genetic effects. The genetic model can also apply to offspring genetically inheriting certain sensitivities or predispositions to behave in a certain manner, which exposes individuals to certain environments which may be adverse (Kendler et al. 1995). This is referred to as gene–environment correlation.

A second model of transmission which should be briefly mentioned is the circumstance in which the environmental conditions, which contribute to prenatal and postnatal depression, also make a contribution to adverse child outcomes. In this case a direct association between perinatal depression and child outcome is actually confounded by a third variable contributing to both. Relevant factors here include low socio-economic status and other perpetuating adversities which create stress, limit opportunities, and possibly contribute to lack of support for new parents. Socio-economic status may imply differences in access to material and social resources for children and their parents (Bradley and Corwyn 2002). Socio-economic status is one of the most widely investigated social determinants of child developmental outcomes and will not be further reviewed here.

There is also clearly a major role for postnatal transmission of maternal mood on offspring outcome. The fetal stress response is rapidly transformed postnatally into a circadian rhythm with a peak around the time of waking which starts to operate within a few months of birth for a term baby (Price et al. 1983). The normal circadian rhythm can facilitate termination of the HPA stress response and conversely disturbances in the daily rhythm may contribute to HPA stress dysregulation (Gunnar and Quevedo 2007). This interaction postnatally between circadian rhythm, stress response and sleep patterns illustrates the hierarchical nature of development where basic bio-behavioural structures established in fetal development can also come to function as the platform for more complex developmental systems. Although these have not been so clearly articulated, similar patterns may exist for the development of interpersonal, emotional, and behavioural responses further into childhood and adolescence (Gluckman and Hanson 2006). Much more could be said on postnatal mechanisms, but the focus in this chapter is on the prenatal period.

5.4   Prenatal Depression and Fetal Programming

The main focus in this chapter is to consider emerging research on the manner in which maternal depression disrupts development through prenatal programming of later development. Animal models of such transmission have been well developed, typically based on inducing either pharmacological or environmental stresses at various times across the perinatal period in rodent models and non-human primates (Darnaudéry and Maccari 2008). Such models have established that the timing of the stress, its intensity and duration, and the gender of the offspring are critical factors influencing offspring outcomes (Field 2011). Such studies also demonstrate neurodevelopmental alterations occurring in the hippocampus, prefrontal cortex, the amygdala, and the nucleus accumbens following maternal stress. The offspring of stress exposed dams go on to display anxious and depressive behaviours (or at least animal analogues of such disorders), but interestingly memory impairments have also been documented (Darnaudéry and Maccari 2008). Such maternal stressors are thought to be transmitted via increases in maternal corticosteroid levels also being transmitted to the fetal brain and thus influencing the development of the offspring HPA system. This programmes later emotional and behavioural disturbances in the offspring such as fearfulness, impulsivity, and substance use, which often become more pronounced when the animal is subjected to a later stressor.

Weinstock has shown in animal studies that offspring outcomes are sex specific which may be due to higher cortisol exposure in males decreasing fetal testosterone, but in females this alters catecholamine activity (Weinstock 2007, 2011). Weinstock suggests that learning deficits are more readily seen in prenatally stressed males while females show anxiety, depression, and an increased response of the HPA axis to stress—findings which are similar to human population studies showing higher vulnerability to attention problems in males and possible links to the well-established rise of depression and anxiety in female adolescents.

There is also a substantial literature on the reversibility of the effects of maternal stress in animal models which cannot be reviewed here. Suffice to say that environmental enrichment and anti-depression treatments appear to ameliorate maternal stress exposures in these animal models. While these models are critical to understanding biological mechanisms and to testing possible interventions, their interpretation needs to be approached with caution. It should be noted that the species-specific ontogeny of the HPA system is important to consider when applying such findings to humans since exposures at different points in fetal and postnatal development may influence various systems involved in neuroendocrine and autonomic responses to stressors and the specific timing and degree of fetal HPA development varies considerably across mammalian species. So too it is difficult to model depression exposure in an animal model given the mood and cognitive components.

5.5   The Role of Glucocorticoids

There has been considerable focus on the early development of the hypothalamic–pituitary–adrenal (HPA) system which is also linked to maturation of other systems responsible for the regulation of circadian rhythms, physical growth, and the integration of limbic-cortical processes. The HPA system plays a critical part in early development, not only in stress regulation, but also in sleep, feeding, emotions, and emotion regulation (Lupien et al. 2009).

Glucocorticoids are responsible for regulation of metabolic functions and the regulation of stress. In normal development glucocorticoids have widespread programming and developmental functions for the fetus across a wide range of tissues such as lung, liver, thymus, and brain and this continues in postnatal development. There are major changes in glucocorticoid function over pregnancy. In the course of a normal pregnancy maternal cortisol increases, reaching a peak during the third trimester, suggesting a gradual upregulation of the maternal HPA axis across pregnancy (Jung et al. 2011). One source is the placenta, another is that maternal adrenal glands show greater sensitivity during pregnancy (Lindsay and Nieman 2005), and another is that increasing oestrogen levels over pregnancy reduce the breakdown of cortisol (Field 2011).

Several lines of evidence suggest that perinatal exposure to maternal depression is associated with deregulation of the child's HPA response to stress, increasing the risk for future stress-related disorders. Higher levels of corticotropin-releasing hormone (CRH) in pregnancy have been associated with higher rates of depression (Rich-Edwards et al. 2008). There is some evidence that higher CRH is transmitted to the offspring. Azak reported that infants of mothers with depression and anxiety had high cortisol production from morning to bedtime and higher bedtime values and the effect was more enduring in children who had mothers with depression (Azak et al. 2013). Naturally this raises the question of whether the child outcomes referred to above, such as emotional and behavioural problems, are a direct effect of fetal programming or are an effect mediated by the offspring's early socio-emotional experiences in the context of a dysregulated stress response.

There are also intriguing effects of patterns of neurotransmitter function which appear to be transmitted from mother to offspring. Over a series of papers Field reported across several monoamines that neonates of depressed women had bio-chemical profiles that mimicked their mothers' antenatal profiles. She identified similar patterns for elevations in noradrenaline and lowered levels of dopamine and serotonin (Field 2011). The relationship between changes in glucocorticoid function and monoamine regulation for antenatally depressed mothers remains a com-pelling question. So too does the functional significance of these changes for early neural development in the fetus and in early childhood social and emotional development.

5.6   Development of the Fetal HPA System

Recent evidence suggests that exposure of the fetus to high maternal levels of glucocorticoids has long-term effects on child neurodevelopment. In a study of intrauterine exposure to synthetic glucocorticoids, Davis et al. showed an impact on development of the anterior cingulate cortex, which was associated with affective symptoms in children 6–10 years of age (Davis et al. 2013). In another study it was found that offspring of postnatally depressed mothers display larger amygdala volumes and have higher cortisol levels which leads to higher levels of internalising problems (Bagner et al. 2010).

The development of the HPA axis in the human fetus is a complex process involving maturation of fetal organs as well as interaction with placental and maternal endocrine systems (Bolt et al. 2002). In late pregnancy, a rise in fetal cortisol levels is necessary to stimulate the development of organ systems such as the lungs. However, as Meaney has discussed, this necessary aspect of fetal development shows that glucocorticoids function differently in distinct fetal tissue.

Across most mammals increased neural exposure to glucocorticoids reduces neurogenesis and synaptic plasticity, suggesting that tissue-specific transcription factors may regulate glucocorticoid receptors, allowing protection for fetal neural development (Meaney 2010). It is also clear that an excess of fetal glucocorticoids may result in growth restriction of the fetus as well as influencing the postnatal adaptation and activity of the pancreas, pituitary–adrenal axis, and cardiovascular activity (Challis et al. 2001).

Postnatally an adaptive stress response occurs via perceptual cues relating to threat, disruption of expectancies, physical pain, infection, or metabolic crisis. Such cues are communicated to the hypothalamus via specific pathways. These signals are integrated in the hypothalamic paraventricular nucleus (PVN) where neurons expressing corticotropin-releasing hormone (CRH), in collaboration with other peptides such as vasopressin (AVP), stimulate the release of corticotropin hormone (ACTH) from the anterior pituitary (De Kloet et al. 2005). When released into circulation from the pituitary ACTH stimulates the adrenal cortices to synthesise and release cortisol. In fetal development the link between pituitary ACTH and adrenal cortisol appears to be established some time after week 20 of gestation (Bolt et al. 2002).

In early gestation, the fetal adrenal cortex produces small amounts of cortisol which gradually increases during the third trimester (Bolt et al. 2002). Across the second trimester placental ACTH, in combination with other placental hormones, regulates fetal production of adrenal steroids. By the third trimester the fetal pituitary gland seems to become integrated with the fetal adrenal cortex (Bolt et al. 2002). By late gestation the human fetal HPA axis is well developed and functions as a stress response system in response to stressors such as hypoxia or nutrient restriction. Therefore, external factors that reduce uterine vascular flow may initiate a fetal stress response similar to that experienced postnatally (Phillips and Jones 2006). Over the third trimester HPA activation begins to function according to its well-known negative feedback mechanism whereby mineralocorticoid and glucocorticoid receptors that are expressed extensively across the hypothalamus and hippocampus operate to inhibit the stress response (De Kloet et al. 2005). However, these two receptors play different roles in modulating both the stress response and the circadian rhythm. [Detailed reviews of HPA system and its fetal development are available in De Kloet et al. (2005)].

5.7   Role of the Placenta

There is a growing interest in the placenta as a critical agent in the transmission of maternal depression and infant outcomes. Placentation is a process which commences with blastocysts attaching to the uterine endometrium. The functioning placenta comes to serve a complex array of functions for the fetus including those of the lungs, intestine, kidney, liver, and a wide range of endocrine functions analogous to the pituitary and gonads (Luckett 1976). The investigation of placental biology in women who are depressed antenatally holds considerable promise in terms of understanding the biological mechanism involved in transmission of risk to offspring (Kaplan et al. 2008). The placenta functions as a temporary endocrine structure which regulates the transfer of nutrients to the fetus, but also protects the fetus from the growth-inhibiting effects of maternal glucocorticoids (Cottrell and Seckl 2009).

The placenta serves as a critical interface between maternal and fetal physiology and, in this respect, regulates the transfer of glucose, amino acids, ketones, and fatty acids. Alterations in maternal hormone levels across pregnancy potentially alter fetal development and conversely the production of placental hormones influences maternal physiology (Haig 1993). This implies a conceptual model where, across gestation, the maternal–fetal dyad is mostly mediated via the placenta which operates in a transactional manner across these two distinct organisms to facilitate fetal development. While it is clear that a proportion of such development is directed in a species typical manner by genomic information, there is also a significant role for input from the intrauterine environment which shapes the trajectory of early development.

There is an increasing research focus on the role of the placenta in the mediation of maternal prenatal distress and its impact on fetal development. Much of this research has focused on the enzyme type 2 isoform of 11beta-hydroxysteroid dehydrogenase (*11β-HSD2*) which specifically inactivates glucocorticoids, is highly expressed within the placenta, and has been suggested to play a role in the ontogeny of the fetal HPA axis (Cottrell and Seckl 2009). The expression level of *11β-HSD2* in the placenta directly influences the exposure of the fetus to circulating maternal stress hormones that cross the fetomaternal interface. Circulating cortisol concentrations in the fetus are typically around 13-fold lower than those in the mother, but there are portions of the placenta with less *11β-HSD2* enzyme allowing the fetus to be exposed to maternal cortisol in proportion to maternal cortisol level over pregnancy (O'donnell et al. 2009). In most cases placental *11β-HSD2* substantially reduces maternal cortisol transfer; however, around 10–20 % of maternal cortisol still contributes to fetal cortisol (Challis et al. 2001). Furthermore, the source of individual variation in placental *11β-HSD2* function remains an area of intense research focus at the present time with maternal stress, diet, and infection during pregnancy under current investigation.

Placental *11β-HSD2* represents a key biomarker of fetal stress biology and one of the earliest indicators that a child is on a pathway of high stress reactivity. Two recent studies have direct relevance. O'Donnell reported a 30 % reduction in placental *11β-HSD2* expression when mothers experienced prenatal anxiety and depression (O'Donnell et al. 2012). A recent paper failed to replicate O'Donnell's findings and also reported no effect of SSRI treatment on levels of placental *11β-HSD2* gene expression (Ponder et al. 2011).

While the placental passage of cortisol is clearly an important mechanism for transmission of the effects of antenatal depression, this supposes that the effect is a direct one. Fetal brain development would need to be directly impacted by increased cortisol exposure. While this is plausible, there is an alternative hypothesis which is that conditions which impose high stress on a pregnant woman such as depression and anxiety have an impact on fetal development via restriction of intrauterine Arterial blood flow which induces hypoxia and limits nutrient supply to the developing fetus. Raised levels of maternal noradrenaline are associated with intrauterine arterial resistance and this mechanism requires additional investigation (Field 2011; Teixeira et al. 1999).

Another possible mechanism to mention is the role of immune function. While one of the adaptive responses to acute stress is to mobilise the immune system, chronic stress and the chronic production of stress-related hormones suppress immune function. At the same time cytokine responses to inflammation are known to activate the HPA axis. A number of studies show that maternal exposure to infection increases the release of pro-inflammatory cytokines into the circulation (Weinstock 2005). Excess levels of these cytokines could induce premature birth and may be linked to the development of asthma and allergies. Again, it remains unclear whether cytokine exposure directly influences fetal neural development, or creates fetal distress via arterial resistance, or the impact on child development occurs via growth restriction and reduced gestational length. Here the timing and type of infection are significant factors. For example, during embryogenesis, the developing embryo is highly sensitive to infections such as rubella which have a direct effect on the development of organs. When maternal circulation is established via the placenta, the rate of fetal growth and development can be influenced by malaria infection (Gluckman et al. 2007).

5.8   Epigenetic Regulation of Fetal Development

Another intriguing aspect of early biological mechanisms is the intrauterine programming by maternal depression of gene expression in the developing fetus. 'Epigenetics' describes the study of all heritable changes in gene expression that are not encoded by the DNA sequence itself (Schroeder et al. 2011). Epigenetic programming of fetal and infant development may be induced by environmental signals transmitted via the mother during prenatal and postnatal development, but it is also increasingly clear that genetic factors also play a role directly programming fetal development and also influencing epigenetic processes. Epigenetics involves changes in the many chromatin functions which regulate tissue- and cell-specific gene expression. These include methylation of CpG sites across the genome, that is, a sequence within DNA where a cytosine nucleotide occurs before a guanine and can be linked by phosphate. The addition of a methyl group to cytosine within the DNA sequence, or more likely multiple methylation of CpG islands leading up to promoter regions, can silence the expression of a particular gene and this effect can be particular to a given cell line or tissue. Another epigenetic mechanism which is increasingly a focus is modification of histone sites which produces the opposite effect of making DNA available for transcription.

In previous studies, prenatal maternal stress and depression have been shown to alter epigenetic programming of genes found in placental tissue and cord blood. Although these tissues are peripheral to fetal brain development, their methylation status may well be an important biomarker for neural development. A number of studies are now providing such evidence of alterations in epigenetic programming as an effect of maternal mental health within specific genes associated with fetal neurodevelopment. For example, one strategy has been the use of high-throughput sequencing techniques to examine genome-wide DNA methylation across initially 27,000 CpG sites, in order to examine the effect of exposure to psychotropic medications and psychiatric illness on the methylation of genes within both placental tissue and umbilical cord blood (Schroeder et al. 2012; Smith et al. 2012). In one such study, numerous sites where the CpG methylation is different between those fetuses exposed to an antiepileptic compared to those who were not exposed have been identified. However, high-throughput sequencing technology is developing rapidly with considerable increases in genomic coverage now available. There is considerable interest in how to best analyse and interpret data on such a massive scale so it is likely such results are preliminary.

Another epigenetic approach is to select genes of known interest to fetal neurodevelopment, so-called candidate genes, and to examine the effect of maternal depression on epigenetic markers and, in some cases, gene expression within tissues of interest. The glucocorticoid receptor gene *NR3C1* is one of the most well-characterised and investigated HPA axis-related genes. Oberlander and colleagues found elevated methylation of *NR3C1* in cord blood samples from infants born to mothers with depression during the third trimester of pregnancy (Oberlander et al. 2008). In this study, infant HPA reactivity was assessed at 3 months of age using a habituation information processing task and levels of *NR3C1* DNA methylation in fetal cord blood predicted infant cortisol response to stress. In a recent study, Radtke and colleagues examined the methylation status of NR3C1 in mothers and their children 10–19 years after birth and remarkably found that in the children methylation status of this gene was associated with their mother's experience of partner violence during pregnancy (Radtke et al. 2011), suggesting that epigenetic processes operating in pregnancy may well have long-term developmental consequences.

The major challenge for epigenetic research seeking to examine the impact of maternal depression is to establish the functional significance and casual pathway for genomic regions where differences in epigenetic profile can be established for specific fetal exposures. For offspring outcomes such as cognition, emotional development, growth, and behavioural development, peripheral tissues can be readily collected such as cord blood, buccal cells, or placental tissue, but establishing their role as biomarkers of relevant outcomes requires carefully controlled studies and replication of associations of these epigenetic markers with later child outcomes. Findings of this kind are beginning to emerge, but this highly promising area is in its infancy.

5.9   Conclusions

5.9.1   The Timing of Exposure to Depression

It is significant that the global definition of perinatal depression includes both prenatal and postnatal maternal depression and therefore does not allow us to differentiate between the effects derived from intrauterine *vs.* postnatal effects. The strong continuity between antenatal and postnatal depression needs to be considered in all study designs of child outcomes. Studies commencing data collection only in the postpartum period are missing important pregnancy factors. Careful consideration of the relative impact of exposure to maternal depression during fetal development and during early childhood is required to understand child developmental outcomes. Exposures in the antenatal and postnatal period may cause different effects and, in many cases, the effect of exposure across both periods may be cumulative or interactive.

The bulk of the evidence, and current practice in perinatal mental health, is concerned with addressing postnatal depression and anxiety so as to improve the chances of more effective parenting postnatally. However, findings emerging from fetal programming research suggest that child stress biology is probably being established during the intrauterine period and that interventions ought to be focused equally on preconception and pregnancy mental health and stress exposure of mothers.

5.9.2   Specific or General Mechanisms

At present it remains unclear whether the mechanism through which depression in pregnancy is transmitted to the child is a general effect of maternal adversity, or may confer highly specific risks to the child's development. The problem is compounded in studies of fetal exposure which consider such exposures in simplistic terms. A good example is the frequently evoked Dutch famine offspring outcomes which are often used as a paradigm of nutritional insufficiency. However, the circumstances of military siege are surely high stress exposures, not to mention the rate of depression and anxiety for these mothers which are unknown. Since antenatal depression is associated with lower birth weight and preterm delivery it is not surprising that associations have also been found with later metabolic disorders such as hypertension and insulin resistance.

While this issue remains elusive, translation of these findings into interventions will also be impeded. At this point the risk factors for child development are well known. However, both exposures and outcomes need to be specific and measureable to enable characterization of biological mechanisms (Waterland and Michels 2007).

5.9.3   Treatment of Antenatal Depression as a Prevention Intervention

Once we understand clearly the effect of each exposure in terms of its discrete mechanisms and probably mechanisms, opportunities will arise for very well-targeted interventions. These may be pharmacological, psychosocial, or lifestyle-based interventions.

There can be little doubt however that higher level functions of cognitive development and skill acquisition depend on, and build on, the more basic functions of emotional regulation and adaptation in the face of challenge. As James Heckman has repeatedly pointed out, investment in interventions targeted at this foundation of human development brings the greatest reward on investment (Knudsen et al. 2006).

While the specific mechanisms for the transmission of antenatal depression require further research, the epidemiological evidence for a clear association between antenatal and postnatal depression and poorer child outcomes is very clear. The evidence is compelling that antenatal depression ought to be a key target in prevention efforts aimed at improving mothers' mental health in the first instance, and with major flow on effects for improvement in maternal health and child development. It is difficult to underestimate the significance of these efforts for ensuring the optimal start to life.

Increasingly economic modelling of interventions targeting early development makes a compelling case that this is the ideal period in which to prevent not only mental health disorders but possibly a range of other metabolic and cardiovascular disorders.

References

Azak S, Murison R, Wentzel-Larsen T, Smith L, Gunnar MR. Maternal depression and infant daytime cortisol. Dev Psychobiol. 2013;55(4):334–51.

Bagner DM, Pettit JW, Lewinsohn PM, Seeley JR. Effect of maternal depression on child behavior: a sensitive period? J Am Acad Child Adolesc Psychiatry. 2010;49(7):699–707.

Bennett HA, Einarson A, Taddio A, Koren G, Einarson TR. Prevalence of depression during pregnancy: systematic review. Obstet Gynecol. 2004;103(4):698–709.

Bennett IM, Coco A, Anderson J, Horst M, Gambler AS, Barr WB, et al. Improving maternal care with a continuous quality improvement strategy: a report from the interventions to minimize preterm and low birth weight infants through continuous improvement techniques (IMPLICIT) network. J Am Board Fam Med. 2009;22(4):380–6.

Bolt R, Van Weissenbruch M, Lafeber H, Delemarre-Van de Waal H. Development of the hypothalamic-pituitary-adrenal axis in the fetus and preterm infant. J Pediatr Endocrinol Metab. 2002;15(6):759–70.

Bradley RH, Corwyn RF. Socioeconomic status and child development. Annu Rev Psychol. 2002;53(1):371–99.

Challis J, Sloboda D, Matthews S, Holloway A, Alfaidy N, Patel F, et al. The fetal placental hypothalamic–pituitary–adrenal (HPA) axis, parturition and post natal health. Mol Cell Endocrinol. 2001;185(1):135–44.

Clavarino AM, Mamun AA, O'Callaghan M, Aird R, Bor W, O'Callaghan F, et al. Maternal anxiety and attention problems in children at 5 and 14 years. J Atten Disord. 2010;13(6):658–67. doi:10.1177/1087054709347203.

Costas J, Gratacòs M, Escaramís G, Martín-Santos R, de Diego Y, Baca-García E, et al. Association study of 44 candidate genes with depressive and anxiety symptoms in post-partum women. J Psychiatr Res. 2010;44(11):717–24.

Cottrell EC, Seckl JR. Prenatal stress, glucocorticoids and the programming of adult disease. Front Behav Neurosci. 2009;3:19.

Darnaudéry M, Maccari S. Epigenetic programming of the stress response in male and female rats by prenatal restraint stress. Brain Res Rev. 2008;57(2):571–85.

Davis EP, Glynn LM, Schetter CD, Hobel C, Chicz-Demet A, Sandman CA. Prenatal exposure to maternal depression and cortisol influences infant temperament. J Am Acad Child Adolesc Psychiatry. 2007;46(6):737–46. doi:10.1097/chi.0b013e318047b775.

Davis EP, Sandman CA, Buss C, Wing DA, Head K. Fetal glucocorticoid exposure is associated with preadolescent brain development. Biol Psychiatry. 2013;74(9):647–55.

Dawson G, Klinger LG, Panagiotides H, Hill D, Spieker S. Frontal lobe activity and affective behavior of infants of mothers with depressive symptoms. Child Dev. 1992;63(3):725–37.

De Kloet ER, Joëls M, Holsboer F. Stress and the brain: from adaptation to disease. Nat Rev Neurosci. 2005;6(6):463–75.

Dennis CL. Psychosocial and psychological interventions for prevention of postnatal depression: systematic review. BMJ. 2005;331(7507):15. doi:10.1136/bmj.331.7507.15.

Doornbos B, Dijck-Brouwer D, Kema IP, Tanke MA, van Goor SA, Muskiet FA, et al. The development of peripartum depressive symptoms is associated with gene polymorphisms of MAOA, 5-HTT and COMT. Prog Neuropsychopharmacol Biol Psychiatry. 2009;33(7):1250–4.

Field T. Maternal depression effects on infants and early interventions. Prev Med. 1998;27(2):200–3.

Field T. Prenatal depression effects on early development: a review. Infant Behav Dev. 2011;34(1):1–14. doi:10.1016/j.infbeh.2010.09.008.

Gaynes BN, Gavin N, Meltzer-Brody S, Lohr KN, Swinson T, Gartlehner G, Brody S, Miller WC. Perinatal depression: prevalence, screening accuracy, and screening outcomes. Evid Rep Technol Assess (Summ). 2005;(119):1–8.

Gluckman PD, Hanson MA. The conceptual basis for the developmental origins of health and disease. In: Gluckman PD, Hanson MA, editors. Developmental origins of health and disease. New York, NY: Cambridge University Press; 2006. p. 33–50.

Gluckman PD, Hanson MA, Beedle AS. Early life events and their consequences for later disease: a life history and evolutionary perspective. Am J Hum Biol. 2007;19(1):1–19.

Gotlib IH, Whiffen VE, Mount JH, Milne K, Cordy NI. Prevalence rates and demographic characteristics associated with depression in pregnancy and the postpartum. J Consult Clin Psychol. 1989;57(2):269–74.

Gunnar M, Quevedo K. The neurobiology of stress and development. Annu Rev Psychol. 2007;58:145–73.

Haig D. Genetic conflicts in human pregnancy. Quart Rev Biol. 1993;68:495–532.

Heron J, O'Connor TG, Evans J, Golding J, Glover V. The course of anxiety and depression through pregnancy and the postpartum in a community sample. J Affect Disord. 2004;80(1):65–73.

Jokela M, Keltikangas-Jarvinen L, Kivimaki M, Puttonen S, Elovainio M, Rontu R, et al. Serotonin receptor 2A gene and the influence of childhood maternal nurturance on adulthood depressive symptoms. Arch Gen Psychiatry. 2007;64(3):356.

Jung C, Ho JT, Torpy DJ, Rogers A, Doogue M, Lewis JG, et al. A longitudinal study of plasma and urinary cortisol in pregnancy and postpartum. J Clin Endocrinol Metab. 2011;96(5):1533–40.

Kaplan LA, Evans L, Monk C. Effects of mothers' prenatal psychiatric status and postnatal caregiving on infant biobehavioral regulation: can prenatal programming be modified? Early Hum Dev. 2008;84(4):249–56.

Kendler KS, Kessler RC, Walters EE, MacLean C, Neale MC, Heath AC, Eaves LJ. Stressful life events, genetic liability, and onset of an episode of major depression in women. Am J Psychiatry. 1995;152:833–42.

Khashan AS, Abel KM, McNamee R, Pedersen MG, Webb RT, Baker PN, et al. Higher risk of offspring schizophrenia following antenatal maternal exposure to severe adverse life events. Arch Gen Psychiatry. 2008;65(2):146–52.

Kinney DK, Miller AM, Crowley DJ, Huang E, Gerber E. Autism prevalence following prenatal exposure to hurricanes and tropical storms in Louisiana. J Autism Dev Disord. 2008;38 (3):481–8. doi:10.1007/s10803-007-0414-0.

Knudsen EI, Heckman JJ, Cameron JL, Shonkoff JP. Economic, neurobiological, and behavioral perspectives on building America's future workforce. Proc Natl Acad Sci. 2006;103 (27):10155–62.

Leigh B, Milgrom J. Risk factors for antenatal depression, postnatal depression and parenting stress. BMC Psychiatry. 2008;8(1):24.

Lewis AJ. A call for an expanded synthesis of developmental and evolutionary paradigms. Behav Brain Sci. 2012;35(5):368–9. doi:10.1017/S0140525X12001021.

Lewis AJ, Olsson CA. Early life stress and child temperament style as predictors of childhood anxiety and depressive symptoms: findings from the longitudinal study of Australian children. Depress Res Treat. 2011;2012:1–9.

Lewis AJ, Bailey C, Galbally M. Anti-depressant use during pregnancy in Australia: findings from the Longitudinal Study of Australian Children. Aust NZ J Public Health. 2012;36(5):487–8. doi:10.1111/j.1753-6405.2012.00917.x.

Lindsay JR, Nieman LK. The hypothalamic-pituitary-adrenal axis in pregnancy: challenges in disease detection and treatment. Endocr Rev. 2005;26(6):775–99.

Loomans EM, van der Stelt O, van Eijsden M, Gemke RJBJ, Vrijkotte T, Van den Bergh BR. Antenatal maternal anxiety is associated with problem behaviour at age five. Early Hum Dev. 2011;87(8):565–70. doi:10.1016/j.earlhumdev.2011.04.014.

Luckett WP. Ontogeny of the fetal membranes and placenta. Springer US: Springer; 1976

Lupien SJ, McEwen BS, Gunnar MR, Heim C. Effects of stress throughout the lifespan on the brain, behaviour and cognition. Nat Rev Neurosci. 2009;10(6):434–45.

Manolio TA, Collins FS, Cox NJ, Goldstein DB, Hindorff LA, Hunter DJ, et al. Finding the missing heritability of complex diseases. Nature. 2009;461(7265):747–53.

Martins C, Gaffan EA. Effects of early maternal depression on patterns of infant-mother attachment: a meta-analytic investigation. J Child Psychol Psychiatry. 2000;41(6):737–46.

Meaney MJ. Epigenetics and the biological definition of gene × environment interactions. Child Dev. 2010;81(1):41–79.

Murray L, Halligan SL, Goodyer I, Herbert J. Disturbances in early parenting of depressed mothers and cortisol secretion in offspring: a preliminary study. J Affect Disord. 2010;122(3):218–23.

Nestler EJ, Barrot M, DiLeone RJ, Eisch AJ, Gold SJ, Monteggia LM. Neurobiology of depression. Neuron. 2002;34(1):13–25.

O'Connor TG, Heron J, Golding J, Beveridge M, Glover V. Maternal antenatal anxiety and children's behavioural/emotional problems at 4 years: report from the Avon Longitudinal Study of Parents and Children. Br J Psychiatry. 2002;180(6):502–8. doi:10.1192/bjp.180.6. 502.

O'Connor TG, Heron J, Golding J, Glover V, the ALSPAC Study Team. Maternal antenatal anxiety and behavioural/emotional problems in children: a test of a programming hypothesis. J Child Psychol Psychiatry. 2003;44(7):1025–36.

O'Donnell K, O'Connor T, Glover V. Prenatal stress and neurodevelopment of the child: focus on the HPA axis and role of the placenta. Dev Neurosci. 2009;31(4):285–92.

O'Donnell KJ, Bugge Jensen A, Freeman L, Khalife N, O'Connor TG, Glover V. Maternal prenatal anxiety and downregulation of placental 11beta-HSD2. Psychoneuroendocrinology. 2012;37(6):818–26.

Oberlander TF, Weinberg J, Papsdorf M, Grunau R, Misri S, Devlin AM. Prenatal exposure to maternal depression, neonatal methylation of human glucocorticoid receptor gene (NR3C1) and infant cortisol stress responses. Epigenetics. 2008;3(2):97–106.

Peerbooms OL, van Os J, Drukker M, Kenis G, Hoogveld L, De Hert M, et al. Meta-analysis of MTHFR gene variants in schizophrenia, bipolar disorder and unipolar depressive disorder: evidence for a common genetic vulnerability? Brain Behav Immun. 2011;25(8):1530–43.

Phillips DI, Jones A. Fetal programming of autonomic and HPA function: do people who were small babies have enhanced stress responses? J Physiol. 2006;572(1):45–50.

Ponder KL, Salisbury A, McGonnigal B, Laliberte A, Lester B, Padbury JF. Maternal depression and anxiety are associated with altered gene expression in the human placenta without modification by antidepressant use: implications for fetal programming. Dev Psychobiol. 2011;53(7):711–23. doi:10.1002/dev.20549.

Price D, Close G, Fielding B. Age of appearance of circadian rhythm in salivary cortisol values in infancy. Arch Dis Child. 1983;58(6):454–6.

Radtke K, Ruf M, Gunter H, Dohrmann K, Schauer M, Meyer A, et al. Transgenerational impact of intimate partner violence on methylation in the promoter of the glucocorticoid receptor. Transl Psychiatry. 2011;1(7):e21.

Rich-Edwards J, Mohllajee A, Kleinman K, Hacker M, Majzoub J, Wright R, et al. Elevated midpregnancy corticotropin-releasing hormone is associated with prenatal, but not postpartum, maternal depression. J Clin Endocrinol Metab. 2008;93(5):1946–51.

Robinson M, Oddy WH, Li J, Kendall GE, de Klerk NH, Silburn SR, et al. Pre- and postnatal influences on preschool mental health: a large-scale cohort study. J Child Psychol Psychiatry. 2008;49(10):1118–28. doi:10.1111/j.1469-7610.2008.01955.x.

Schlotz W, Phillips DI. Fetal origins of mental health: evidence and mechanisms. Brain Behav Immun. 2009;23(7):905–16. doi:10.1016/j.bbi.2009.02.001.

Schroeder JW, Conneely KN, Cubells JF, Kilaru V, Newport DJ, Knight BT, et al. Neonatal DNA methylation patterns associate with gestational age. Epigenetics. 2011;6(12):1498–504.

Schroeder JW, Smith AK, Brennan PA, Conneely KN, Kilaru V, Knight BT, et al. DNA methylation in neonates born to women receiving psychiatric care. Epigenetics. 2012;7(4):409–14.

Shonkoff JP. Building a new biodevelopmental framework to guide the future of early childhood policy. Child Dev. 2010;81(1):357–67.

Smith AK, Conneely KN, Newport DJ, Kilaru V, Schroeder JW, Pennell PB, et al. Prenatal antiepileptic exposure associates with neonatal DNA methylation differences. Epigenetics. 2012;7(5):458–63.

Spauwen J, Krabbendam L, Lieb R, Wittchen HU, van Os J. Early maternal stress and health behaviours and offspring expression of psychosis in adolescence. Acta Psychiatr Scand. 2004;110:356–64.

Sullivan PF, Neale MC, Kendler KS. Genetic epidemiology of major depression: review and meta-analysis. Am J Psychiatry. 2000;157(10):1552–62.

Swanson JD, Wadhwa PM. Developmental origins of child mental health disorders. J Child Psychol Psychiatry. 2008;49(10):1009–19. doi:10.1111/j.1469-7610.2008.02014.x.

Talge NM, Neal C, Glover V. Antenatal maternal stress and long-term effects on child neurodevelopment: how and why? J Child Psychol Psychiatry. 2007;48(3–4):245–61. doi:10.1111/j.1469-7610.2006.01714.x.

Teixeira J, Fisk NM, Glover V. Association between maternal anxiety in pregnancy and increased uterine artery resistance index: cohort based study. BMJ. 1999;318(7177):153–7.

Van Den Bergh BRH, Van Calster B, Smits T, Van Huffel S, Lagae L. Antenatal maternal anxiety is related to HPA-axis dysregulation and self-reported depressive symptoms in adolescence: a prospective study on the fetal origins of depressed mood. Neuropsychopharmacology. 2008;33(3):536–45.

Waterland RA, Michels KB. Epigenetic epidemiology of the developmental origins hypothesis. Annu Rev Nutr. 2007;27:363–88.

Watson JB, Mednick SA, Huttunen M, Wang X. Prenatal teratogens and the development of adult mental illness. Dev Psychopathol. 1999;11(3):457–66.

Weinstock M. The potential influence of maternal stress hormones on development and mental health of the offspring. Brain Behav Immun. 2005;19(4):296–308.

Weinstock M. Gender differences in the effects of prenatal stress on brain development and behaviour. Neurochem Res. 2007;32(10):1730–40.

Weinstock M. Sex-dependent changes induced by prenatal stress in cortical and hippocampal morphology and behaviour in rats: an update. Stress. 2011;14(6):604–13.

Pharmacological Management of Major Depression in Pregnancy

6

Philip Boyce, Megan Galbally, Martien Snellen, and Anne Buist

Abstract

Depression is now recognised as a common complication of pregnancy and the postpartum period. If untreated this mental illness has implications for maternal morbidity and foetal, infant and child outcomes. Most treatment guidelines recommend for moderate to severe depression the consideration of pharmacological treatment and this includes guidelines developed for the perinatal period. This chapter will provide an overview of depression in pregnancy, risks and benefits of antidepressant treatment in pregnancy and suggestions for management should pharmacological treatment be instigated or maintained in pregnancy.

Keywords

Major depression • Prevalence • EPDS • Assessment • Treatment • Antidepressants • SSRI • Malformations • Miscarriage • Obstetric complications • Risk benefit analysis • Poor neonatal adaptation syndrome • Persistent pulmonary hypertension of the newborn

P. Boyce (✉)
Discipline of Psychiatry, Sydney Medical School, University of Sydney, Sydney, NSW, Australia

Department of Psychiatry, Westmead Hospital, Wentworthville, NSW 2145, Australia
e-mail: philip.boyce@sydney.edu.au

M. Galbally
Department of Obstetrics and Gynaecology, University of Melbourne, Melbourne, VIC, Australia

Perinatal Mental Health, Mercy Hospital for Women, Heidelberg, VIC, Australia
e-mail: mgalbally@mercy.com.au

M. Snellen
Mercy Hospital for Women, Heidelberg, VIC, Australia
e-mail: msnellen@iprimus.com.au

A. Buist
Women's Mental Health, University of Melbourne, Austin Health and Northpark,
West Heidelberg, VIC, Australia
e-mail: a.buist@unimelb.edu.au

M. Galbally et al. (eds.), *Psychopharmacology and Pregnancy*,
DOI 10.1007/978-3-642-54562-7_6, © Springer-Verlag Berlin Heidelberg 2014

6.1   Introduction

Major depression is a common and distressing mental disorder that carries with it considerable disease burden (Murray et al. 2012), making it a major public health issue. Its particular relevance in perinatal mental health is that major depression is more common among women than men and has its highest prevalence levels during the childbearing years (Kessler et al. 2003; Slade et al. 2009) making it likely that women could be depressed prior to conception or over the course of their pregnancy. There is also building evidence that maternal depression can have adverse effects on infant development making it critically important to recognise and treat depression over the perinatal period (Chaudron 2013).

There has been interest in an association between childbirth and mental illness since antiquity, with the recognition that severe mental illness, leading to hospital admission or even suicide, can arise following childbirth. A series of studies linking obstetric and psychiatric data demonstrated the elevated risk of the onset of psychosis, especially puerperal psychosis (a variant of bipolar disorder) following childbirth (Kendell et al. 1981, 1987) with 1–2 women per 1,000 confinements having such an illness (Boyce and Barriball 2010). Severe depression following childbirth also occurred, but the rate was considered to be low based upon hospital admissions (Tod 1964). These studies also found that the risk of psychosis onset and admission to hospital was low during pregnancy with suggestions that pregnancy had a protective effect. The idea that pregnancy was protective probably stalled efforts into examining mental disorders, particularly depression, occurring during pregnancy.

It was not until community-based studies were conducted that there was a recognition that there were high rates of depression arising following childbirth (Kumar and Robson 1984; Pitt 1968; O'Hara et al. 1984; Watson et al. 1984). These studies, examining the prevalence of postnatal depression and its risk factors, highlighted that many women with postnatal depression often did not have their illness recognised and thus went without treatment (Boyce and Stubbs 1994). Major efforts were then made to develop instruments to screen for, and identify, postnatal depression (Buist et al. 2002) so that women could access treatment and minimise against any possible adverse effects of depression upon infant development (Murray 1992; Boyce and Stubbs 1994). In response to the potential adverse effects of postnatal depression, there was an increased effort to identify at-risk women earlier, ideally during pregnancy. A number of risk factors are known to predict postnatal depression (Boyce and Hickey 2005; O'Hara and Swain 1996) and scales developed to assess them (Appleby et al. 1994; Austin et al. 2005); however, one of the best predictors of postnatal depression was found to be depressive symptoms during pregnancy (O'Hara and Swain 1996). Identifying depressive symptoms in pregnancy then seemed to be a strategy to identify women at risk of developing postnatal depression. When screening tools, such as the Beck Depression Inventory (BDI) (Beck et al. 1961) and the Edinburgh Postnatal Depression Scale (EPDS) (Cox et al. 1987), were used during pregnancy high levels of depressive symptoms were found to be present. Not only that, using cut-off scores to identify major depression (generally developed for postnatal samples) the rates of depression were found to be much higher than previously thought. This was clearly demonstrated in the influential Avon longitudinal study (Evans et al. 2001). Here 14,541 pregnant women completed the EPDS at 18 and 32 weeks gestation (and at 8 weeks and 8 months postpartum). The women's scores on the EPDS were significantly higher at 18 weeks (6.62) and 32 weeks (6.72) gestation than the postpartum scores of 5.84 and 5.25. Using the standard cut-off score on the EPDS of greater than 12, 13.5 % of women scored above the threshold for probable depression at 32 weeks of pregnancy compared to only 9.1 % at 8 weeks postpartum.

Subsequent studies confirmed the high levels of depressive symptoms and depression in pregnancy; these were reviewed by Bennett et al. (2004b). They examined findings from studies that used self-report measures; mainly the EPDS and the BDI. Studies that used structured diagnostic instruments were also reviewed, where the rates were much lower than those found using questionnaires. The highest rates of depression were found when the BDI was used (see Fig. 6.1), especially in the first trimester, whereas the highest rates of depression were found in the third trimester when the EPDS was used as the case finding measure. The EPDS was developed specifically for assessing postnatal depression and did not focus on the somatic symptoms associated with depression. This would account for the lower rates of depression identified using the EPDS rather than the BDI which includes the common somatic symptoms of depression that could be accounted for by pregnancy itself.

Structured clinical instruments had lower rates of depression, with the highest rates in the second (9.1 %) and third trimesters (8.9 %), a rate not much higher than the rate of depression among women identified in community epidemiological studies and consistent with the findings of the National Epidemiologic Survey on Alcohol and Related Conditions (NESARC) in which data from 14,549 women were examined using a validated structured interview (Vesga-Lopez et al. 2008). The prevalence rate of major depression for non-pregnant women was 8.1 % and similar to the rate of depression among women who had been pregnant in the past year (8.4 %), whereas the rate of major depression was significantly higher for postpartum women (9.3 %).

Women with recurrent episodes of depression (recurrent unipolar disorder or bipolar disorder) are of particular interest in that they are at high risk of having a relapse of the illness postpartum. Viguera et al. assessed episodes of illness, using DSM-IV criteria, during pregnancy or up to 6 months postpartum in a cohort of women who had been diagnosed with bipolar I, bipolar II or unipolar depressive disorder (Viguera et al. 2011). An episode of major depressive disorder occurred in 2.7 % of the 1,132 women with unipolar disorder during pregnancy (1.89 % reported an episode of anxiety or panic), with the rate of depression being 16.1 % in the first 6 months postpartum.

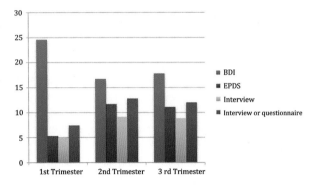

Fig. 6.1 Prevalence of depression during pregnancy assessed by questionnaire or interview. *Notes*: Edinburgh Postnatal Depression Scale (EPDS) cut-off score greater than or equal to 1.0 Beck Depression Inventory (BDI) cut-off score greater than or equal to 9. Adapted from Bennett et al. (2004b)

6.2 Impact of Depression

These studies make it clear that major depression occurs during pregnancy with a prevalence rate of between 3 and 9 %. They also demonstrate that a significant proportion of women will report high levels of depressive symptoms. Major depression and depressive symptoms may cause significant distress and impairment for women over an important life transition, as well as potentially having an adverse effect on pregnancy outcomes and the developing foetus. Maternal depression has been associated with increased risk of premature delivery, low birth weight, gestational hypertension (Grote et al. 2010a; Grigoriadis et al. 2013c) and perinatal death (Howard et al. 2007). It is not clear, however, whether this is a direct result of the depression or behaviours associated with depression such as poor diet and smoking and greater use of prescription drugs such as hypnotics, anti-emetics and opioid analgesics (Newport et al. 2012). It is also associated with a low uptake of breastfeeding (Grote et al. 2010a; Grigoriadis et al. 2013c), which could have an adverse impact on infant development and well-being.

Depression in pregnancy may have an adverse impact on infant emotional and cognitive development (Deave et al. 2008; Field 2011; Chaudron 2013). It has been proposed that the mechanism of that is the result of the biological substrates of depression, such as activation of the HPA axis that primes the foetus itself to depression in later life, and that activation of the maternal HPA axis leading to placental hypersecretion of corticotropin-releasing factor with adverse effects of the foetus and on labour (Field 2011; Chaudron 2013). Such findings emphasise the importance of recognising, and treating, depression in pregnancy.

6.3 Relapse Risk of Major Depression in Pregnancy

Relapse rates have been examined in those women who continue or cease antidepressants during pregnancy. Cohen et al. (2006) found that patients with major depression who ceased antidepressant treatment during pregnancy showed significantly higher relapse rates than those who remained on their preconception dose of medication throughout pregnancy (68 % vs. 26 %) (Cohen et al. 2006). However, a more recent study by Yonkers et al. (2011) found no difference at all. Significant methodological differences, which include patient population and severity of illness factors, limit our ability to form firm conclusions regarding risk (Yonkers et al. 2011). However, an earlier study of women who abruptly discontinued antidepressants on becoming pregnant found 31 % developed suicidal ideation (Einarson et al. 2001). This is of particular concern given the high rates of cessation found in community samples when pregnancy is diagnosed (Ververs et al. 2006).

The biological mechanisms of exposure to antidepressant medication are further discussed in Chap. 4 and the literature regarding untreated maternal mental illness, including depression, in Chap. 5.

6.4 Assessment of Depression in Pregnancy

The key to successful management of depression in pregnancy is a careful assessment. It is important to distinguish between women with distressing depressive symptoms and those that meet the full diagnostic criteria for a major depressive disorder. That is not to say that these symptoms should be ignored; their origin should be explored, the relevant stressors identified and their worries dealt with through supportive counselling. Making a diagnosis of major depressive disorder in pregnancy is complicated by the fact that there are overlapping symptoms between major depression and pregnancy-related symptoms. Yonkers et al. (2009a) found that some of the typical somatic depressive symptoms such as appetite, sleep and energy level disturbance did not differentiate well between depressed and non-depressed pregnant women. By contrast, the more cognitive symptoms of depression, such as feeling guilty or worthless and having trouble concentrating, were much more discriminatory. The assessment process needs to take this into account. The same has been found using questionnaires such as the EPDS, as a diagnostic tool (it was not designed to be used as a diagnostic tool but as a screening tool). Scores on the EPDS are often inflated on the first administration (especially if it is administered at the first antenatal visit when women are naturally apprehensive) and it is recommended that women who score high should complete the instrument a week or two later to give a more valid result (Matthey and Ross-Hamid 2012). Asking about the attribution of endorsed symptoms on the EPDS will also alter the rate of depression, (identified using a structured interview) when symptoms that were attributable to the normal physical changes of pregnancy are excluded (Matthey and Ross-Hamid 2011).

When assessing women in pregnancy it is necessary to enquire about the woman's attribution for the symptom and not merely use a "checkbox" approach to make a diagnosis; otherwise there is a risk of making a spurious diagnosis and leading to overpathologising.

The woman's previous history of depression should also be elicited as well as her treatment response as this will give an indication of what will be beneficial for her current episode of depression. The possibility of bipolar depression should also be considered, so asking about possible episodes of hypomania or mania is essential, especially when there is a family history of bipolar disorder.

The assessment of depression should include an assessment of the severity and type of depression. The treatment approach for a more severe, melancholic type of depression will be very different from the treatment that is offered to a woman with mild depression arising as a consequence of psychosocial difficulties in which psychosocial intervention is preferable.

6.5   Treatment of Depression in Pregnancy

Antidepressants are a mainstay for the treatment of moderate to severe depression in adults. Guidelines which are specific to the perinatal period suggest the consideration of their use where there has been a failure of response to psychosocial interventions or significant and debilitating symptoms of depression (Yonkers et al. 2009c; Austin et al. 2011). There is evidence from studies in the US, Canada and Denmark of the increasing use of antidepressants in pregnancy with rates between 3.2 % and 13.4 % shown in these studies (Cooper et al. 2007; Jimenez-Solem et al. 2013; Andrade et al. 2008; Oberlander et al. 2006), although studies from both the Netherlands and Australia show lower rates of use of around 2 % (Lewis et al. 2012; Ververs et al. 2006).

There is an absence of specific evidence examining the effectiveness of antidepressant medication for depression in pregnancy. The absence of evidence regarding the efficacy of antidepressants in pregnancy is not surprising as pregnant women are routinely excluded from clinical trials (Coverdale et al. 2008). However, given the absence of evidence it is reasonable to make use of the treatment approaches for depression in general as the clinical presentation of depression in pregnancy is not different from other forms of depression (Yonkers et al. 2009b; Bennett et al. 2004a). Broadly speaking this would mean that women with mild-to-moderate depression be preferentially offered psychosocial treatments such as interpersonal therapy (Spinelli 1997) or cognitive behaviour therapy; however, there is a lack of evidence to recommend their use.

What is essential, especially if antidepressant medication is being considered, is to conduct a careful risk:benefit analysis. The essence of this is shown in the figure below (Fig. 6.2).

First, no antidepressant medications are used because of concerns about the possible adverse effects on the developing foetus. Many women will not contemplate taking medication during pregnancy because of fears that it could harm the developing foetus and a significant number stop their antidepressant in the first trimester of pregnancy (Ververs et al. 2006). The consequence of this is that the depression will persist and that the depression could have an adverse effect on pregnancy outcome. The foetus, meanwhile, will not be exposed to the antidepressant, but will be exposed to any adverse consequences of the woman's depression.

	No medication	Taking medication
Woman	Persistent depression	Maternal wellbeing
	Distress	Side-effects of medication
	Adverse effect on pregnancy outcome	
Developing foetus	No risk of harm from medication	Reduced risk of effects of severe depression on foetal
	Possible adverse impact on foetal development	development
		Risk of harm from exposing foetus to medication

Fig. 6.2 Risks vs. benefits of medication during pregnancy

If, however, the woman takes an antidepressant her depression will remit (though not in all cases) but she may experience significant side effects from the medication, and effects of the medication on obstetric outcome, and a possible risk of gestational hypertension (Toh et al. 2009). Care, therefore, has to be taken to provide an antidepressant that is both efficacious and well tolerated (Malhi et al. 2013). When an antidepressant is used, the foetus will be exposed to the medication and potential harmful effects. These have been reviewed and there have now been eight meta-analyses examining this (Galbally 2013), which show a small increased risk of foetal abnormality. The major adverse effects of antidepressant medications in pregnancy include foetal malformations, persistent pulmonary hypertension and poor neonatal adaptation syndrome.

6.6 Pregnancy and Neonatal Complications of Antidepressant Medication

6.6.1 Malformations

There has been considerable debate as a result of conflicting findings for an association with SSRI antidepressant exposure and a range of malformations. In addition to numerous conflicting studies there have now been eight meta-analyses in an attempt to resolve this question; however, these too have produced varied results (Rahimi et al. 2006; Addis and Koren 2000; Einarson and Einarson 2005; O'Brien et al. 2008; Myles et al. 2013). Of the eight meta-analyses four have found no association between antidepressant exposure and malformation and three have found an association between paroxetine and heart defects (Wurst et al. 2010; Bar-Oz et al. 2007). The two most recent meta-analyses also found an association between fluoxetine and an increased malformation risk (Grigoriadis et al. 2013b; Myles et al. 2013). Both tricyclic antidepressants (TCAs) and the newer antidepressants such as Selective Noradrenaline Reuptake Inhibitors (SNRIs) have not been associated with malformation, although the literature is far more limited (Lennestal and Kallen 2007; Simon et al. 2002).

The challenge with the original research and with the subsequent meta-analyses is the considerable variation in methodology. The larger studies which have examined this question have tended to be retrospective studies based on population-based registries or reviews of medical files with variables analysed which were not originally collected for research projects. Many of these studies have unverified data on exposure, such as measuring exposure as the provision of a prescription, not adequately accounting for key confounding variables and a lack of measures of maternal mental illness that in itself has the potential to be a teratogen.

The issue of confounding variables is important, given that studies such as Malm et al. and Lewis et al. both show higher alcohol and cigarette exposure, especially the latter as well as other prescribed medications in women taking antidepressants (Malm et al. 2011; Lewis et al. 2012). Given that women with mental illness, including depression, have higher rates of vitamin deficiencies, such as vitamin D, poorer nutrition, obesity and unplanned pregnancy (Warner et al. 1996)' the latter is significant given the importance of folate, ideally preconception, and early pregnancy, to prevent malformations such as neural tube defects, but also potentially for cardiac malformation (Scanlon et al. 1998; Leanza et al. 2013). Another important potential confounder that has been mostly unexamined is maternal obesity. Depression is associated with a higher incidence of co-morbid obesity (Onyike et al. 2003) and in turn maternal obesity is associated with an increased risk of malformations (Stothard et al. 2009). What has not been adequately investigated is whether specific maternal mental illnesses are associated with increased risk of malformations. Other maternal illnesses such as Rubella, Diabetes Mellitus and Gestational Diabetes are regarded as teratogenic (Balsells et al. 2012). There is now a volume of research particularly in maternal anxiety which has shown an association with effects on specific foetal outcomes as well as longer term child development (Van den Bergh et al. 2005). Whether either depression or anxiety, are in themselves, teratogenic, and therefore associated with structural or neurodevelopmental teratogenicity, is yet to be explored.

The basic premise of teratology is that exposure during early pregnancy to a specific agent results in a specific malformation. This risk inherently must be above the baseline risk for malformation of 2–3 %. While there is concerning data about a potential small increase in malformation risk from exposure to antidepressants in pregnancy, particularly specific SSRIs such as paroxetine, there have not yet been data that are conclusive as to this risk. Future studies, which clearly account for important key confounding variables, accurately document exposure and maternal mental illness and are needed in order to elucidate any association between antidepressant exposure and malformation.

6.6.2 Miscarriage

Two previous meta-analyses that examined the rate of spontaneous abortion and antidepressant exposure both found an increased risk (Hemels et al. 2005; Rahimi et al. 2006). However, the authors could not account for maternal depression as a variable across the identified studies. Interestingly, a more recent meta-analysis found no association between spontaneous abortion and antidepressant exposure (Ross et al. 2013).

6.6.3 Delivery Complications: Birth Weight, Preterm Delivery and Neonatal Adaptation

Around the time of delivery two major issues have been raised for infants exposed to antidepressants; one is that of potential growth effects and the other of neonatal adaption. The latter in particular is relevant to the clinical management of the mother and whether reducing the medication prior to delivery reduces negative effects in the infant and how this is weighed up against the risk of mother's depression recurring.

Prematurity and low birth weight, even when adjusted for gestation, were noted in early evaluations of the first use of SSRI in pregnancy. In Kallen's meta-analysis (2004) he estimated the risk of this to be increased two- to threefold (Kallen 2004). Our study (Galbally et al. 2009; Lewis et al. 2010) of a prospective case-controlled comparison of women treated and not treated with antidepressants showed the former group to be significantly more likely to have infants with a low birth weight (BW), be shorter and have a decreased head circumference. Davidson et al. (2009) had similar findings and proposed a correlation to lower cortisol, higher TSH and increased placental I GF-1 receptor expression. Wisner et al. (2009) found similar rates of prematurity between those on SSRIs (21 %) and those depressed but not on SSRIs (23 %) compared to only 6 % of those women with neither, but found no differences between these three groups with respect to length, weight and head circumference (Wisner et al. 2009).

Wisner's comparison groups highlight one of the key areas of difficulties in this research, being a lack in many studies of an adequate or appropriate control group, as well as taking into account maternal symptoms and confounding variables. Grote et al. (2010) concluded that women with depression were more likely to have poor obstetric care, be isolated, smoke, have poor nutrition and use illicit substances, all of which may affect foetal growth as well as neonatal adaption (Grote et al. 2010). They found a 39 % increased risk of preterm birth associated with maternal depression, a 49 % increase in low birth weight and a 45 % increase in intrauterine growth retardation. They proposed possible mechanisms of deregulation of the HPA axis, increased uterine artery resistance with placental hyperperfusion secondary to maternal stress or an inflammatory response.

Wisner et al. (2013) in an attempt to resolve the issue of depression versus SSRI causation completed a detailed prospective study of 97 women with no SSRI exposure, 46 women with SSRI exposure and 31 women with depression but no SSRI exposure, from 20 weeks gestation to 52 weeks postpartum (Wisner et al. 2013). They found no significant association between either of the study groups and birth weight, length or head circumference. Prematurity was associated with SSRI exposure compared to no SSRIs, but not when compared to the depressed group. These findings may relate to the relatively small depressed study group, but anxiety was also calculated for and the infant ratings were blind, strengthening these results and certainly suggesting that there is not a good evidence base to advise women to stop taking medication in order to prevent these outcomes.

After delivery these infants have been noted to have an increased risk of poor neonatal adaption (PNAS), characterised by jitteriness, decreased muscle tone and cry, respiratory distress, hypoglycaemia, low APGAR and seizures (Koren et al. 2005). These authors concluded in their review of six studies that the absolute risk was up to 30 % (compared to 6–9 % in those not exposed or exposed early in pregnancy) and a 2–10-fold increase if the exposure was around the time of delivery. Warburton et al. (2010) in a large population data study found that neonates with exposure in the previous 14 days had higher rates of respiratory distress compared to those with earlier exposures, but not when confounding variables were controlled for (Warburton et al. 2010). They concluded that unlike previous assumptions of it being a toxicity or withdrawal, the phenomena may not be an acute pharmacological issue.

Byatt et al, in a literature review found PNAS in up to 30 % of infants, but criticised the data because of a lack of systematic infant evaluation and blind raters, as well as the inappropriate control groups and lack of consideration of maternal variables (Byatt et al. 2013). As for the possible mechanisms, besides serotonin toxicity or overstimulation, infant genotype was also considered. Given the lack of clear associations, and the relatively minor self-limiting nature of the symptoms, and the risk to the mother of relapse, and to the infant through untreated depression (antenatal and postnatal), recommendations for management tend towards keeping the mother well and treating the infant conservatively, but with observation and intervention best suited to a specialised neonatal unit. Koren et al. (2005) comment that earlier recommendations to taper may in fact be ill-conceived and even potentially dangerous. A recent meta-analysis identified 12 studies that met their inclusion criteria and found evidence for an increased risk of PNAS in neonates exposed to antidepressants in pregnancy (Grigoriadis et al. 2013a).

6.6.4   Persistent Pulmonary Hypertension of the Newborn

Persistent Pulmonary Hypertension of the Newborn (PPHN) occurs in 1–2 per 1,000 babies. It represents the failure to transition to newborn circulatory functioning during delivery. PPHN is associated with increased rates of morbidity and mortality and hence is of significant concern. There have been seven studies investigating the potential association between SSRI exposure in pregnancy and

PPHN. Of these, four, have found an association of variable magnitude and three have not found any association (Galbally et al. 2012a).

The concerns, until the two most recent studies (Wilson et al. 2011; Kieler et al. 2012) were the considerable methodological variation between studies and the failure to account for known confounding variables such as caesarean delivery (Galbally et al. 2012a). These two recent studies have had conflicting findings with Wilson et al. finding no association and Kieler et al. finding a small association (Kieler et al. 2012). The latter was a combined study of the Scandinavian national health registers and this allowed an adequately powered study to investigate a relatively rare condition. They found a general incidence of PPHN of 1.2 per 1,000, and with exposure to any of the SSRIs this increased to 3 per 1,000. While this is an increased risk this is far lower than previously reported.

Kieler et al. also examined a range of other antidepressants including tricyclic antidepressants (TCAs) and Selective Noradrenaline Reuptake Inhibitors (SNRIs) and found that exposure in late pregnancy was also associated with an elevated risk. A recent meta-analysis found evidence for a small increase in PPHN with exposure to antidepressants in pregnancy (Grigoriadis et al. 2014).

6.6.5 Longer Term Complications

There are only a limited number of studies that have examined child development outcomes following antidepressant exposure in utero and none have followed children beyond early childhood (Gentile and Galbally 2010; Galbally et al. 2012b). These studies have predominantly been done on SSRIs with some including TCAs. Studies have predominantly examined children under 12 months of age using measures with low predictive validity (Gentile and Galbally 2010). There have been seven studies that have used more comprehensive measures of development such as the Bayleys Scales of Infant Development or the Wechsler measures in children over 12 months of age. The majority of these studies have not found any association with poorer child development. However, three found poorer motor development (Galbally et al. 2011; Casper et al. 2003, 2011). Whether this represents a 'real' finding and why antidepressants could potentially effect the developing motor system are still unanswered questions. What is known is that serotonin acts as a developmental signal during neural development (Whitaker-Azmitia et al. 1996; Whitaker-Azmitia 1999). Animal models such as Jacob's studies on cats have shown that the serotonergic system does regulate motor activity (Jacobs and Fornal 1997).

Like most of the published research on the effects of exposure to antidepressants in pregnancy the studies on child development are hampered by variable methodology, verification of exposure and adequate measures of key confounding variables including maternal mental illness. The reassuring finding is that in the 21 published studies there have been none that have found an effect on global cognition (Galbally et al. 2012b).

6.7   Specific Clinical Considerations and Recommended Monitoring

Given the high risk of unrecognised physical comorbidity in women who suffer from major depression it is recommended that a baseline organic screen be performed as a matter of course. Investigations should include full blood examination, renal, thyroid and hepatic function testing, estimations of iron, vitamin B12, folate and vitamin D, fasting glucose and serum lipids, in addition to the usual obstetric investigations. Consideration should also be given to ECG examination if a patient is taking a medication that could compromise the QT interval (e.g. TCA's and citalopram/escitalopram in high dose).

Antidepressants vary in their placental passage (in part due to molecular size and degree of protein binding) and extent of breast milk excretion. Placental passage studies for the SSRIs, in which cord blood estimations were measured, have found variable concentrations; however, all were much lower than maternal levels (Hendrick et al. 2003). Such data should influence the choice of antidepressant used, as well as the knowledge base regarding its potential to cause teratogenicity or adverse neonatal outcome.

Changes in gastric emptying, increased volume of distribution, decreased gastrointestinal motility, decreased drug-binding capacity and increased hepatic metabolism during pregnancy frequently alter the therapeutic dose of antidepressants. Increased frequency of psychiatric review is essential and medication doses may need to be increased in order to maintain efficacy (especially during the third trimester).

Consideration should be given to the administration of folate at a dose of 0.5–5 mg daily depending on a woman's risk for neural tube defect, preferably from 3 months before conception and throughout pregnancy, as it may reduce the risk of various birth defects. Similarly, given the high rates of inadequate nutrition and self-care in this patient population, multivitamins specifically formulated for pregnancy may also be recommended.

Given that both depression and its pharmacological treatment have been (in some studies) associated with preterm labour, growth restriction and intrauterine growth retardation, adequate obstetric monitoring above and beyond usual care may be necessary.

A written individualised Perinatal Mental Health Care Plan should be prepared for each mother and baby and placed in a prominent position within the case file. It should outline the current treatment team, all pharmacological and other treatments, a plan for mode of infant feeding, recommendations for support, minimum length of stay, plans for regular psychiatric and paediatric review and a comprehensive discharge plan that ideally includes support for the mother, partner, mother–infant relationship, early parenting skills and establishment of pathways to care should relapse occur.

6.8   Recommendations for the Treatment of Women with Major Depression in Pregnancy

1. Careful and considered diagnostic assessment utilising a bio-psycho-social-cultural model.
2. Organise a baseline organic screen.
3. Wherever possible, taking into account the potential for pregnancy, preconception consideration should be given to the most appropriate form of treatment in women who suffer from depression. Illness of mild severity should be treated first and foremost utilising psychosocial interventions with established efficacy. Pharmacotherapy should be reserved for moderately to severely depressed women and those not responsive to psychotherapeutic interventions alone.
4. Optimise the therapeutic alliance and non-pharmacological treatments.
5. Address lifestyle factors such as exercise, diet, sleep, sunlight exposure, stress, smoking, substance abuse and support structures.
6. Make an active, rather than passive, decision regarding the continuation of established antidepressant treatment during pregnancy following consideration of personal risk factors for relapse.
7. Should antidepressant medication be initiated in pregnancy consider the data regarding placental passage, breast milk excretion, teratogenic risk, obstetric risks and the potential for adverse neonatal or longer term outcomes.
8. Aim for monotherapy wherever possible.
9. Use the lowest effective dose of any antidepressant utilised; however, the emphasis needs to be on *effective* rather than *lowest* as partial treatment exposes mother and the foetus to both the risks of treatment and illness.
10. Consider prescribing folate daily from 3 months preconception and throughout pregnancy as well as multivitamins.
11. Ensure that a process of obtaining informed consent is followed in which all available information regarding risks and benefits of treatment and non-treatment in the perinatal setting are detailed.
12. Establish a close liaison relationship between all disciplines involved: psychiatry, obstetrics, paediatrics, general practice, midwifery, social work and maternal and child health-care nursing.
13. Ensure that adequate monitoring throughout pregnancy occurs of foetal development, obstetric physiology and maternal mental state.
14. At delivery commence observation for evidence of neonatal withdrawal, toxicity, sedation, persistent pulmonary hypertension or other adverse effects and ensure that a careful morphological examination is undertaken.
15. Create and implement a Mental Health Care Plan for the post-delivery maternity setting that encourages a close liaison between all health-care providers and allows an extended maternity stay in which observations can be made for any neonatal compromise secondary to exposure to antidepressant medications in utero.

16. Establish early warning signs for relapse and pathways to care should this occur.
17. When treating all women of childbearing age for depression consideration should be paid to the fact that she could conceive. If an antidepressant is prescribed ensure she is aware of the potential risks and advised to have a medical review, especially when planning to conceive.

Conclusion

Given maternal depression is now recognised as one of the most common complications of childbirth understanding the risks and benefits of specific treatments for this condition is relevant to a range of clinical disciplines. There is evidence of increasing use of antidepressant medications, and given that SSRIs are one of the most commonly prescribed psychotropic medication, this is of no surprise. The challenge to researchers is to clarify the mechanisms by which maternal depression may impact on child development. In clarifying this it may be clearer which treatment options are most effective at ameliorating this risk for offspring of women with depression. Given the potential for treatments to both improve maternal morbidity and prevent poorer child outcomes this is an important future area for public health research (Lewis et al. 2014).

References

Addis A, Koren G. Safety of fluoxetine during the first trimester of pregnancy: a meta-analytical review of epidemiological studies. Psychol Med. 2000;30(1):89–94.

Andrade SE, Raebel MA, Brown J, Lane K, Livingston J, Boudreau D, et al. Use of antidepressant medications during pregnancy: a multisite study. Am J Obstet Gynecol. 2008;198(2):194.e1–5. doi:10.1016/j.ajog.2007.07.036. S0002-9378(07)00915-5 [pii].

Appleby L, Gregoire A, Platz C, Prince M, Kumar R. Screening women for high risk of postnatal depression. J Psychosom Res. 1994;38(6):539–45.

Austin MP, Hadzi-Pavlovic D, Saint K, Parker G. Antenatal screening for the prediction of postnatal depression: validation of a psychosocial Pregnancy Risk Questionnaire. Acta Psychiatr Scand. 2005;112(4):310–7. doi:10.1111/j.1600-0447.2005.00594.x.

Austin M, Highet N, GEA Committee. The beyondblue clinical practice guidelines for depression and related disorders – anxiety, bipolar disorder and puerperal psychosis – in the perinatal period. A guideline for primary care health professionals providing care in the perinatal period. Melbourne: beyondblue: the national depression initiative; 2011.

Balsells M, Garcia-Patterson A, Gich I, Corcoy R. Major congenital malformations in women with gestational diabetes mellitus: a systematic review and meta-analysis. Diabetes Metab Res Rev. 2012;28(3):252–7.

Bar-Oz B, Einarson T, Einarson A, Boskovic R, O'Brien L, Malm H, et al. Paroxetine and congenital malformations: meta-analysis and consideration of potential confounding factors. Clin Ther. 2007;29(5):918–26. doi:10.1016/j.clinthera.2007.05.003. S0149-2918(07)00121-X [pii].

Beck AT, Ward CH, Mendelson M, Mock J, Erbaugh J. An inventory for measuring depression. Arch Gen Psychiatry. 1961;4:561–71.

Bennett HA, Einarson A, Taddio A, Koren G, Einarson TR. Depression during pregnancy: overview of clinical factors. Clin Drug Investig. 2004a;24(3):157–79. doi:2434 [pii].

Bennett HA, Einarson A, Taddio A, Koren G, Einarson TR. Prevalence of depression during pregnancy: systematic review. Obstet Gynecol. 2004b;103(4):698–709. doi:10.1097/01.AOG. 0000116689.75396.5f. 103/4/698 [pii].

Boyce P, Barriball E. Puerperal psychosis. Arch Womens Ment Health. 2010;13(1):45–7. doi:10. 1007/s00737-009-0117-y.

Boyce P, Hickey A. Psychosocial risk factors to major depression after childbirth. Soc Psychiatry Psychiatr Epidemiol. 2005;40(8):605–12.

Boyce PM, Stubbs JM. The importance of postnatal depression. Med J Aust. 1994;161(8):471–2.

Buist AE, Barnett BEW, Milgrom J, Pope S, Condon JT, Ellwood DA, et al. To screen or not to screen–that is the question in perinatal depression. Med J Aust. 2002;177(Suppl):S101–5.

Byatt N, Deligiannidis KM, Freeman MP. Antidepressant use in pregnancy: a critical review focused on risks and controversies. Acta Psychiatr Scand. 2013;127(2):94–114. doi:10.1111/ acps.12042.

Casper RC, Fleisher BE, Lee-Ancajas JC, Gilles A, Gaylor E, DeBattista A, et al. Follow-up of children of depressed mothers exposed or not exposed to antidepressant drugs during pregnancy. J Pediatr. 2003;142(4):402–8. doi:10.1067/mpd.2003.139.

Casper RC, Gilles AA, Fleisher BE, Baran J, Enns G, Lazzeroni LC. Length of prenatal exposure to selective serotonin reuptake inhibitor (SSRI) antidepressants: effects on neonatal adaptation and psychomotor development. Psychopharmacology (Berl). 2011;217:211–9.

Chaudron LH. Complex challenges in treating depression during pregnancy. Am J Psychiatry. 2013;170(1):12–20. doi:10.1176/appi.ajp.2012.12040440.

Cohen LS, Altshuler LL, Harlow BL, Nonacs R, Newport DJ, Viguera AC, et al. Relapse of major depression during pregnancy in women who maintain or discontinue antidepressant treatment. JAMA. 2006;295(5):499–507. doi:10.1001/jama.295.5.499. 295/5/499.

Cooper WO, Willy ME, Pont SJ, Ray WA. Increasing use of antidepressants in pregnancy. Am J Obstet Gynecol. 2007;196(6):544.e1–5. doi:10.1016/j.ajog.2007.01.033. S0002-9378(07) 00144-5 [pii].

Coverdale JH, McCullough LB, Chervenak FA. The ethics of randomized placebo-controlled trials of antidepressants with pregnant women: a systematic review. Obstet Gynecol. 2008;112 (6):1361–8. doi:10.1097/AOG.0b013e31818c2a27.

Cox JL, Holden JM, Sagovsky R. Detection of postnatal depression: development of the 10-item Edinburgh Postnatal Depression Scale. Br J Psychiatry. 1987;150:782–6.

Davidson S, Prokonov D, Taler M, Maayan R, Harell D, Gil-Ad I, et al. Effect of exposure to selective serotonin reuptake inhibitors in utero on fetal growth: potential role for the IGF-I and HPA axes. Pediatr Res. 2009;65(2):236–41.

Deave T, Heron J, Evans J, Emond A. The impact of maternal depression in pregnancy on early child development. BJOG. 2008;115(8):1043–51. doi:10.1111/j.1471-0528.2008.01752.x.

Einarson TR, Einarson A. Newer antidepressants in pregnancy and rates of major malformations: a meta-analysis of prospective comparative studies. Pharmacoepidemiol Drug Saf. 2005;14 (12):823–7. doi:10.1002/pds.1084.

Einarson A, Selby P, Koren G. Discontinuing antidepressants and benzodiazepines upon becoming pregnant. Beware of the risks of abrupt discontinuation. Can Fam Physician. 2001;47:489–90.

Evans J, Heron J, Francomb H, Oke S, Golding J. Cohort study of depressed mood during pregnancy and after childbirth. BMJ. 2001;323(7307):257–60.

Field T. Prenatal depression effects on early development: a review. Infant Behav Dev. 2011;34 (1):1–14. doi:10.1016/j.infbeh.2010.09.008.

Galbally M. Teratology: more than malformations. Aust N Z J Psychiatry. 2013;47(11):1082–4. doi:10.1177/0004867413495931.

Galbally M, Lewis AJ, Lum J, Buist A. Serotonin discontinuation syndrome following in utero exposure to antidepressant medication: prospective controlled study. Aust N Z J Psychiatry. 2009;43(9):846–54. doi:10.1080/00048670903107583. 913775190 [pii].

Galbally M, Lewis AJ, Buist A. Developmental outcomes of children exposed to antidepressants in pregnancy. Aust N Z J Psychiatry. 2011;45(5):393–9. doi:10.3109/00048674.2010.549995.

Galbally M, Gentile S, Lewis AJ. Further findings linking SSRIs during pregnancy and persistent pulmonary hypertension of the newborn. CNS Drugs. 2012a;26(10):813–22.

Galbally M, Lewis AJ, Gentile S, Buist A, Walker S. The biology of fetal exposure to serotonin reuptake inhibitors: implications for neurodevelopment. In: Migne LJ, Post JW, editors. Antidepressants: pharmacology, health effects and controversy. New York: Nova; 2012b. p. 1–26.

Gentile S, Galbally M. Prenatal exposure to antidepressant medications and neurodevelopmental outcomes: a systematic review. J Affect Disord. 2010;128(1–2):1–9. doi:10.1016/j.jad.2010. 02.125. S0165-0327(10)00262-4 [pii].

Grigoriadis S, VonderPorten EH, Mamisashvili L, Eady A, Tomlinson G, Dennis CL, et al. The effect of prenatal antidepressant exposure on neonatal adaptation: a systematic review and meta-analysis. J Clin Psychiatry. 2013a;74(4):e309–20. doi:10.4088/JCP.12r07967.

Grigoriadis S, VonderPorten EH, Mamisashvili L, Roerecke M, Rehm J, Dennis CL, et al. Antidepressant exposure during pregnancy and congenital malformations: is there an association? A systematic review and meta-analysis of the best evidence. J Clin Psychiatry. 2013b;74(4):e293–308. doi:10.4088/JCP.12r07966.

Grigoriadis S, Vonderporten EH, Mamisashvili L, Tomlinson G, Dennis CL, Koren G, et al. The impact of maternal depression during pregnancy on perinatal outcomes: a systematic review and meta-analysis. J Clin Psychiatry. 2013c;74(4):e321–41. doi:10.4088/JCP.12r07968.

Grigoriadis S, Vonderporten EH, Mamisashvili L, Tomlinson G, Dennis CL, Koren G, et al. Prenatal exposure to antidepressants and persistent pulmonary hypertension of the newborn: systematic review and meta-analysis. BMJ. 2014;348:f6932.

Grote NK, Bridge JA, Gavin AR, Melville JL, Iyengar S, Katon WJ. A meta-analysis of depression during pregnancy and the risk of preterm birth, low birth weight, and intrauterine growth restriction. Arch Gen Psychiatry. 2010;67(10):1012–24. doi:10.1001/archgenpsychiatry.2010. 111.

Hemels ME, Einarson A, Koren G, Lanctot KL, Einarson TR. Antidepressant use during pregnancy and the rates of spontaneous abortions: a meta-analysis. Ann Pharmacother. 2005;39 (5):803–9. doi:10.1345/aph.1E547. aph.1E547.

Hendrick V, Stowe ZN, Altshuler LL, Hwang S, Lee E, Haynes D. Placental passage of antidepressant medications. Am J Psychiatry. 2003;160(5):993–6.

Howard LM, Kirkwood G, Latinovic R. Sudden infant death syndrome and maternal depression. J Clin Psychiatry. 2007;68(8):1279–83.

Jacobs BL, Fornal CA. Serotonin and motor activity. Curr Opin Neurobiol. 1997;7(6):820–5.

Jimenez-Solem E, Andersen JT, Petersen M, Broedbaek K, Andersen NL, Torp-Pedersen C, et al. Prevalence of antidepressant use during pregnancy in Denmark, a nation-wide cohort study. PLoS One. 2013;8(4):e63034.

Kallen B. Neonate characteristics after maternal use of antidepressants in late pregnancy. Arch Pediatr Adolesc Med. 2004;158(4):312–6. doi:10.1001/archpedi.158.4.312. 158/4/312 [pii].

Kendell RE, Rennie D, Clarke JA, Dean C. The social and obstetric correlates of psychiatric admission in the puerperium. Psychol Med. 1981;11:341–50.

Kendell RE, Chalmers JC, Platz C. Epidemiology of puerperal psychoses. Br J Psychiatry. 1987;150:662–73.

Kessler RC, Berglund P, Demler O, Jin R, Koretz D, Merikangas KR, et al. The epidemiology of major depressive disorder: results from the National Comorbidity Survey Replication (NCS-R). JAMA. 2003;289(23):3095–105. doi:10.1001/jama.289.23.3095.

Kieler H, Artama M, Engeland A, Ericsson O, Furu K, Gissler M, et al. Selective serotonin reuptake inhibitors during pregnancy and risk of persistent pulmonary hypertension in the newborn: population based cohort study from the five Nordic countries. BMJ. 2012;344:d8012.

Koren G, Matsui D, Einarson A, Knoppert D, Steiner M. Is maternal use of selective serotonin reuptake inhibitors in the third trimester of pregnancy harmful to neonates? CMAJ. 2005;172 (11):1457–9. doi:10.1503/cmaj.1041100. 172/11/1457.

Kumar R, Robson KM. A prospective study of emotional disorders in childbearing women. Br J Psychiatry. 1984;144:35–47.

Leanza V, Stracquadanio M, Ciotta L, Pafumi C, Giannone T, Giunta M, et al. Folates and prevention of neural-tube diseases. Science. 2013;2(2):47–51.

Lennestal R, Kallen B. Delivery outcome in relation to maternal use of some recently introduced antidepressants. J Clin Psychopharmacol. 2007;27(6):607–13. doi:10.1097/jcp. 0b013e31815ac4d2. 00004714-200712000-00009 [pii].

Lewis AJ, Galbally M, Opie G, Buist A. Neonatal growth outcomes at birth and one month postpartum following in utero exposure to antidepressant medication. Aust N Z J Psychiatry. 2010;44(5):482–7. doi:10.3109/00048670903559593.

Lewis A, Galbally M, Bailey C. Perinatal mental health, antidepressants and neonatal outcomes: findings from the Longitudinal Study of Australian Children. Neonatal Paediatr Child Health Nurs. 2012;15(3):22–8.

Lewis A, Galbally M, Gannon T, Symeonides C. Early life programming as a target for prevention of child and adolescent mental disorders. BMC Med. 2014;12(1):33.

Malhi GS, Hitching R, Berk M, Boyce P, Porter R, Fritz K. Pharmacological management of unipolar depression. Acta Psychiatr Scand Suppl. 2013;443:6–23. doi:10.1111/acps.12122.

Malm H, Artama M, Gissler M, Ritvanen A. Selective serotonin reuptake inhibitors and risk for major congenital anomalies. Obstet Gynecol. 2011;118(1):111.

Matthey S, Ross-Hamid C. The validity of DSM symptoms for depression and anxiety disorders during pregnancy. J Affect Disord. 2011;133(3):546–52. doi:10.1016/j.jad.2011.05.004.

Matthey S, Ross-Hamid C. Repeat testing on the Edinburgh Depression Scale and the HADS-A in pregnancy: differentiating between transient and enduring distress. J Affect Disord. 2012;141 (2–3):213–21. doi:10.1016/j.jad.2012.02.037.

Murray L. The impact of postnatal depression on infant development. J Child Psychol Psychiatry. 1992;33(3):543–61.

Murray CJ, Vos T, Lozano R, Naghavi M, Flaxman AD, Michaud C, et al. Disability-adjusted life years (DALYs) for 291 diseases and injuries in 21 regions, 1990–2010: a systematic analysis for the Global Burden of Disease Study 2010. Lancet. 2012;380(9859):2197–223. doi:10.1016/ S0140-6736(12)61689-4.

Myles N, Newall H, Ward H, Large M. Systematic meta-analysis of individual selective serotonin reuptake inhibitor medications and congenital malformations. Aust N Z J Psychiatry. 2013;47 (11):1002–12. doi:10.1177/0004867413492219. 0004867413492219 [pii].

Newport DJ, Ji S, Long Q, Knight BT, Zach EB, Smith EN, et al. Maternal depression and anxiety differentially impact fetal exposures during pregnancy. J Clin Psychiatry. 2012;73(2):247–51. doi:10.4088/JCP.10m06783.

O'Hara MW, Swain AM. Rates and risk of postpartum depression – a meta-analysis. Int Rev Psychiatry. 1996;8:37–54.

O'Hara MW, Neunaber J, Zekoski EM. Prospective study of postpartum depression: prevalence, course and predictive factors. J Abnorm Psychol. 1984;93:158–71.

Oberlander TF, Warburton W, Misri S, Aghajanian J, Hertzman C. Neonatal outcomes after prenatal exposure to selective serotonin reuptake inhibitor antidepressants and maternal depression using population-based linked health data. Arch Gen Psychiatry. 2006;63(8):898–906. doi:10.1001/archpsyc.63.8.898. 63/8/898 [pii].

O'Brien L, Einarson TR, Sarkar M, Einarson A, Koren G. Does paroxetine cause cardiac malformations? J Obstet Gynaecol Can. 2008;30(8):696–701.

Onyike CU, Crum RM, Lee HB, Lyketsos CG, Eaton WW. Is obesity associated with major depression? Results from the Third National Health and Nutrition Examination Survey. Am J Epidemiol. 2003;158(12):1139–47.

Pitt B. 'Atypical' depression following childbirth. Br J Psychiatry. 1968;114:1325–35.

Rahimi R, Nikfar S, Abdollahi M. Pregnancy outcomes following exposure to serotonin reuptake inhibitors: a meta-analysis of clinical trials. Reprod Toxicol. 2006;22(4):571–5. doi:10.1016/j. reprotox.2006.03.019. S0890-6238(06)00099-2 [pii].

Ross LE, Grigoriadis S, Mamisashvili L, VonderPorten EH, Roerecke M, Rehm J, et al. Selected pregnancy and delivery outcomes after exposure to antidepressant medication: a systematic review and meta-analysis outcomes after antidepressant use in pregnancy. JAMA Psychiatry. 2013;70:1–8.

Scanlon KS, Ferencz C, Loffredo CA, Wilson PD, Correa-Villaseñor A, Khoury MJ, et al. Preconceptional folate intake and malformations of the cardiac outflow tract. Epidemiology. 1998;9(1):95–8.

Simon GE, Cunningham ML, Davis RL. Outcomes of prenatal antidepressant exposure. Am J Psychiatry. 2002;159(12):2055–61.

Slade T, Johnston A, Oakley Browne MA, Andrews G, Whiteford H. 2007 National Survey of Mental Health and Wellbeing: methods and key findings. Aust N Z J Psychiatry. 2009;43 (7):594–605. doi:10.1080/00048670902970882.

Spinelli MG. Interpersonal psychotherapy for depressed antepartum women: a pilot study. Am J Psychiatry. 1997;154(7):1028–30.

Stothard KJ, Tennant PW, Bell R, Rankin J. Maternal overweight and obesity and the risk of congenital anomalies. JAMA. 2009;301(6):636–50.

Tod ED. Puerperal depression. A prospective epidemiological study. Lancet. 1964;2(7372):1264–6.

Toh S, Mitchell AA, Louik C, Werler MM, Chambers CD, Hernandez-Diaz S. Selective serotonin reuptake inhibitor use and risk of gestational hypertension. Am J Psychiatry. 2009;166(3):320–8. doi:10.1176/appi.ajp.2008.08060817.

Van den Bergh BRH, Mulder EJH, Mennes M, Glover V. Antenatal maternal anxiety and stress and the neurobehavioural development of the fetus and child: links and possible mechanisms. A review. Neurosci Biobehav Rev. 2005;29(2):237–58.

Ververs T, Kaasenbrood H, Visser G, Schobben F, de Jong-van den Berg L, Egberts T. Prevalence and patterns of antidepressant drug use during pregnancy. Eur J Clin Pharmacol. 2006;62 (10):863–70. doi:10.1007/s00228-006-0177-0.

Vesga-Lopez O, Blanco C, Keyes K, Olfson M, Grant BF, Hasin DS. Psychiatric disorders in pregnant and postpartum women in the United States. Arch Gen Psychiatry. 2008;65(7):805–15. doi:10.1001/archpsyc.65.7.805.

Viguera AC, Tondo L, Koukopoulos AE, Reginaldi D, Lepri B, Baldessarini RJ. Episodes of mood disorders in 2,252 pregnancies and postpartum periods. Am J Psychiatry. 2011;168(11):1179–85. doi:10.1176/appi.ajp.2011.11010148.

Warburton W, Hertzman C, Oberlander TF. A register study of the impact of stopping third trimester selective serotonin reuptake inhibitor exposure on neonatal health. Acta Psychiatr Scand. 2010;121(6):471–9. doi:10.1111/j.1600-0447.2009.01490.x. ACP1490 [pii].

Warner R, Appleby LS, Whitton A, Faragher BA. Demographic and obstetric risk factors for postnatal psychiatric morbidity. Br J Psychiatry. 1996;168(5):607–11.

Watson JP, Elliott SA, Rugg AJ, Brough DI. Psychiatric disorder in pregnancy and the first postnatal year. Br J Psychiatry. 1984;144:453–62.

Whitaker-Azmitia PM. The discovery of serotonin and its role in neuroscience. Neuropsychopharmacology. 1999;21(2 Suppl):2S.

Whitaker-Azmitia PM, Druse M, Walker P, Lauder JM. Serotonin as a developmental signal. Behav Brain Res. 1996;73(1–2):19.

Wilson KL, Zelig CM, Harvey JP, Cunningham BS, Dolinsky BM, Napolitano PG. Persistent pulmonary hypertension of the newborn is associated with mode of delivery and not with maternal use of selective serotonin reuptake inhibitors. Am J Perinatol. 2011;28(1):19.

Wisner KL, Sit DK, Hanusa BH, Moses-Kolko EL, Bogen DL, Hunker DF, et al. Major depression and antidepressant treatment: impact on pregnancy and neonatal outcomes. Am J Psychiatry. 2009;166(5):557–66. doi:10.1176/appi.ajp.2008.08081170. appi.ajp.2008.08081170 [pii].

Wisner KL, Bogen DL, Sit D, McShea M, Hughes C, Rizzo D, et al. Does fetal exposure to SSRIs or maternal depression impact infant growth? Am J Psychiatry. 2013;170(5):485–93. doi:10.1176/appi.ajp.2012.11121873. 1669748.

Wurst KE, Poole C, Ephross SA, Olshan AF. First trimester paroxetine use and the prevalence of congenital, specifically cardiac, defects: a meta-analysis of epidemiological studies. Birth Defects Res A Clin Mol Teratol. 2010;88(3):159–70. doi:10.1002/bdra.20627.

Yonkers KA, Smith MV, Gotman N, Belanger K. Typical somatic symptoms of pregnancy and their impact on a diagnosis of major depressive disorder. Gen Hosp Psychiatry. 2009a;31 (4):327–33. doi:10.1016/j.genhosppsych.2009.03.005. S0163-8343(09)00050-4 [pii].

Yonkers KA, Wisner KL, Stewart DE, Oberlander TF, Dell DL, Stotland N, et al. The management of depression during pregnancy: a report from the American Psychiatric Association and the American College of Obstetricians and Gynecologists. Gen Hosp Psychiatry. 2009b;31 (5):403–13. doi:10.1016/j.genhosppsych.2009.04.003.

Yonkers KA, Wisner KL, Stewart DE, Oberlander TF, Dell DL, Stotland N, et al. The management of depression during pregnancy: a report from the American Psychiatric Association and the American College of Obstetricians and Gynecologists. Obstet Gynecol. 2009c;114(3):703–13. doi:10.1097/AOG.0b013e3181ba0632. 00006250-200909000-00044 [pii].

Yonkers KA, Gotman N, Smith MV, Forray A, Belanger K, Brunetto WL, et al. Does antidepressant use attenuate the risk of a major depressive episode in pregnancy? Epidemiology. 2011;22 (6):848–54. doi:10.1097/EDE.0b013e3182306847.

Anxiety and Sleep Disorders, Psychopharmacology, and Pregnancy

7

Salvatore Gentile

Abstract

Antenatal anxiety may adversely impact on several aspects of fetal maturation, pregnancy, the puerperium, and child development, thus demonstrating an intrinsic teratogenic structural, gestational, and neurobehavioral liability. Moreover, insomnia during the first trimester of pregnancy is quite common and is usually a result of associated hormonal changes. Insomnia is also common during the third trimester of pregnancy. There are a number of reasons for this, but by far the most common is the discomfort as the mother gets bigger and her baby begins to place more pressure on her internal organs, making it more difficult to find a comfortable position to sleep in. However, when possible, benzodiazepines should be avoided in both the first trimester and third trimester of pregnancy because of possible structural teratogenicity (especially, anal atresia and other gastrointestinal tract anomalies, and oral cleft), ascertained gestational teratogenity (spontaneous abortion) when taken in overdose, and ascertained perinatal teratogenicity (neonatal withdrawal syndromes). As regards hypnotic agents, preliminary data, although apparently encouraging, are too limited to confirm or exclude a potential structural teratogenic liability. Above all, concordant safety signals seem to discourage the use of hypnotic agents during pregnancy because of an increase in the risk of gestational teratogenicity (preterm birth, low birth weight, and babies small for gestational age). Given these considerations, interventions alternative to pharmacological treatments should be considered first-line options for managing anxiety and sleep disorders in pregnancy.

S. Gentile (✉)
Department of Mental Health, ASL Salerno, Mental Health Center n. 63, Piazza Galdi 84013, Cava de' Tirreni, Salerno, Italy

Department of Neurosciences, Medical School "Federico II", University of Naples, Naples, Italy
e-mail: salvatore_gentile@alice.it

M. Galbally et al. (eds.), *Psychopharmacology and Pregnancy*,
DOI 10.1007/978-3-642-54562-7_7, © Springer-Verlag Berlin Heidelberg 2014

Keywords

Benzodiazepines • Pregnancy • Teratogenicity • Pregabalin • Zaleplon •
Zolpidem • Zopiclone

7.1   Anxiety Disorders and Motherhood

7.1.1   Epidemiology of Antenatal Anxiety Disorders

Antenatal clinics can expect at least one in five pregnant women to experience
mental health problems, especially depression and anxiety (Qiao et al. 2012). In
fact, pregnancy is a period highly vulnerable to the onset of anxiety symptoms.

"Health anxiety" is particularly elevated in pregnancy, especially in women who
have experienced earlier obstetric complications (Collingwood 2012). Miscarriage,
fetal death, and preterm birth indeed reduce women's quality of life scores and
significantly raise their anxiety scores during subsequent pregnancies.

The prevalence of specific anxiety disorders in pregnancy is highly variable.
Panic disorder (PD) has a reported prevalence of 1.3–2.0 %. Although an increased
risk of relapse and new-onset PD has been reported in the postpartum period, the
risk in pregnancy per se is not known (Vythilingum 2008).

Few studies have examined the prevalence of obsessive–compulsive disorder
(OCD) in pregnant women, with reported prevalences varying between 0.2 and
3.5 % (Ross and McLean 2006; Uguz et al. 2007). There is no data on the course of
preexisting posttraumatic stress disorder (PTSD) during pregnancy (Vythilingum
2008). Perinatal PTSD (i.e., PTSD related to medical procedures, childbirth, or
other obstetric events) has been reported (Beck 2004). One study found that 20 % of
women reported traumatic pregnancy-related procedures. Of these, 6 % met criteria
for PTSD (Menage 1993).

To diagnose generalized anxiety disorder (GAD) symptoms must be present for
at least 6 months (APA 1994). Thus, it is unlikely that criteria for new-onset GAD
will be met in pregnancy (Vythilingum 2008). Indeed, limited data exist on the
epidemiology of GAD in pregnancy. Only one study investigated the prevalence of
GAD in pregnancy. It found a rate of 8.5 % in the third trimester (Shear and
Oommen 1995). No information is available on the course of preexisting GAD in
pregnancy.

7.1.2   Hormonal Changes in Pregnancy and Their Relationship
with the Onset of Anxiety Disorders

Hormonal changes in pregnancy may facilitate the onset of anxiety disorders
(Miller 2011). Progesterone, metabolized into pregnanolone and allopregnanolone
in the brain, is neuroactive gamma-aminobutyric acid (GABA) agonist. As levels of
these hormones increase during pregnancy, GABA receptors are downregulated,

and this phenomenon may confer the increased vulnerability of the expectant mothers (Smith et al. 2007; Parízek et al. 2005; Altemus et al. 2004; Hill et al. 2001; Maes et al. 2001).

Moreover, abrupt estrogen reduction can reduce serotonergic functioning. Tryptophan is an amino acid that is a "building block" of serotonin (Miller 2011). In pregnancy, serum tryptophan is reduced, especially relative to other amino acids that compete to cross into the brain (Miller 2011). The fall in serum tryptophan levels may also contribute to the onset of anxiety disorders (Smith et al. 2007; Parízek et al. 2005; Maes et al. 2001; Altemus et al. 2004; Hill et al. 2001).

7.1.3 Anxiety Disorders in Pregnancy: Antenatal and Postnatal Effects

Antenatal anxiety may adversely impact on several aspects of fetal maturation, pregnancy, the puerperium, and child development, thus demonstrating an intrinsic "teratogenic structural, gestational, and neurobehavioral liability" (Gentile 2012).

As noted by Glover and O'Connor (2002) in an interesting editorial, studies of the effects of antenatal stress and anxiety in humans found that women who experience severe life events in the first trimester of pregnancy have a 50 % increase in the rate of congenital abnormalities, especially cleft palate (Hansen et al. 2000).

Reports from the pre-ultrasound era had suggested that prenatal maternal stress, anxiety, and emotions might affect fetal functioning, as evidenced by increased fetal heart rate and mobility (Van den Bergh 1992). A review describing results obtained during the post-ultrasound era confirms that good evidence exists for a direct link between antenatal anxiety/stress and abnormal fetal behavior (Van den Bergh et al. 2005).

Moreover, interesting research indicates that severe maternal anxiety in late (but not early) pregnancy might be associated with impaired blood flow or raised resistance index to the fetus through the maternal uterine arteries (Teixeira et al. 1999). High resistance is associated with adverse obstetric outcomes, particularly intrauterine growth restriction and pre-eclampsia, and could therefore help to explain why anxious mothers are likely to have babies small for gestational age (Glover and O'Connor 2002). In fact, preterm labor and low birth weight are the outcomes linked most consistently with antenatal stress or anxiety in humans (Hedegaard et al. 1993; Lou et al. 1992). These findings are relatively robust across different measures of stress/anxiety (Glover and O'Connor 2002).

In addition, well-designed studies have shown a relationship between antenatal stress or anxiety and behavioral/emotional disturbance in the child. The Avon Longitudinal Study of Parents and Children (ALSPAC) suggests a strong link between maternal anxiety in the third trimester and behavioral/emotional problems in 4-year-old children (O'Connor et al. 2002). Analyses from the ALSPAC cohort also found evidence of an impact of antenatal anxiety on neurological development. High levels of maternal anxiety at 18 weeks gestation may indeed predict atypical laterality (i.e., mixed handedness) in the child, independently of maternal and paternal handedness and obstetric and other antenatal risks.

Furthermore, a recent study demonstrated that neurocognitive functioning at 5 years of age is impaired in those children whose mothers had suffered from anxiety symptoms during the gestational period (Loomans et al. 2012). At the same age, such children show behavior and hyperactivity/inattention problems, emotional symptoms, peer relationship impairment, and conduct disturbances (Loomans et al. 2011). Of note, in boys exposure to antenatal anxiety is associated with a stronger increase in overall problem behavior compared to girls. Moreover, high levels of maternal state anxiety during pregnancy enhances the offspring's susceptibility for developing childhood disorders, such as attention-deficit hyperactivity disorder (ADHD) symptoms, externalizing problems, and anxiety at 8–9 years of age (Van den Bergh and Marcoen 2004). Impaired patterns of decision-making processes may persist up to 17 years of age (Mennes et al. 2009).

Several plausible mechanisms linking antenatal stress/anxiety and disturbances in offspring have been suggested. Preterm birth is the single largest perinatal risk factor for later morbidity, including ADHD and schizophrenia, and being small for gestational age is associated with similar adverse mental and behavioral problems (Hultman et al. 1999). Research supporting a mechanism involving the maternal hypothalamic–pituitary–adrenal (HPA) axis is also increasing. Gitau et al. (2001) suggested that high levels of maternal cortisol levels (due to chronic anxiety) can cross the placenta to significantly alter fetal exposure.

It should also be highlighted that, after accounting for the presence of other antenatal anxiety disorders, antenatal depression, maternal age at child's birth, socioeconomic status, and ethnicity in the models, antenatal GAD independently predicts depression at all time points after delivery (Coelho et al. 2011).

Therefore, anxiety disorders at onset or worsening during pregnancy may require pharmacological treatment to obtain a prompt remission of maternal mental impairment and, thus, to prevent potential serious complications to the mother–infant pair (Gentile 2011).

7.2   Benzodiazepines and Pregnancy

Benzodiazepines (BDZs) are the class of medication most frequently prescribed in pregnant women to treat anxiety symptoms (Daw 2012). They have been on the market for more than 40 years and it is estimated that at least 3–15 % of any adult population in the world is using prescribed BDZs (Bendtsen et al. 1999). Pharmacoepidemiological data suggest that not only are women are more likely to be prescribed such medications compared to men (Taylor et al. 1998), but women are also more likely to be prescribed BDZs for longer periods of time (Jorm et al. 2000). Women are also more likely than men to be prescribed BDZs and sleeping pills for nonmedical reasons such as coping with grief or stress (Currie 2004). They are also prescribed these drugs when adjusting to natural processes such as childbirth (Morales-Suárez-Varela et al. 1997).

Worldwide, an estimated 85 % of all psychotropic medicines prescribed to pregnant women are for BDZs (Marchetti et al. 1993). The incidence of BDZ use during pregnancy is unclear (Bncc.org.uk 2012), and figures varying from 1–3 % to 40 % have been suggested (Ormond and Guttmacher 1995; McElhatton 1994). These figures do not include women who misuse BDZs, 90 % of whom are of childbearing age (Institute for the Study of Drug Addiction 2012).

However, the safety of their use during pregnancy remains controversial because there have been conflicting results regarding their teratogenicity. Thus, the risk/benefit ratio of using such medications is still unclear.

7.2.1 Structural Teratogenicity

Studies Suggesting an Increase in the Risk of Birth Defects

A significantly higher risk of cardiovascular malformations (OR 2.5) was observed in 201 newborns whose mother was exposed to chlordiazepoxide during pregnancy (Czeizel et al. 2004). However, it should be noted that more than 90 % of cases were exposed concomitantly to other drugs (promethazine, prevalently). In an analysis by Milkovich and Van den Berg (1974) of 19,044 live births, severe congenital anomalies (including spastic diplegia, microcephaly, duodenal atresia, and mental deficiency) occurred more often among infants of mothers who took chlordiazepoxide during the first 42 days of pregnancy than among infants of mothers who took other drugs or no drugs (11.4 % compared with 4.6 % and 2.6 %, respectively).

In a sample of 262 newborns with a congenital birth defect, those antenatally exposed to either lorazepam or bromazepam were at a statistically significant increased risk of anal atresia and digestive tract anomalies (OR 6.19 and 6.15, respectively) compared to newborns exposed to other BDZs (Bonnot et al. 2001). Godet et al. (1995) described a study in which 187 malformed infants were observed among 100,000 births that involved exposure to BDZs, including lorazepam, during the first trimester of pregnancy. A significant association was found between lorazepam and anal atresia (five cases, $p < 0.001$).

Two studies investigating the reproductive safety of diazepam analyzed the rate of birth defects recorded in the Hungarian Case-Control Surveillance of Congenital Abnormalities (HCCSCA). The first of these studies found a statistically significant increase in the risk of limb malformations, rectal–anal stenosis/atresia, cardiovascular malformations, and multiple congenital abnormalities (Czeizel et al. 2003). In the second study, Kjaer et al. (2007) examined data from the HCCSCA according to a case-time-control design. The results confirmed that antenatal diazepam exposure may significantly increase the risk of birth defects (OR 1.2).

Other studies had already suggested that the use of diazepam during the first trimester of pregnancy was significantly greater among mothers of children born with oral cleft. Aarskog (1975) found that 6.3 % of 30 infants born with cleft palate in the USA between 1967 and 1971 had been exposed to diazepam in the first trimester, compared with 1.1 % of control infants. Such results were confirmed by the contemporaneous study by Saxen (1975a). Safra and Oakley (1975) also reported that mothers of infants with cleft lip, cleft palate, or both had used diazepam four times more frequently than mothers of control infants.

A review of 599 oral clefts by Saxen and Saxen (1975) showed a significant association ($p < 0.05$) between ingestion of anxiolytics, mostly diazepam, during the first trimester of pregnancy. Many other epidemiological studies have shown an association between the use of diazepam in the first trimester and oral clefts (Rosenberg et al. 1983; Entman and Vaughn 1984; Czeizel 1976; Saxen 1975b). In prospective studies of the effect on the infant of maternal use of psychoactive drugs during pregnancy, an embryofetopathy that resembles the fetal alcohol syndrome (Olegård et al. 1979) has been associated with antenatal maternal use of BDZs (Laegreid et al. 1987). The authors reported a specific BDZ syndrome among 7 infants with dysmorphism in a prospective study in which 36 mothers of 37 infants regularly took such medications during pregnancy. Five of these mothers had taken diazepam.

An association with BDZ exposure following suicidal attempts by overdose and increased rates of birth defects was confirmed for nitrazepam (Gidai et al. 2010).

Studies Suggesting No Increase in the Risk of Birth Defects

Short-term exposure to 10 mg b.i.d. of diazepam during the first trimester of pregnancy for hyperemesis gravidarum was not associated with higher risks of birth defects (Tasci et al. 2009).

Two studies considered exposure to clonazepam monotherapy during pregnancy. In the study by Lin et al. (2004), 73 newborns had been exposed antenatally to clonazepam at doses up to 2 mg/day during the first trimester. No increased rates of birth defects were recorded. In the second study no significant variations in birth weight-adjusted head circumference were observed in 71 newborns after intrauterine clonazepam exposure (Almgren et al. 2008). However, the specific risk of microcephaly was not investigated.

In several studies, the frequency of congenital anomalies was not greater than expected amongst infants of women who took chlordiazepoxide during the first trimester of pregnancy (Czeizel 1988; Bracken and Holford 1981; Kullander and Källén 1976; Crombie et al. 1975; Hartz et al. 1975).

In a prospective study conducted between 1982 and 1992, St Clair and Schirmer (1992) evaluated the pregnancy outcomes of 542 women who were exposed to alprazolam during the first trimester of pregnancy. They noted neither a pattern of defects, nor excess of congenital anomalies in 411 infants who were exposed to alprazolam during the first trimester. Another study prospectively identified 236 women who were exposed to therapeutic dosages of alprazolam during the first trimester and found only five cases of congenital malformations (Schick-Boschetto and Zuber 1992). These data do not support an association between antenatal alprazolam exposure and congenital defects.

7.2.2 Gestational Teratogenicity

Studies Suggesting an Increase in the Risk of Miscarriage

Some studies investigated the reproductive safety of BDZs in women who took high doses of such medications as suicide attempts.

A small sample of women who were exposed to high doses of alprazolam (mean 29.8 mg; range 7.5–100 mg) showed an increase in the rate of spontaneous abortion (7 out of 30 pregnancies: 23.3 %), but no increased risk of birth defects was observed (Gidai et al. 2008a).

High rates of spontaneous abortions, as well as low birth weight, were also found in women who ingested chlordiazepoxide or diazepam as overdoses (Gidai et al. 2008b, c). Exposure to both medazepam and nitrazepam confirmed that BDZ overdose is strongly associated with an increased risk of miscarriage (Gidai et al. 2008d, 2010).

7.2.3 Perinatal Teratogenicity

Studies Suggesting an Increase in the Risk of Perinatal Teratogenicity

If used during pregnancy, *all BDZs* have been associated with an increased risk of inducing neonatal withdrawal symptoms (Iqbal et al. 2002). Symptoms of neonatal withdrawal, which may also include signs resembling the "floppy infant syndrome", are summarized in Table 7.1. This neonatal withdrawal can appear within a few days to 21 weeks (depending on the half-life of the specific BDZ used) after birth and can last up to several months. This syndrome is best minimized by gradually tapering the BDZ dose before delivery and usually infants who develop BDZ withdrawal symptoms will recover without any long-lasting sequelae (Iqbal et al. 2002).

7.2.4 Neurobehavioral Teratogenicity

Studies Suggesting an Increase in the Risk of Neurobehavioral Teratogenicity

A small and so far unreplicated study (which did not explore the role of potential confounders and the effects of specific medications) found a combination of delayed mental development and neuropsychological symptoms in 18-month-old children prenatally exposed to *various BDZs* (Viggedal et al. 1993).

Studies Suggesting No Increase in the Risk of Neurobehavioral Teratogenicity

In contrast, reassuring results emerged from a study performed on a large number of children exposed prenatally to chlordiazepoxide (Hartz et al. 1975). In fact, such children showed normal motor, mental, and IQ scores at 3 years of age.

Table 7.1 The benzodiazepine neonatal withdrawal syndrome

Hypo/hypertonia	Hyperreflexia	Tremors	Sleep disturbances
Cyanosis	Bradycardia	Apnea	Feed aspiration
Vomiting	Diarrhea	Suckling difficulties	Growth retardation

Preschool children exposed to diazepam during the last stages of their intrauterine life showed no neurodevelopmental problems (Gidai et al. 2008c).

Even if taken in overdose (for maternal suicidal attempts), BDZs (specifically, alprazolam) were devoid of effects on the principal neurodevelopmental milestones (Gidai et al. 2008a).

7.3 Pregabalin and Pregnancy

Pregabalin (PGB) is an anticonvulsant drug used for neuropathic pain and as an adjunct therapy for partial seizures with or without secondary generalization in adults. It has also been found effective for GAD and is (as of 2007) approved for this use in the European Union.

7.3.1 Structural, Gestational, Perinatal, and Behavioral Teratogenicity

No published information is available on PGB use during pregnancy. A single case report found that passage of the drug into breast milk is extensive, but low concentrations were measured in the infant (Ohman et al. 2011).

7.4 Insomnia and Pregnancy

Pregnancy is a time of great change in a woman's life. Likewise, sleep is altered and may not return to pre-pregnancy quality for several years after the birth of the child (Sharma and Franco 2004). Some sleep disturbances are a harbinger of sleep disorders (Sharma and Franco 2004). If they are not recognized and treated, there can be negative effects for the patient and her unborn child (Sharma and Franco 2004).

Insomnia during the first trimester of pregnancy is quite common and is usually a result of the hormonal changes (Pregnancy Calendar 2012). One of the main causes of insomnia is a result of the progesterone that is released. Progesterone is a natural sedative, which leads to women feel tired and often fall asleep at hours which are not in their normal sleeping cycle, which leaves them wide awake when they are supposed to be sleeping (Pregnancy Calendar 2012). This also explains why fatigue is a common symptom of pregnancy (Pregnancy Calendar 2012). Furthermore, progesterone has been shown to increase non-REM sleep (Friess et al. 1997).

Indeed, studies on the sleep architecture of pregnant women demonstrate increased light sleep (stage 1 sleep) and suppression of dream sleep (REM sleep), as well as more awakenings (Driver and Shapiro 2002).

Insomnia is also common during the third trimester of pregnancy. There are a number of reasons for this, but by far the most common is obviously discomfort as the mother gets bigger and her baby begins to place more pressure on her internal organs, making it more difficult to find a comfortable sleeping position (Pregnancy Calendar 2012). Add to that the constant pressure on the bladder from the baby; the expectant mother will need to urinate more frequently throughout the night (Pregnancy Calendar 2012). Also, many pregnant women report that it is hard to sleep due to leg cramps (BabyCenter Medical Advisory Board 2012).

With so many physical and emotional changes happening, it is no surprise that 8 out of 10 women have insomnia and other sleep problems during pregnancy (BabyCenter Medical Advisory Board 2012).

7.5   Hypnotic Agents and Pregnancy

Hypnotic BDZ receptor agonists (HBRAs: zolpidem, zopiclone, and zaleplon) are widely used in the treatment of insomnia.

7.5.1   Structural Teratogenicity

Studies Suggesting an Increased Risk of Birth Defects
To date, no reports are available suggesting that hypnotic agent exposure during pregnancy may increase the rate of fetal malformations.

Studies Suggesting No Increase in the Risk of Birth Defects
Data from the Swedish Medical Birth Registry from July 1, 1995, up to 2007 were used to identify 1,318 women who reported the use of HBRAs in early pregnancy (Wikner and Källén 2011). Such drugs were not associated with an increased risk of congenital malformations.

Zolpidem crosses the human placenta and rapidly clears the fetal circulation. The ratio of umbilical cord to maternal plasma zolpidem concentrations ranges from 0.48 to 2.75 (Juric et al. 2009). Although the use of zolpidem has not been associated with teratogenic effects in usual clinical doses, a case of fetal neural tube defect has been reported following high dose exposure in the first trimester of pregnancy (Sharma et al. 2011).

7.5.2 Gestational Teratogenicity

Studies Suggesting an Increase in the Risk of Gestational Teratogenicity

To examine the extent and clinical sequelae of fetal exposure to zolpidem, pregnant women with psychiatric illness participated in a study of psychotropic pharmacokinetics (Juric et al. 2009). Outcomes were compared between the zolpidem-exposed group and a 1:1-matched comparator group. Forty-five women taking zolpidem during pregnancy were studied. Rates of preterm delivery and low birth weight were 26.7 % and 15.6 %, respectively, in the zolpidem-exposed group versus 13.3 % and 4.4 % in the matched comparator group, but no significant differences were found. However, pregnant women with psychiatric illness treated with zolpidem may have less optimal obstetrical outcome, though it is unclear if this was related to the medication (Juric et al. 2009).

A nationwide population-based study was carried out in Taiwan with the aim of comparing the risk of adverse pregnancy outcomes in women who received zolpidem treatment for insomnia during pregnancy with women who did not (Wang et al. 2010). The adverse outcomes identified and assessed were delivery of low-birth-weight (LBW) infants, preterm deliveries, delivery of small for gestational age (SGA) infants, delivery of infants with congenital anomalies, and cesarean delivery. The incidences of these were compared between the groups after adjusting for other characteristics of the mothers and infants. The study used the Taiwan National Health Insurance Research Dataset (NHIRD) and Birth-Certificate Registry. In total, the data from 2,497 mothers who received zolpidem treatment during pregnancy and those from 12,485 randomly selected mothers who did not receive the drug were included in the analysis. The results show that the adjusted odds ratios (ORs) for adverse pregnancy outcomes (LBW infants, preterm deliveries, SGA infants, and cesarean delivery) were all higher in mothers who received zolpidem treatment during pregnancy, relative to the randomly selected controls (1.39 (95 % confidence interval (CI) = 1.17–1.64), 1.49 (95 % CI = 1.28–1.74), 1.34 (95 % CI = 1.20–1.49), and 1.74 (95 % CI = 1.59–1.90), respectively).

7.5.3 Perinatal and Neurobehavioral Teratogenicity

To date, there have been no reports of perinatal complications and neurobehavioral impairment associated with in utero exposure to HBRAs.

7.6 Management of Anxiety Disorders in Pregnancy

Women with antenatal anxiety disorders require timely and efficient management that aims to reduce all such symptoms that may adversely impact on baby's health.

7.6.1   Pharmacological Treatments

Benzodiazepines

When possible, BDZs should be avoided in both the first trimester and third trimester of pregnancy due to:

1) Possible structural teratogenicity (especially anal atresia and other gastrointestinal tract anomalies, and oral cleft)
2) Ascertained gestational teratogenity (spontaneous abortion) when taken in overdose
3) Ascertained perinatal teratogenicity (neonatal withdrawal syndromes). To minimize the risk of neonatal withdrawal, BDZs should be tapered gradually before delivery, and because the baby's due date is calculated to be ±2 weeks before delivery, tapering should begin 3–4 weeks before the due date and BDZ treatment should be discontinued at least 1 week before delivery (Vythilingum 2009).

Pregabalin

Since no information is available about the outcomes of pregnancies exposed to PGB, the drug should be avoided during pregnancy.

Hypnotic BDZ receptor agonists

Preliminary data, although apparently encouraging, are too limited to confirm or exclude a potential structural teratogenic liability. Above all, however, concordant safety signals seem to discourage the use of hypnotic agents during pregnancy because of an increase in the risk of gestational teratogenicity (preterm birth, low birth weight, and babies small for gestational age).

7.6.2   Antidepressants

Antidepressants have been shown to be an effective treatment for a range of Anxiety Disorders including OCD (Insel and Murphy 1981) and GAD (Ballenger et al. 2001). Details regarding the risks of antidepressant treatment in pregnancy are outlined in Chap. 6: Depression, Pharmacology and Pregnancy.

7.6.3   Non-pharmacological Interventions

Given these considerations, alternative interventions to pharmacological treatments should be considered first-line options.

Mild to moderate symptoms of anxiety are highly treatable using Cognitive Behavioral Therapy (CBT), an evidence-based, short-term, and focused treatment, in which patients learn to identify their distorted thinking, increase awareness of triggers, and modify maladaptive behaviors (Butler et al. 2006). Guidelines issued by the National Institute for health and Clinical Excellence recommend CBT as a first-line intervention especially for managing antenatal GAD and PD, whereas pharmacological treatment should be preferred for severe OCD (NICE 2007). Trauma-focused psychological therapy, for example, eye movement desensitization and reprocessing therapy, should be offered to those patients diagnosed with antenatal PTSD (NICE 2007). In contrast, insufficient evidence exists to determine if interpersonal psychotherapy is truly effective (Dennis et al. 2007).

Stress reduction techniques such as meditation, modified deep breathing for pregnant women (Wiegartz and Gyoerkoe 2009), and exercising (when medical conditions allow) may complement other forms of treatment (Avni-Barron 2001).

Similarly, treatments such as acupuncture and biofeedback (where patients learn to use their own bodily responses to monitor and control their anxiety) show promise, but their effectiveness is not conclusive (Avni-Barron 2001).

Another treatment evaluated by Chinese researchers is music therapy, a safe and inexpensive method to reduce antenatal anxiety. They explored whether this approach could relieve anxiety in pregnant women confined to bed. They recruited 120 women and gave them music therapy for 30 min on 3 consecutive days. Anxiety levels fell significantly in this group, compared to another group given usual health care (Yang et al. 2009).

Preliminary information seems to suggest that both aromatherapy and massage may be successful in producing clinically significant reductions in anxiety (Bastard and Tiran 2006).

References

Aarskog D. Association between maternal intake of diazepam and oral clefts [letter]. Lancet. 1975;2:921.

Almgren M, Källén B, Lavebratt C. Population-based study of antiepileptic drug exposure in utero-influence on head circumference in newborns. Seizure. 2008;18:672–5.

Altemus M, Fong J, Yang R, Damast S, Luine V, Ferguson D. Changes in cerebrospinal fluid neurochemistry during pregnancy. Biol Psychiatry. 2004;56(6):386–92.

American Psychiatric Association. Diagnostic and statistical manual of mental disorders. 4th ed. Washington, DC: American Psychiatric Association; 1994.

Avni-Barron O. Anxious for two: assessing and treating antenatal anxiety disorders. 2001. http://hcp.obgyn.net/blog/content/article/1760982/1974839. Accessed 26 Oct 2012.

BabyCenter Medical Advisory Board. Sleep problem: insomnia during pregnancy. 2012. http://www.babycenter.com/0_sleep-problem-insomnia-during-pregnancy_7521.bc. Accessed 6 Oct 2012.

Ballenger JC, Davidson JR, Lecrubier Y, Nutt DJ, Borkovec TD, Rickels K, et al. Consensus statement on generalized anxiety disorder from the International Consensus Group on Depression and Anxiety. J Clin Psychiatry. 2001;62 Suppl 13:47–55.

Bastard J, Tiran D. Aromatherapy and massage for antenatal anxiety: its effect on the fetus. Complement Ther Clin Pract. 2006;12(1):48–54.

Bcnc.org.uk. Benzodiazepine use in pregnancy. 2012. http://www.bcnc.org.uk/BZ_pregnancy.pdf. Accessed 6 Oct 2012.

Beck CT. Post-traumatic stress disorder due to childbirth: the aftermath. Nurs Res. 2004;53:216–24.

Bendtsen P, Honsing G, McKenzie L, Strideman A. Prescribing benzodiazepines – a critical incident study of a physician dilemma. Soc Sci Med. 1999;49:459–67.

Bonnot O, Vollset SE, Godet PF, D'Amato T, Robert E. Maternal exposure to lorazepam and anal atresia in newborns: results from a hypothesis-generating study of benzodiazepines and malformations. J Clin Psychopharmacol. 2001;21:456–8.

Bracken MB, Holford TR. Exposure to prescribed drugs in pregnancy and association with congenital malformations. Obstet Gynecol. 1981;58:336–44.

Butler AC, Chapman JE, Forman EM, Beck AT. The empirical status of cognitive-behavioral therapy: a review of meta-analyses. Clin Psychol Rev. 2006;26:17–31.

Coelho HF, Murray L, Royal-Lawson M, Cooper PJ. Antenatal anxiety disorder as a predictor of postnatal depression: a longitudinal study. J Affect Disord. 2011;129(1–3):348–53.

Collingwood J. Anxiety in pregnancy. 2012. http://psychcentral.com/lib/2010/anxiety-in-pregnancy/. Accessed 26 Oct 2012.

Crombie DL, Pinsent RJ, Fleming DM, Rumeau-Rouquette C, Goujard J, Huel G. Letter: fetal effects of tranquilizers in pregnancy. N Engl J Med. 1975;293:198–9.

Currie JC. British Columbia Centre of excellence for women's health. Policy Series. Manufacturing addiction. The over-prescription of benzodiazepines and sleeping pills to women in Canada. 2004. http://www.cwhn.ca/en/node/39526. Accessed 24 Sept 2012.

Czeizel A. Diazepam, phenytoin, and aetiology of cleft lip and/or cleft palate [letter]. Lancet. 1976;1:810.

Czeizel A. Lack of evidence of teratogenicity of benzodiazepine drugs in Hungary. Reprod Toxicol. 1988;1:183–8.

Czeizel AE, Eros E, Rockenbauer M, Sorensen HT, Olsen J. Short-term oral diazepam treatment during pregnancy: a population-based teratological case-control study. Clin Drug Investig. 2003;23:451–62.

Czeizel AE, Rockenbauer M, Sorensen HT, Olsen J. A population-based case-control study of oral chlordiazepoxide use during pregnancy and risk of congenital abnormalities. Neurotoxicol Teratol. 2004;26:593–8.

Daw RJ. Prescription drug use in pregnancy: a retrospective, population-based study in British Columbia, Canada (2001–2006). Clin Ther. 2012;34(1):239–49.e2.

Dennis CL, Ross LE, Grigoriadis S. Psychosocial and psychological interventions for treating antenatal depression. Cochrane Database Syst Rev. 2007;18(3), CD006309.

Driver HS, Shapiro CM. A longitudinal study of sleep stages in young women during pregnancy and postpartum. Sleep. 2002;15(5):877–85.

Entman SS, Vaughn WK. Lack of relation of oral clefts to diazepam use in pregnancy [letter]. N Engl J Med. 1984;310:1121–2.

Friess E, Tagaya H, Trachsel L, Holsboer F, Rupprecht R. Progesterone-induced changes in sleep in male subjects. Am J Physiol. 1997;272(5 Pt 1):E885–91.

Gentile S. Drug treatment for mood disorders in pregnancy. Curr Opin Psychiatry. 2011;24:34–40.

Gentile S. Bipolar disorder and pregnancy: to treat or not to treat? Br Med J. 2012;345:e7367.

Gidai J, Acs N, Bánhidy F, Czeizel AE. An evaluation of data for 10 children born to mothers who attempted suicide by taking large doses of alprazolam during pregnancy. Toxicol Ind Health. 2008a;24:53–60.

Gidai J, Acs N, Bánhidy F, Czeizel AE. A study of the teratogenic and fetotoxic effects of large doses of chlordiazepoxide used for self-poisoning by 35 pregnant women. Toxicol Ind Health. 2008b;24:41–51.

Gidai J, Acs N, Bánhidy F, Czeizel AE. No association found between use of very large doses of diazepam by 112 pregnant women for a suicide attempt and congenital abnormalities in their offspring. Toxicol Ind Health. 2008c;24:29–39.

Gidai J, Acs N, Bánhidy F, Czeizel AE. A study of the effects of large doses of medazepam used for self-poisoning in 10 pregnant women on fetal development. Toxicol Ind Health. 2008d;24:61–8.

Gidai J, Acs N, Bánhidy F, Czeizel AE. Congenital abnormalities in children of 43 pregnant women who attempted suicide with large dose of nitrazepam. Pharmacoepidemiol Drug Saf. 2010;19:175–82.

Gitau R, Fisk NM, Teixeira JM, Cameron A, Glover V. Fetal HPA stress responses to invasive procedures are independent of maternal responses. J Clin Endocrinol Metabol. 2001;86:104–9.

Glover V, O'Connor TG. Effects of antenatal stress and anxiety. Implications for development and psychiatry. Br J Psychiatry. 2002;180:389–91.

Godet PF, Damato T, Dalery J, Robert E. Benzodiazepines in pregnancy: analysis of 187 exposed infants drawn from a population based birth defects registry. Reprod Toxicol. 1995;9:585.

Hansen D, Lou HC, Olsen J. Serious life events and congenital malformations: a national study with complete follow-up. Lancet. 2000;356:875–80.

Hartz SC, Heinonen OP, Shapiro S, Siskind V, Slone D. Antenatal exposure to meprobamate and chlordiazepoxide in relation to malformations, mental development, and childhood mortality. N Engl J Med. 1975;292:726–8.

Hedegaard M, Henriksen TB, Sabroe S, Secher NJ. Psychological distress in pregnancy and preterm delivery. BMJ. 1993;307:234–9.

Hill M, Bicíková M, Parízek A, Havlíková H, Klak J, Fajt T, et al. Neuroactive steroids, their precursors and polar conjugates during parturition and postpartum in maternal blood: 2. Time profiles of pregnanolone isomers. J Steroid Biochem Mol Biol. 2001;78(1):51–7.

Hultman CM, Sparen P, Takei N, Murray RM, Cnattingius S. Prenatal and perinatal risk factors for schizophrenia, affective psychosis, and reactive psychosis of early onset: case-control study. Br Med J. 1999;318:421–6.

Insel TR, Murphy DL. The psychopharmacological treatment of obsessive-compulsive disorder: a review. J Clin Psychopharmacol. 1981;1(5):304–11.

Institute for the Study of Drug Addiction (ISDD). Drug situation in the UK – trends and update, 24.01.2000. 2012. www.bcnc.org.uk.

Iqbal MM, Tanveer Sobhan T, Ryals T. Effects of commonly used benzodiazepines on the fetus, the neonate, and the nursing infant. Psychiatr Serv. 2002;53:39–49.

Jorm AF, Grayson D, Creasey H, Waite L, Broe GA. Long-term benzodiazepine use by elderly people living in the community. Aust N Z J Public Health. 2000;24(1):7–10.

Juric S, Newport DJ, Ritchie JC, Galanti M, Stowe ZN. Zolpidem (Ambien) in pregnancy: placental passage and outcome. Arch Womens Ment Health. 2009;12(6):441–6.

Kjaer D, Horvath-Puhó E, Christensen J, Vestergaard M, Czeizel AE, Sørensen HT, et al. Use of phenytoin, phenobarbital, or diazepam during pregnancy and risk of congenital abnormalities: a case–time–control study. Pharmacoepidemiol Drug Saf. 2007;16:181–8.

Kullander S, Källén B. A prospective study of drugs and pregnancy: I. Psychopharmaca. Acta Obstet Gyn Scand. 1976;55:25–33.

Laegreid L, Olegård R, Wahlström J, Conradi N. Abnormalities in children exposed to benzodiazepines in utero. Lancet. 1987;1:108–9.

Lin AE, Peller AJ, Westgate MN, Houde K, Franz A, Holmes LB. Clonazepam use in pregnancy and the risk of malformations. Birth Defects Res A Clin Mol Teratol. 2004;70:534–6.

Loomans EM, van der Stelt O, van Eijsden M, Gemke RJ, Vrijkotte T, Van den Bergh BR. Antenatal maternal anxiety is associated with problem behaviour at age five. Early Hum Dev. 2011;87(8):565–70.

Loomans EM, van der Stelt O, van Eijsden M, Gemke RJ, Vrijkotte TG, Van den Bergh BR. High levels of antenatal maternal anxiety are associated with altered cognitive control in five-year-old children. Dev Psychobiol. 2012;54(4):441–50.

Lou HC, Nordentoft M, Jensen F, Pryds O, Nim J, Hemmingsen R. Psychosocial stress and severe prematurity. Lancet. 1992;340:54.

Maes M, Ombelet W, Verkerk R, Bosmans E, Scharpé S. Effects of pregnancy and delivery on the availability of plasma tryptophan to the brain: relationships to delivery-induced immune activation and early post-partum anxiety and depression. Psychol Med. 2001;31(5):847–58.

Marchetti F, Romero M, Bonati M, Tognoni G, CGDUP. Use of psychotropic drugs during pregnancy. Eur J Clin Pharmacol. 1993;45:495–501.

McElhatton PR. The Effects of benzodiazepine use during pregnancy and lactation. Reprod Toxicol. 1994;8(6):461–75.

Menage J. Post-traumatic stress disorders in women who have undergone obstetric and/or gynaecological procedures. J Reprod Infant Psychol. 1993;11:221–8.

Mennes M, Van den Bergh B, Lagae L, Stiers P. Developmental brain alterations in 17 year old boys are related to antenatal maternal anxiety. Clin Neurophysiol. 2009;120(6):1116–22.

Milkovich L, Van den Berg BJ. Effects of prenatal meprobamate and chlordiazepoxide hydrochloride on human embryonic and fetal development. N Engl J Med. 1974;291:1268–71.

Miller LJ. Treating perinatal anxiety disorder. 2011. http://www.cmellc.com/psychcongress/2011/syllabi/309.pdf. Accessed 5 Oct 2012.

Morales-Suárez-Varela M, Jaén-Martinez F, Llopis-Gonzalez A, Sobrecases B. Sociodemographic characteristics of female habitual benzodiazepine consumers in the catchment area of a health care centre. Scand J Soc Med. 1997;3:176–9.

NICE guidelines. Antenatal and postnatal mental health. Clinical management and service guidance. 2007. http://www.nice.org.uk/nicemedia/live/11004/30433/30433.pdf. Accessed 10 Jan 2013

O'Connor TG, Heron J, Golding J, Beveridge M, Glover V. Maternal antenatal anxiety and children's behavioural/emotional problems at 4 years. Report from the Avon Longitudinal Study of Parents and Children. Br J Psychiatry. 2002;180:502–8.

Ohman I, de Flon P, Tomson T. Pregabalin kinetics in the neonatal period, and during lactation. Epilepsia. 2011;52 Suppl 6:249–50.

Olegård R, Sabel KG, Aronsson M, Sandin B, Johansson PR, Carlsson C, et al. Effects on the child of alcoholic abuse during pregnancy. Retrospective and prospective studies. Acta Paediatr Scand. 1979;275:112–21.

Ormond KE, Guttmacher MD. Vermont pregnancy risk information service. 1995. www.bcnc.org.uk.

Parízek A, Hill M, Kancheva R, Havlíková H, Kancheva L, Cindr J, et al. Neuroactive pregnanolone isomers during pregnancy. J Clin Endocrinol Metab. 2005;90(1):395–403.

Pregnancy Calendar. Insomnia during pregnancy. 2012. http://www.pregnancy-calendars.net/insomnia.aspx. Accessed 6 Oct 2012.

Qiao Y, Wang J, Li J, Wang JJ. Effects of depressive and anxiety symptoms during pregnancy on pregnant, obstetric and neonatal outcomes: a follow-up study. Obstet Gynecol. 2012;32 (3):237–40.

Rosenberg L, Mitchell AA, Parsells JL, Pashayan H, Louik C, Shapiro S. Lack of relation of oral clefts to diazepam use during pregnancy. N Engl J Med. 1983;309:1282–5.

Ross LE, McLean LM. Anxiety disorders during pregnancy and the postpartum period: a systematic review. J Clin Psychiatry. 2006;67:1285–98.

Safra MD, Oakley GP. Association between cleft lip with or without cleft palate and prenatal exposure to diazepam. Lancet. 1975;2:478–80.

Saxen I. Associations between oral clefts and drugs taken during pregnancy. Int J Epidemiol. 1975a;4:37–44.

Saxen I. Epidemiology of cleft lip and palate: an attempt to rule out chance correlations. Br J Prev Soc Med. 1975b;29:103–10.

Saxen I, Saxen L. Association between maternal intake of diazepam and oral clefts. Lancet. 1975;2:498.

Schick-Boschetto B, Zuber C. Alprazolam exposure during early human pregnancy [abstract]. Teratology. 1992;45:460.

Sharma S, Franco R. Sleep and its disorders in pregnancy. Wiscon Med J. 2004;103(5):48–52.

Sharma A, Sayeed N, Khees CR, Akhtar S. High dose zolpidem induced fetal neural tube defects. Curr Drug Saf. 2011;6(2):128–9.

Shear KM, Oommen M. Anxiety disorders in pregnant and postpartum women. Psychopharmacol Bull. 1995;31:693–703.

Smith SS, Shen H, Gong QH, Zhou X. Neurosteroid regulation of GABA(A) receptors: focus on the alpha4 and delta subunits. Pharmacol Ther. 2007;116(1):58–76.

St Clair SM, Schirmer RG. First trimester exposure to alprazolam. Obstet Gynecol. 1992;80:843–6.

Tasci Y, Demir B, Dilbaz S, Haberal A. Use of diazepam for hyperemesis gravidarum. J Matern Fetal Neonatal Med. 2009;22:353–6.

Taylor S, McCracken CF, Wilson KC, Copeland JR. Extent and appropriateness of benzodiazepine use: results from an elderly community. Br J Psychiatry. 1998;173:433–8.

Teixeira JM, Fisk NM, Glover V. Association between maternal anxiety in pregnancy and increased uterine artery resistance index: cohort based study. Br Med J. 1999;318:153–7.

Uguz F, Gezginc K, Zeytinci IE, Karatayli S, Askin R, Guler O, et al. Obsessive-compulsive disorder in pregnant women during the third trimester of pregnancy. Compr Psychiatry. 2007;48:441–5.

Van den Bergh BRH. Maternal emotions during pregnancy and fetal and neonatal behavior. In: Nijhuis JG, editor. Fetal behaviour: developmental and perinatal aspects. Oxford: Oxford University Press; 1992. p. 157–78.

Van den Bergh BRH, Marcoen A. High Antenatal maternal anxiety is related to ADHD symptoms, externalizing problems, and anxiety in 8- and 9-year-olds. Child Dev. 2004;75(4):1085–97.

Van den Bergh BRH, Mulder EJH, Mennes M, Glover V. Antenatal maternal anxiety and stress and the neurobehavioural development of the fetus and child: links and possible mechanisms. A review. Neurosci Biobehav Rev. 2005;29:237–58.

Viggedal G, Hagberg BS, Laegreid L, Aronsson M. Mental development in late infancy after prenatal exposure to benzodiazepines – a prospective study. J Child Psychol Psychiatry. 1993;3:295–305.

Vythilingum B. Anxiety disorders in pregnancy. Curr Psychiatry Rep. 2008;10:331–5.

Vythilingum B. Anxiety disorders in pregnancy and the postnatal period. CME. 2009;27 (10):450–2.

Wang LH, Lin HC, Lin CC, Chen YH, Lin HC. Increased risk of adverse pregnancy outcomes in women receiving zolpidem during pregnancy. Clin Pharmacol Ther. 2010;88(3):369–74.

Wiegartz PS, Gyoerkoe KL. The pregnancy and postpartum anxiety workbook: practical skills to help you overcome anxiety, worry, panic attacks, obsessions and compulsions. Oakland, CA: New Harbinger; 2009.

Wikner BN, Källén B. Are hypnotic benzodiazepine receptor agonists teratogenic in humans? J Clin Psychopharmacol. 2011;3:356–9.

Yang M, Li L, Zhu H, Alexander IM, Liu S, Zhou W. Music therapy to relieve anxiety in pregnant women on bedrest: a randomized, controlled trial. Am J Matern Child Nurs. 2009;34:316–23.

Bipolar Disorder, Psychopharmacology, and Pregnancy

8

Martien Snellen and Gin S. Malhi

Abstract

The antenatal management of women with bipolar disorder presents a major challenge for both obstetric and mental health services due to the inherent risks associated with both the condition and its treatment: each of which can be considered to be teratogenic in their own right. The possibility of pregnancy in all women of reproductive age should be considered when making treatment decisions from the outset, especially given that unplanned pregnancy is particularly common in this patient group. For all women with bipolar disorder it is essential that specific considerations be attended to, and monitoring systems established and followed perinatally.

Keywords

Bipolar disorder • Psychophamacology • Pregnancy • Guidelines

The antenatal management of women with bipolar disorder presents a major challenge for both obstetric and mental health services due to the inherent risks associated with both the condition and its treatment: each of which can be considered to be teratogenic in their own right. The possibility of pregnancy in all women of reproductive age should be considered when making treatment decisions from the outset, especially given that unplanned pregnancy is particularly common in this patient group. For all women with bipolar disorder it is essential that specific

M. Snellen (✉)
Mercy Hospital for Women, Heidelberg, Australia
e-mail: msnellen@iprimus.com.au

G.S. Malhi
Department of Psychiatry, University of Sydney, Sydney, Australia

CADE Clinic, Royal North Shore Hospital, Sydney, Australia

Mood Disorders Unit, Northside Clinic, Ramsay Healthcare, Sydney, Australia

M. Galbally et al. (eds.), *Psychopharmacology and Pregnancy*,
DOI 10.1007/978-3-642-54562-7_8, © Springer-Verlag Berlin Heidelberg 2014

considerations be attended to, and monitoring systems established and followed perinatally.

With a lifetime prevalence for bipolar disorder of around 1 %, increasing fertility rates within this population due in part to both the success of modern treatments and the prolactin sparing options available, and the tendency to manifest during the reproductive years, all clinicians will at some time need to consider the inherent risks of treatment and non-treatment in the perinatal setting. Specifically, prevalence differs across age cohorts peaking in the 18–24 age group (0.9 %) and dropping to its lowest in those 55 and over (0.1 %).

Bipolar disorder is frequently a recurrent, disabling illness with most people suffering many episodes (an average of 0.4–0.7 per year), each lasting 3–6 months (Angst and Selloro 2000), with only 50 % achieving syndromic recovery, 25 % symptomatic and functional recovery (Keck et al. 1998), and a suicide rate 15 times that of the general population (Harris and Barraclough 1997). High rates of serious comorbid medical conditions that go unrecognised (Feldman et al. 2012) and high treatment noncompliance rates (Colom et al. 2000) confound the risks further.

The perinatal period has long been recognised to represent a period of significant relapse risk for women who suffer from bipolar disorder; however, increasingly we are becoming aware that this is not only due to inherent risks, but also to precipitous cessation of pharmacological treatment during pregnancy and breastfeeding. Treatment guidelines written for the general population frequently ignore these risks by advising tapered medication withdrawal if a pregnancy is contemplated or confirmed, possibly due to medico-legal considerations as well as a desire to avoid potential adverse foetal development effects. With the average pregnancy taking up to 1 year to conceive, and pregnancy lasting around 9 months, this leaves open a significant window of opportunity for relapse or psychosocial deterioration to occur. More recent publications focus more on the process of obtaining informed consent and adequate obstetric and psychiatric monitoring in recognition of the fact that most women with bipolar disorder require maintenance treatment during their pregnancies (Galbally et al. 2010a, b).

8.1   Bipolar Disorder in Women

About 65 % of patients with bipolar disorder have a co-morbid psychiatric or physical condition (Sasson et al. 2003) and it has been reported that this is 2.7 times more likely to be the case in women than men (Strakowski et al. 1992). Gender differences have also been reported that suggest women are also more likely to experience a rapid cycling pattern of illness and mixed episodes, have a greater latency before treatment with maintenance treatment, and follow a depressive diathesis in their illness course (Barnes and Mitchel 2005). All of which potentially elevate the overall risks within the perinatal setting.

Furthermore, there is considerable evidence that cessation of lithium is associated with a significantly elevated risk of relapse in the general bipolar population (Biel et al. 2007) and that the majority of relapses occur within 3 months of discontinuation (Suppes et al. 1991; Cavanagh et al. 2004) and that this phenomenon extends to withdrawal of other mood stabilisers (Franks et al. 2008).

8.2 Bipolar Disorder in Pregnant Women

Unfortunately, there remains a distinct lack of clarity regarding the natural course of bipolar disorder in pregnancy. It has been proposed that this altered physiological and psychological state may exert a favourable effect on the course of the illness (Grof et al. 2000); however, more recent studies suggest an elevated recurrence rate (Freeman et al. 2002; Viguera et al. 2011). Others have found that up to a half of women with bipolar disorder report an exacerbation of their symptoms during pregnancy (Blehar et al. 1998). This likely reflects a number of pathophysiological processes and alterations in oestrogen levels and inflammatory processes, and fluctuations in biorhythms and functioning are currently under investigation as potential aetiological triggers.

In a prospective study that examined the effects of mood stabiliser cessation during pregnancy those women with bipolar disorder were more than twice as likely to relapse in pregnancy (85.5 % vs. 37 %), with the majority of episodes being either depressive or mixed dysphoric states, and were unwell for five times longer than those who continued their medication (Viguera et al. 2007). These observations suggest that pregnancy needs to be regarded as a high-risk period for relapse, particularly in the setting of discontinuation of maintenance treatment, and that perhaps the very "nature" of bipolar disorder, as it manifests in women, further complicates matters.

But in practice how do we differentiate those women with bipolar disorder who need pharmacological intervention in pregnancy and those who do not? A number of pharmacological treatment guidelines have been established in order to inform decision-making. However, methodological differences between evidence-based and consensus-based guidelines add as much confusion as they do clarity. Furthermore, the suggested algorithms can change dramatically when evidence regarding teratogenicity is prioritised over evidence for treatment efficacy. For instance, the National Institute for Health and Clinical Excellence (NICE) guidelines support the use of anticonvulsants and lithium as first-line treatment agents in the non-pregnant population due to their established evidence base, but withdraw this recommendation in the pregnant population where they prefer second-generation antipsychotics that have a less established evidence base for efficacy (NICE 2006). Given that the overall success rate for pharmacological treatment in bipolar disorder is moderate at best, we suggest that the best treatment option is usually the one that works for any particular patient. This also raises the issue of whether the mother's health should take precedence over that of the child? However, should discontinuation of mood stabilising medication be contemplated, there is universal acceptance that it should be slowly tapered and abrupt withdrawal avoided.

Bipolar disorder is not only heterogeneous in its acute manifestations, but also in its longitudinal course. A clinician will need to consider many individual factors prior to making any recommendations regarding prophylactic treatment: number and severity of relapses, severity of psychotic episodes, co-morbidity, previous treatment response or non-response to any particular agent, side effects, family history of bipolar disorder, previous suicidality, residual symptoms, ongoing stressful life events or poor social support, age of onset, and time intervals between episodes. There also remains a lack of consensus as to the duration of long-term treatment with the NICE guidelines recommending maintenance for up to 5 years for patients with risk factors for relapse, whereas the other evidence-based guidelines such as those developed by the World Federation of Societies of Biological Psychiatry (WFSBP), the British Association for Psychopharmacology (BAP), and the Canadian Network for Mood and Anxiety Treatments (CANMAT) recommend lifelong treatment (Samalin et al. 2013).

A recent publication has added significantly in our endeavour to prevent postpartum psychosis and mania in women at high risk by recommending prophylactic treatment immediately postpartum in those women who have a history of psychosis limited to the postpartum period, to avoid in utero foetal exposure to medication, and continuous prophylaxis throughout pregnancy and the postpartum period to reduce peripartum relapse risk in women with bipolar disorder (Bergink et al. 2012). What has in effect been achieved here is a realisation that *not all* episodes of puerperal psychosis are necessarily an episode of bipolar disorder.

Given that it is now clear that in the majority of cases treatment with maintenance psychotropics throughout pregnancy is required, it has been suggested that the question is not whether "to treat or not to treat?" but instead "how to treat optimally?"(Gentile 2012a). With this in mind we consider the treatment of bipolar disorder in pregnancy.

8.3 Treatment of Bipolar Disorder in Pregnancy

The Developmental Origins of Health and Disease paradigm (DOHaD) suggests that pregnancy and infancy are critical periods of growth and development that have lifelong implications (Gluckman et al. 2008). Untreated bipolar disorder has been linked with increased risks of pregnancy complications such as preterm birth, low birth weight and Apgar scores, induced labour, caesarean section, and instrumental delivery, and neonatal microcephaly and hypoglycaemia (Jablensky et al. 2005; Lee and Lin 2010; Bodén et al. 2012). Offspring of women with bipolar disorder have been shown to have increased rates of memory and attention disturbance as well as emotional, social, and behavioural problems. It has been proposed that both microcephaly and recurrent neonatal hypoglycaemia may be aetiological in this regard (Gentile 2012a). It remains unclear as to whether adequate maintenance treatment throughout pregnancy attenuates these risks. Of greatest concern, however, is the fact that within the obstetric setting there is an extremely low rate of case identification (Spitzer et al. 2000).

Standard treatment of bipolar disorder includes lithium, the anticonvulsants sodium valproate, carbamazepine, and lamotrigine, and increasingly second-generation antipsychotics. The aim is always to achieve the minimum effective dose; however, the emphasis needs to be on *effective* rather than *minimal*, and this is often not the case. It can be argued that "half treatment" represents the worst possible scenario as it exposes the foetus to both the risks of treatment and maternal mental illness. Despite evidence that polypharmacy increases the overall teratogenic risk (Burt et al. 2010); many patients who would otherwise remain symptomatic cannot afford the luxury of monotherapy. There is also the possibility that increased dosing frequency can offer advantage through minimising peak plasma levels, although compliance issues need to be taken into consideration. Essentially, a risk-free scenario does not exist. It is rather a matter of harm minimisation, informed consent, and careful monitoring of mental health as well as maternal physiological and foetal anatomical parameters.

Psychotherapy remains an essential adjunct to pharmacotherapy in the treatment of all forms of mental illness. Despite the paucity of research into the direct and indirect effects of non-pharmacological treatments for bipolar disorder, it is widely accepted that psychotherapy assists overall improved psychosocial functioning (Scott 2006) and a healthy therapeutic alliance is an essential component of care. Attention needs to be paid to life and lifestyle stressors, sleep preservation, the establishment of realistic expectations, early warning signs for relapse, support structures, and pathways to care.

8.4   Safety of Specific Treatments for Bipolar Disorder in Pregnancy

Inevitably, at some point, difficult decisions need to be made and ideally these should involve a collaborative approach between clinician and patient. It is essential that a process of obtaining informed consent be followed and patient preference be involved in the decision-making process. A comprehensive risk:benefit analysis needs to consider both the risks of treatment and also those associated with non-treatment for both mother and child. Consideration needs to be given to the risks of teratogenesis, obstetric complications, impairment of neonatal adaption, and negative long-term neurodevelopmental or other health outcome. Once decisions are made and enacted a comprehensive plan for obstetric, paediatric, and psychiatric monitoring needs to be put in place that considers the unique challenges that exist within the perinatal setting.

It has been estimated that at least 500 cases are needed to determine differences in occurrence of major malformation and larger numbers are required to adequately control for other variables (Meador et al 2008). To date, only some of the anticonvulsants have been adequately investigated in this regard. There is a reasonable body of data regarding the potential risks associated with the use of lithium in pregnancy; however, much of our comfort in prescribing antipsychotics during pregnancy comes from the absence of negative data rather than the presence of positive data. The issue is further complicated by the fact that the majority of studies that aim to evaluate and clarify teratogenic risk associated with antenatal exposure to psychotropic medications were not designed to control for possible teratogenic effects of the underlying bipolar disorder. We eagerly await further clarity from current prospective registry studies that include a non-treatment control group.

8.5   Lithium Safety in Pregnancy

Lithium remains a gold standard treatment for bipolar disorder; however, initial retrospective reports identified an elevated risk of cardiac malformation, in particular Ebstein's anomaly that is characterised by downward displacement of the tricuspid valve into the right ventricle and variable levels of right ventricular hypoplasia (Schou et al. 1973). More recent research has downgraded the overall concern with the estimated incidence being 0.05–0.1 % which represents 20–40 times the general population risk (Cohen et al. 1994). There is also some suggestion that lithium may be associated with a slightly increased risk of neural tube defect (Gentile 2012b). However, a recent systematic review and meta-analysis of lithium's toxicity profile recorded no significant increased risk of congenital malformation (McKnight et al. 2012).

Lithium demonstrates complete placental passage and equilibrates between maternal and foetal circulations, and adverse perinatal outcomes are more extensive when concentrations are higher at delivery (Newport et al. 2005). Exposure has been associated with an increased risk of diabetes insipidus, polyhydramnios, thyroid dysfunction, floppy baby syndrome and cardiac rhythm disturbances in the newborn (Llewellen et al. 1998; Gentile 2012b); however, most of these concerns arise from case reports. Lithium-exposed babies are more likely to be large for dates and this does not appear to be a dose-related effect (Jacobson et al. 1992; Troyer et al. 1993).

There is extremely sparse information regarding infant neurodevelopmental outcomes following in utero exposure to lithium; however, that which is available is reassuring in that no difference has been identified between exposed and non-exposed infants (Jacobson et al. 1992; Schou 1976; van der Lugt et al. 2012).

Whilst certain guidelines recommend that lithium exposure during the first trimester is a contraindication (e.g. NICE 2006) it is now widely acknowledged that the actual overall teratogenic risk is both significantly less than first presumed and certainly less in comparison to a number of alternatives (i.e. the anticonvulsants sodium valproate and carbamazepine). In a highly select patient population first trimester exposure can be avoided only after a clinical judgment is made regarding the potential risk of relapse secondary to discontinuation.

8.6 Anticonvulsant Safety in Pregnancy

Most studies into structural malformation and neurocognitive development in women receiving anticonvulsants have focused on women treated for epilepsy rather than bipolar disorder and this introduces potential confounding factors such as genetic predisposition and an independent effect of seizures. Hence, it is only in the last decade or so that some clarity has emerged regarding such risk.

Anticonvulsants are clear teratogens and a recent review of prospective registry data suggests malformation rates of 2.7 % for lamotrigine, 2.9 % for carbamazepine, and 8.7 % for sodium valproate (Walker et al. 2009). The majority of structural abnormalities relate to central nervous system anomalies, particularly neural tube defects (5–9 % for sodium valproate and 0.5–1 % for carbamazepine), as well as cardiac, facial, limb, and urogenital malformations (Yonkers et al. 2004). With sodium valproate there appears to be a dose-related effect with the risk of malformation rising most dramatically with doses above 1,000 mg per day (Morrow et al. 2006); however, this is potentially the case with all anticonvulsants (Tomson et al. 2011). A pattern of specific facial abnormalities has been suggested for both sodium valproate and carbamazepine with mid-face hypoplasia, short nose with anteverted nostrils, and long upper lip (Jones et al. 1989). Carbamazepine has also been associated with reductions in birth weight (of about 250g) and mean head circumference (Diav-Citrin et al. 2001; Hiilesmaa et al. 1981). There have also been conflicting reports regarding a slightly elevated risk of orofacial cleft with lamotrigine (Hunt et al. 2009).

Neonatal complications appear to be most problematic with sodium valproate with reports of elevated risks for heart rate decelerations, withdrawal symptoms such as irritability, jitteriness, abnormal tone, feeding difficulties, and hepatotoxicity, hypoglycaemia, and reduction in fibrinogen. Carbamazepine and lamotrigine have been associated with hepatotoxicity and the latter with the potential for Stevens–Johnson syndrome in the infant (Yonkers et al. 2004).

The anticonvulsants are increasingly being studied with regard to their potential to cause adverse neurodevelopmental outcomes following in utero exposure. Both carbamazepine and lamotrigine have not been associated with any later developmental delay or IQ reduction; however, sodium valproate is clearly teratogenic in this regard and a clear association has been demonstrated between in utero exposure and reduced IQ scores, impaired verbal acquisition, increased frequency of maladaptive behaviour, as well as global neurodevelopmental delay (Meador et al. 2007; Bromley et al. 2013). The risk of adverse neurodevelopmental outcome appears to be dose dependent and further worsened when used in combination with other anticonvulsants.

Essentially, unless absolutely necessary, sodium valproate should be avoided throughout pregnancy as well as first trimester exposure to the other mood stabilising anticonvulsants. Whilst this represents the ideal, it needs to be recognised that not all patients can be afforded this luxury given the high risk of relapse in those women with bipolar disorder who discontinue maintenance treatment during pregnancy.

8.7 Antipsychotic Safety in Pregnancy

At this point in time any comfort we may have in prescribing antipsychotics during pregnancy comes from the absence of negative data rather than the presence of positive data. Slowly, encouraging data is emerging from pregnancy registries that follow a prospective design. A recent review identified only seven studies on pregnancy outcomes and antipsychotic exposure and no clear association with any specific malformation has emerged (Einarson and Boskovic 2009). However, a further systematic review of antipsychotic therapy during early and late pregnancy concluded that presently we are unable to adequately advise regarding malformation risk secondary to in utero exposure to atypicals (Gentile 2010).

Antipsychotic medications have been associated with both low birth weight and large-for-dates babies, the latter mainly associated with exposure to atypicals (Newham et al. 2008). Hypertonicity, tremulousness, and poor motor maturity in neonates have been observed in typical antipsychotics (Auerbach et al. 1992). However, it remains unclear to what extent atypical antipsychotics may complicate the neonatal period and it is recommended that observation should occur for transient extra-pyramidal side effects, withdrawal, and sedation (Galbally et al. 2010a, b).

Recent studies that follow prospective case-controlled designs have found an association between in utero exposure to atypical antipsychotics and reduced neuromotor performance; in particular delays were observed in cognition, motor skill, and social-emotional and adaptive behavioural domains (Peng et al. 2013; Johnson et al. 2012). Encouragingly the suggestion is that exposure increases the risk of delay not permanent impairment; however, further studies with longer follow-up periods are required. Infant outcomes were also negatively associated with indices of maternal mental illness and it is likely that adverse effects on subsequent infant neurodevelopment are influenced by both maternal mental illness and foetal exposure to antipsychotics, and these effects may be additive.

8.8 Specific Clinical Considerations and Recommended Monitoring

Unless otherwise referenced the following recommendations have been derived from previous publications by Galbally et al. (2010a, b, 2011):

Given the high risk of unrecognised physical comorbidity in women who suffer from bipolar disorder it is recommended that a baseline organic screen be performed as a matter of course. Investigations should include full blood examination, renal, thyroid, and hepatic function testing, estimations of iron, vitamin B12, folate, and vitamin D, fasting glucose, and serum lipids, in addition to the usual obstetric investigations. Consideration should also be given to ECG examination if a patient is taking a medication that could compromise the QT interval.

As most medications used to treat bipolar disorder carry an elevated risk of foetal malformation it is recommended that high-resolution ultrasounds that focus in particular on neural tube and cardiac and facial structures be performed at 12 and 20 weeks gestation.

Changes in gastric emptying, increased volume of distribution, decreased gastrointestinal motility, decreased drug-binding capacity, and increased hepatic metabolism during pregnancy frequently alter the therapeutic dose of all psychotropic medications. Increased frequency of serum level estimation of lithium and the anticonvulsants is recommended as well as increased frequency of psychiatric review.

Folate, administered at a dose of 5 mg daily, is recommended for all pregnant women who take mood stabilisers or antipsychotics, or those contemplating pregnancy as it may reduce the risk of various birth defects: although this suggestion remains controversial (Lassi et al. 2013; Sotres-Alvarez et al. 2013). Ideally it should be commenced 3 months prior to conception and continued throughout pregnancy, particularly in women who take anticonvulsants that can adversely influence folate metabolism. Similarly, given the high rates of inadequate nutrition and self-care in this patient population, multivitamins specifically formulated for pregnancy are also recommended.

A written individualised Perinatal Mental Health Care Plan should be prepared for each mother and baby and placed in a prominent position within the case file. It should outline: the current treatment team, all pharmacological and other treatments (including dose recommendations across the peripartum), a plan for mode of infant feeding and avoidance of pharmacological lactation suppressants (as they may precipitate relapse), recommendations for support, rest and sleep preservation within a low stimulus environment, recommendations regarding minimum length of stay, plans for regular psychiatric and paediatric review, and a comprehensive discharge plan that ideally includes support for the mother, partner, mother–infant relationship, early parenting skills, and establishment of pathways to care should relapse occur.

8.9   Lithium: Monitoring in Pregnancy

Given the physiological changes that occur in pregnancy lithium levels require careful monitoring throughout, but particularly in the third trimester and this is over and above the usual requirements (Malhi et al. 2012). This should include monthly serum estimations throughout pregnancy increasing to weekly after 36 weeks gestation. Thyroid and renal function should also be measured during each trimester as well as serum calcium early in pregnancy. In order to be consistent with the table presented later.

Ultrasound assessment that focuses on nuchal translucency should be performed at 12 weeks, followed by high-resolution ultrasound and Doppler flow studies for early cardiac assessment at 16 weeks, and a morphological scan with specific attention to foetal echocardiography performed at 20 weeks gestation. As there is an increased risk of babies being large for dates all lithium-exposed pregnancies should be monitored for growth through scanning during the third trimester.

Wherever possible, lithium should be ceased 24–48 h prior to delivery and reinstated post delivery at pre-pregnancy dose. Adequate hydration needs to be ensured during labour and consideration given to intravenous hydration when necessary. Nephrotoxins such as aminoglycosides and nonsteroidal anti-inflammatory drugs need to be avoided, and cord blood taken for lithium level and renal and thyroid function estimation. The neonate needs to be carefully monitored for any evidence of lithium toxicity or withdrawal. It is further recommended that a mother does not breastfeed whilst taking lithium.

8.10 Anticonvulsants: Monitoring in Pregnancy

Women treated with sodium valproate, carbamazepine, and lamotrigine should have an ultrasound at around 12 weeks gestation. Early signs of anencephaly should be recognised at this gestation and the nuchal translucency measurement further offers a useful screening for cardiac and other structural malformations. A mid-trimester morphology scan that pays particular attention to the neural axis, heart, and face should be performed in preference to maternal serum alpha-fetoprotein estimation that is much less reliable. Similarly, adequate review of foetal growth (preferably through growth scanning at 28 and 34 weeks and further as indicated) is recommended.

Serum level estimations of anticonvulsants should be performed monthly throughout pregnancy. In particular, lamotrigine levels are highly variable during pregnancy and clinically significant fluctuations in drug concentrations have been observed (Patsalos et al. 2008; Clark et al 2013). Similarly, serum lamotrigine levels can rise dramatically postpartum, introducing the possibility of toxicity if dose adjustments are not made (Clark et al. 2013). Hepatic function estimations should also be performed each trimester for those women who take sodium valproate and carbamazepine, as well as a platelet count for those on sodium valproate.

At birth Konakion should be administered to all newborns exposed to the enzyme inducers carbamazepine and sodium valproate in order to minimise the risk of neonatal bleeding and the neonate observed for any evidence of toxicity or withdrawal, and a careful morphological examination performed.

8.11 Antipsychotics: Monitoring in Pregnancy

Given the potential for increased risk of metabolic syndrome and gestational diabetes with atypical antipsychotics it has been suggested that glucose tolerance testing, rather than glucose challenge testing, should be performed early in the second trimester (14–16 weeks) and at 28 weeks gestation. Similarly, adequate review of foetal growth (preferably through growth scanning at 28 and 34 weeks and further as indicated) is essential given the increased risk of abnormal birth weight.

Ultrasound assessment that focuses on nuchal translucency should be performed at 12 weeks, followed by a high-resolution morphology scan performed at 20 weeks gestation. As there is an increased risk of babies being either large for dates or small for dates all antipsychotic-exposed pregnancies should be monitored for growth through scanning during the third trimester.

Neonates should be observed for any evidence of toxicity, withdrawal, sedation, and extra-pyramidal side effects.

8.12 Summary of Pregnancy Monitoring for Mood Stabilisers and Antipsychotics (Adapted from Galbally et al. 2010a, b, 2011)

	All mood stabilisers and antipsychotics	Lithium carbonate	Anticonvulsants	Antipsychotics
First trimester	FBE, U&E, LFT, TFT, iron studies, vitamin D, B12, folate High-resolution ultrasound with focus on NT at 12 weeks gestation	Monthly serum level Calcium	Monthly serum level	BMI, fasting glucose, and lipids, ECG
Second trimester	High-resolution morphology scan at 20 weeks gestation. Growth monitoring	Monthly serum level Fetal Echocardiography and Doppler Flow Studies at 16 weeks gestation. U&E, TFT	Monthly serum level Platelet count, LFT	Early GTT at 14–16 weeks gestation Weight, BP
Third trimester	Growth Scans at 28 and 34 weeks gestation	Monthly serum level and then weekly from 36 weeks U&E, TFT	Monthly serum level Platelet count, LFT	Weight, BP Repeat GTT at 28 weeks gestation
After delivery	Observe neonate for toxicity, withdrawal, and sedation Careful morphological examination	Maternal serum level, U&E, TFT Cord blood lithium level, TFT, U&E	Serum level Platelet count, LFT Administer Konakion to valproate- or carbamazepine-exposed neonates	Observe neonate for EPSE

8.13 Recommendations for the Treatment of Women with Bipolar Disorder in Pregnancy

1. Wherever possible, taking into account the potential for pregnancy, preconception consideration should be given to the most appropriate form of pharmacological treatment in women who suffer from bipolar disorder.
2. Optimise the therapeutic alliance and non-pharmacological treatments.
3. Establish a close liaison relationship between all disciplines involved: psychiatry, obstetrics, paediatrics, midwifery, social work, and maternal and child health-care nursing.
4. Obtain baseline measures of biological parameters that could be compromised by both illness and its treatment.
5. Ensure that a process of obtaining informed consent is followed in which all available information regarding risks and benefits of treatment and non-treatment in the perinatal setting are detailed.
6. Prescribe 5 mg of folate daily from 3 months preconception and throughout pregnancy as well as multivitamins.
7. Aim for monotherapy where possible and minimise peak plasma levels of psychotropics through more frequent dosing so long as compliance can be maintained.
8. Insist that a treatment team that specialises in high-risk scenarios undertake the obstetric care.
9. Ensure that adequate monitoring throughout pregnancy occurs of foetal development, obstetric physiology, drug levels, and maternal mental state.
10. At delivery commence observation for evidence of neonatal withdrawal, toxicity, sedation, or other adverse effect and ensure that a careful morphological examination is undertaken.
11. Create and implement a Mental Health Care Plan for the post-delivery maternity setting that encourages a low stimulus environment and sleep preservation, and close liaison between all health-care providers and allows an extended maternity stay in which observations can be made for any neonatal compromise secondary to exposure to psychotropic medications in utero.
12. Establish early warning signs for relapse and pathways to care should this occur.

References

Angst J, Selloro R. Historical perspectives and natural history of bipolar disorder. Biol Psychiatry. 2000;48:445–57.

Auerbach JG, Hans SL, Marcus J, Maeir S. Maternal psychotropic medication and neonatal behavior. Neurotoxicol Teratol. 1992;14(6):399–406.

Barnes C, Mitchel P. Considerations in the management of bipolar disorder in women. Aust N Z J Psychiatry. 2005;39:662–73.

Bergink V, Bouvy PF, Jeren SP, Koorengevel KM, Steegers EA, Kushner SA. Prevention of postpartum psychosis and mania in women at high risk. Am J Psychiatry. 2012;169(6):609–15.

Biel MG, Peselow E, Mulcare L, Case BG, Fieve R. Continuation versus discontinuation of lithium in recurrent bipolar illness: a naturalistic study. Bipolar Disord. 2007;9:435–42.

Blehar MC, DePaulo Jr JR, Gershon ES, Reich T, Simpson SG, Nurnberger Jr JI. Women with bipolar disorder: findings from the NIMH genetics initiative sample. Psychopharmacol Bull. 1998;34:239–43.

Bodén R, Lundgren M, Brandt L, Reutfors J, Andersen M, Kieler H. Risks of adverse pregnancy and birth outcomes in women treated or not treated with mood stabilisers for bipolar disorder: population based cohort study. Br Med J. 2012;345:e7085.

Bromley RL, Mawer GE, Briggs M, Cheyne C, Clayton-Smith J, García-Fiñana M, Liverpool and Manchester Neurodevelopment Group, et al. The prevalence of neurodevelopmental disorders in children prenatally exposed to antiepileptic drugs. J Neurol Neurosurg Psychiatry. 2013;84:637–43.

Burt VK, Bernstein C, Rosenstein WS, Altshuler LL. Bipolar disorder and pregnancy: maintaining psychiatric stability in the real world of obstetric and psychiatric complications. Am J Psychiatry. 2010;167:892–7.

Cavanagh J, Smyth R, Goodwin GM. Relapse into mania or depression following lithium discontinuation. Acta Psychiatr Scand. 2004;109:91–5.

Clark CT, Klein AM, Perel JM, Helsel J, Wisner KL. Lamotrigine dosing for pregnant patients with bipolar disorder. Am J Psychiatry. 2013;170:1240–7.

Cohen LS, Friedman JM, Jefferson JW, Johnson EM, Weiner ML. A re-evaluation of risk of in utero exposure to lithium. JAMA. 1994;271:146–50.

Colom F, Vieta E, Martínez-Arán A, Reinares M, Benabarre A, Gastó C. Clinical factors associated with treatment noncompliance in euthymic bipolar patients. J Clin Psychiatry. 2000;61(8):549–55.

Diav-Citrin O, Shechtman S, Arnon J, Ornoy A. Is carbamazepine teratogenic? A prospective controlled study of 210 pregnancies. Neurology. 2001;57:321–4.

Einarson A, Boskovic R. Use and safety of antipsychotic drugs during pregnancy. J Psychiatr Pract. 2009;15:183–92.

Feldman NS, Gwizdowski IS, Fischer EG, Yang H, Suppes T. Co-occurrence of serious or undiagnosed medical conditions with bipolar disorder preventing clinical trial randomization: a case series. J Clin Psychiatry. 2012;73:874–7.

Franks M, Macritchie KA, Mahmood T, Young AH. Bouncing back: is the bipolar rebound phenomenon peculiar to lithium? A retrospective naturalistic study. J Psychopharmacol. 2008;22(4):452–6.

Freeman MP, Smith KW, Freeman SA, McElroy SL, Kmetz GE, Wright R, et al. The impact of reproductive events on the course of bipolar disorder in women. J Clin Psychiatry. 2002;63:284–7.

Galbally M, Roberts M, Buist A, Perinatal Psychotropic Review Group. Mood stabilisers in pregnancy: a systematic review. Aust N Z J Psychiatry. 2010a;44:967–77.

Galbally M, Snellen M, Walker S, Permezel M. Management of antipsychotic and mood stabilizer medication in pregnancy: recommendations for antenatal care. Aust N Z J Psychiatry. 2010b;44:99–108.

Galbally M, Snellen M, Lewis AJ. A review of the use of psychotropic medication in pregnancy. Curr Opin Obstet Gynecol. 2011;23(6):408–14.

Gentile S. Antipsychotic therapy during early and late pregnancy. A systematic review. Schizophr Bull. 2010;36:518–44.

Gentile S. Bipolar disorder in pregnancy: to treat or not to treat? Br Med J. 2012a;345:e7367.

Gentile S. Lithium in pregnancy: the need to treat, the duty to ensure safety. Expert Opin Drug Saf. 2012b;11(3):425–37.

Gluckman PD, Hanson MA, Cooper C, Thornburg KL. Effect of in utero and early-life conditions on adult health and disease. N Engl J Med. 2008;359(1):61–73.

Grof P, Robbins W, Alda M, Berghoefer A, Vojtechovsky M, Nilsson A, et al. Protective effects of pregnancy in women with lithium-responsive bipolar disorder. J Affect Disord. 2000;61:31–9.

Harris EC, Barraclough B. Suicide as an outcome for mental disorders: a meta-analysis. Br J Psychiatry. 1997;170:205–28.

Hiilesmaa VK, Teramo K, Granstrom ML, Bardy AH. Fetal head growth retardation associated with maternal antiepileptic drugs. Lancet. 1981;2:165–7.

Hunt SJ, Craig JJ, Morrow CJ. Increased frequency of isolated cleft palate in infants exposed to lamotrigine during pregnancy. Neurology. 2009;72:1108–9.

Jablensky AV, Morgan V, Zubrick SR, Bower C, Yellachich LA. Pregnancy, delivery and neonatal complications in a population cohort of women with schizophrenia and major affective disorders. Am J Psychiatry. 2005;162:79–91.

Jacobson SJ, Jones K, Johnson K, Ceolin L, Kaur P, Sahn D, et al. Prospective multicentre study of pregnancy outcome after lithium exposure during first trimester. Lancet. 1992;339:530–3.

Johnson KC, LaPrairie JL, Brennan PA, Stowe ZN, Newport DJ. Prenatal antipsychotic exposure and neuromotor performance during infancy. Arch Gen Psychiatry. 2012;69(8):787–94.

Jones KL, Lacro RV, Johnson KA, Adams J. Pattern of malformations in the children of women treated with carbamazepine during pregnancy. N Engl J Med. 1989;320:1661–6.

Keck Jr PE, McElroy SL, Strakowski SM, West SA, Sax KW, Hawkins JM, et al. 12-month outcome of patients with bipolar disorder following hospitalization for a manic or mixed episode. Am J Psychiatry. 1998;155:646–52.

Lassi ZS, Salam RA, Haider BA, Bhutta ZA. Folic acid supplementation during pregnancy for maternal health and pregnancy outcomes. Cochrane Database Syst Rev. 2013; (28);3.

Lee HC, Lin HC. Maternal bipolar disorder increased low birthweight and preterm births: a nationwide population based study. J Affect Disord. 2010;121:100–5.

Llewellen A, Stowe ZN, Strader Jr JR. The use of lithium and management of women with bipolar disorder during pregnancy and lactation. J Clin Psychiatry. 1998;59 Suppl 6:57–64.

Malhi GS, Tanious M, Das P, Berk M. The science and practice of lithium therapy. Aust N Z J Psychiatry. 2012;46(3):192–211.

McKnight RF, Adida M, Budge K, Stockton S, Goodwin GM, Geddes JR. Lithium toxicity profile: a systematic review and meta-analysis. Lancet. 2012;379(9817):721–8.

Meador KJ, Baker G, Cohen MJ, Gaily E, Westerveld M. Cognitive/behavioral teratogenetic effects of antiepileptic drugs. Epilepsy Behav. 2007;11:292–302.

Meador KJ, Pennell PB, Harden CL, Gordon JC, Tomson T, Kaplan PW, et al. Pregnancy registries in epilepsy. A consensus statement on health outcomes. Neurology. 2008;71: 1109–17.

Morrow J, Russell A, Guthrie E, Parsons L, Robertson I, Waddell R, et al. Malformation risks of antiepileptic drugs in pregnancy: a prospective study from the UK Epilepsy and Pregnancy Register. J Neurol Neurosurg Psychiatry. 2006;77(2):193–8.

Newham JJ, Thomas SH, MacRitchie K, McElhatton PR, McAllister-Williams RH. Birth weight of infants after maternal exposure to typical and atypical antipsychotics: prospective comparison study. Br J Psychiatry. 2008;192:333–7.

Newport DJ, Viguera AC, Beach AJ, Ritchie JC, Cohen LS, et al. Lithium placental passage and obstetric outcome: implications for clinical management during late pregnancy. Am J Psychiatry. 2005;162:2162–70.

NICE (National Institute for Health and Care Excellence). The management of bipolar disorder in adults, children and adolescents, in primary and secondary care. 2006; http://www.nice.org.uk/CG38

Patsalos PN, Berry DJ, Bourgeois BF, Cloyd JC, Glauser TA, Johannessen SI, et al. Antiepileptic drugs–best practice guidelines for therapeutic drug monitoring: a position paper by the subcommission on therapeutic drug monitoring, ILAE Commission on Therapeutic Strategies. Epilepsia. 2008;49:1239–76.

Peng M, Gao K, Ding Y, Ou J, Calabrese JR, Wu R, et al. Effects of prenatal exposure to atypical antipsychotics on postnatal development and growth of infants: a case-controlled, prospective study. Psychopharmacology (Berl). 2013;228(4):577–84.

Samalin L, Guillaume S, Courtet P, Abbar M, Lancrenon S, Llorca PM. Methodological differences between pharmacological treatment guidelines for bipolar disorder: what to do for the clinicians? Compr Psychiatry. 2013;54:309–20.

Sasson Y, Chopra M, Harrari E, Amitai K, Zohar J. Bipolar comorbidity: from diagnostic dilemmas to therapeutic challenge. Int J Neuropsychopharmacol. 2003;6(2):139–44.

Schou M. What happened later to the lithium babies? A follow up study of children born without malformations. ACTA Psychiatr Scand. 1976;54:193–7.

Schou M, Goldfield MD, Weinstein MR, Villeneuve A. Lithium and pregnancy, I: report from the Register of Lithium Babies. Br Med J. 1973;2:135–6.

Scott J. Psychotherapy for bipolar disorders—efficacy and effectiveness. J Psychopharmacol. 2006;20(2 Suppl):46–50.

Sotres-Alvarez D, Siega-Riz AM, Herring AH, Carmichael SL, Feldkamp ML, Hobbs CA, National Birth Defects Prevention Study, et al. Maternal dietary patterns are associated with risk of neural tube and congenital heart defects. Am J Epidemiol. 2013;177(11):1279–88.

Spitzer RL, Williams JB, Kroenke K, Hornyak R, McMurray J. Validity and utility of the PRIME-MD patient health questionnaire in assessment of 3000 obstetric-gynecologic patients: the PRIME-MD Patient Health Questionnaire Obstetrics-Gynecology Study. Am J Obstet Gynecol. 2000;183(3):759–69.

Strakowski SM, Tohen M, Stoll A, Faedda GL, Goodwin DC. Comorbidity in mania at first hospitalization. Am J Psychiatry. 1992;149:554–6.

Suppes T, Baldessarini RJ, Faedda GL, Tohen M. Risk of recurrence following discontinuation of lithium treatment in bipolar disorder. Arch Gen Psychiatry. 1991;48:1082–8.

Tomson T, Battino D, Bonizzoni E, Craig J, Lindhout D, Sabers A et al.; EURAP study group. Dose-dependent risk of malformations with antiepileptic drugs: an analysis of data from the EURAP epilepsy and pregnancy registry. Lancet Neurol. 2011;10:609–17.

Troyer WA, Percira GR, Lannon RA, Belik J, Yoder MC. Association of maternal lithium exposure and premature delivery. J Perinatol. 1993;13:123–7.

van der Lugt NM, van de Matt JS, van Kamp IL, Knoppert-van der Klein EA, Hovens JG, Walther FJ. Fetal, neonatal and developmental outcomes of lithium exposed pregnancies. Early Hum Dev. 2012;88:375–8.

Viguera AC, Whitfield T, Baldessarini RJ, Newport DJ, Stowe Z, Reminick A, et al. Risk of recurrence in women with bipolar disorder during pregnancy: prospective study of mood stabilizer discontinuation. Am J Psychiatry. 2007;164:1817–24.

Viguera AC, Tondo L, Koukopoulos AE, Reginaldi D, Lepri B, Baldessarini RJ. Episodes of mood disorders in 2252 pregnancies and postpartum periods. Am J Psychiatry. 2011;168(11):1179–85.

Walker SP, Permezel M, Berkovic SF. The management of epilepsy in pregnancy. Br J Obstet Gynaecol. 2009;116:758–67.

Yonkers KA, Wisner KL, Stowe Z, Leibenluft E, Cohen L, Miller L, et al. Management of bipolar disorder during pregnancy and the postpartum period. Am J Psychiatry. 2004;161:608–20.

Schizophrenia, Psychopharmacology, and Pregnancy

9

Kathryn M. Abel, Katie Au, and Louise M. Howard

Abstract

Most women with schizophrenia have children at some point in their lives despite reduced fertility compared with the general population. They often stop psychotropic medication due to concerns about harming their infant and it is not clear to what extent they are at risk of relapse in pregnancy, though there is good evidence that the postpartum period is a time of increased risk. Their pregnancies are at increased risk of adverse outcomes including pre-eclampsia, poor fetal growth, preterm birth, low birth weight, still births, and neonatal and post-neonatal deaths. Lifestyle risk factors, such as smoking and nutritional deficiencies, are likely to explain many of these outcomes. Current evidence suggests that most antipsychotics are unlikely to be major teratogens, and it is unclear to what extent other adverse outcomes, including developmental outcomes, are related to medication or confounders. Pregnancy in women with a diagnosis of schizophrenia should be considered high risk and managed accordingly. A focus on reducing modifiable risk factors, such as obesity and smoking, ideally before conception, as well as optimising antenatal care using the lowest effective medication doses with appropriate monitoring through pregnancy, is key to improving the long-term outcomes in these vulnerable families.

K.M. Abel
Centre for Women's Mental Health, The University of Manchester, 3rd Floor East, Jean McFarlane Building, Oxford Rd, Manchester M13 9PL, UK

K. Au
South London and Maudsley NHS Foundation Trust, London, UK

L.M. Howard (✉)
Section of Women's Mental Health, Institute of Psychiatry, King's College London, London SE5 8AF, UK
e-mail: louise.howard@kcl.ac.uk

M. Galbally et al. (eds.), *Psychopharmacology and Pregnancy*,
DOI 10.1007/978-3-642-54562-7_9, © Springer-Verlag Berlin Heidelberg 2014

Keywords

antipsychotic • schizophrenia • psychosis

9.1 Schizophrenia: An Overview

Schizophrenia is a major psychiatric disorder characterised by distortions of thought, perception, affect, and behaviour. Symptoms of schizophrenia are conventionally divided into positive symptoms such as delusions, hallucinations, and formal thought disorder, and negative symptoms such as loss of volition, blunting of affect, and poverty of thought and speech. Cognitive difficulties are also an important feature, especially in more severe illness. It is a relatively uncommon disorder, with a lifetime risk of 7.2 per 1,000 and is significantly more common in men than in women (1.4:1) (McGrath et al. 2004). Symptoms usually start in adolescence or young adulthood, but can occur at any age. For the majority, the first acute episode resolves with pharmacological treatment (Emsley et al. 2007), but the course of schizophrenia varies widely with some individuals making a complete recovery, others having a chronic course with severe, persistent disorder and disability, and for others an episodic course, with complete or partial resolution of symptoms between acute episodes with substantial disability (Emsley et al. 2007). Each relapse significantly increases the risk of chronicity, as well as worsening of personal, social, and occupational functioning (Wiersma et al. 1998; Wiersma et al. 2000). Risk of relapse is linked to non-adherence with antipsychotic treatment, substance misuse, carers' critical comments. and poor premorbid adjustment (Alvarez-Jimenez et al. 2012). There is a high prevalence of comorbid problems including substance and alcohol misuse, depressive and anxiety disorders, obesity, smoking, and physical health problems such as hypertension, cardiovascular disease, and diabetes (Buckley et al. 2009; Wildgust and Beary 2010).

Pharmacological intervention, specifically antipsychotic medications, remains the primary treatment at least for the positive symptoms of schizophrenia. Antipsychotic drugs are effective for the treatment of acute episodes, for relapse prevention, for the emergency treatment of acute behavioural disturbance, and for symptom reduction. A recent systematic review and meta-analysis (Leucht et al. 2012) (65 trials, $n = 6,493$ patients) reported that antipsychotic drugs compared with placebo significantly reduced relapse rates at 1 year (drugs 27 % vs. placebo 64 %; risk ratio [RR] 0.40, 95 % CI 0.33–0.49; number needed to treat to benefit [NNTB] 3, 95 % CI 2–3) and re-admission rates (10 % vs. 26 %; RR 0.38, 95 % CI 0.27–0.55; NNTB 5, 4–9), with some evidence of better quality of life and fewer aggressive acts. More patients given antipsychotic drugs than placebo gained weight (10 % vs. 6 %; RR 2.07, 95 % CI 2.31–3.25), had movement disorders (16 % vs. 9 %; 1.55, 1.25–1.93), and experienced sedation (13 % vs. 9 %; 1.50, 1.22–1.84). Depot preparations reduced relapse (RR 0.31, 95 % CI 0.21–0.41) more than oral drugs (0.46, 0.37–0.57; $p = 0.03$). A systematic review and meta-analysis by the same group (Leucht et al. 2009) comparing "second-generation" versus "first-generation" antipsychotic drugs for schizophrenia (150 RCTs; $n = 21,533$ participants) reported better overall efficacy for four of these drugs, with small to medium effect sizes (amisulpride −0.31 [95 % CI −0.44 to −0.19, $p < 0.0001$], clozapine −0.52 [−0.75 to −0.29, $p < 0.0001$], olanzapine −0.28 [−0.38 to −0.18, $p < 0.0001$], and risperidone −0.13 [−0.22 to −0.05, $p = 0.002$]). The other second-generation drugs were not more efficacious than the first-generation drugs, even for negative symptoms. Second-generation antipsychotic (SGA) drugs were associated with fewer extrapyramidal side effects than haloperidol (even at low doses) and other than aripiprazole and ziprasidone SGA drugs were associated with more weight gain, in various degrees, than haloperidol.

Recognition of the poor effectiveness of antipsychotics for negative and cognitive symptoms has led to research into psychological and psychosocial interventions for schizophrenia offered as adjunctive therapy. There is some evidence for effectiveness of cognitive behavioural therapy (CBT), particularly for the affective problems associated with the illness (Pharoah et al. 2010; Jones et al. 2011), cognitive remediation therapy for cognition and function (Wykes et al. 2011), and family interventions which reduce hospitalisation rates and global symptom severity (Pharoah et al. 2010).

9.2   Natural History of Schizophrenia in the Perinatal Period

Women with schizophrenia have lower fertility rates compared with women in the general population, though recent studies suggest fertility has increased since the advent of antipsychotics that are not associated with persistent hyperprolactinaemia (Howard et al. 2002; Vigod et al. 2012). The nature of schizophrenia can also affect a women's ability to make and sustain relationships (Howard 2005) which will also affect general fertility rates. However, most women with schizophrenia have children (Howard et al. 2001), value motherhood highly, and often describe motherhood as central to their existence (Dolman et al. 2013). Nevertheless, pregnancies of women with schizophrenia are more likely to be unplanned and unwanted (Miller and Finnerty 1996) than women in the general population for whom around 50 % of pregnancies are unplanned.

There are few studies published investigating the impact of pregnancy on schizophrenia. One of the few prospective studies is now three decades old but reported that two-thirds of pregnant women with a history of psychosis were not in contact with psychiatric services during pregnancy, despite the presence of active mental disturbance (McNeil et al. 1984). There is little evidence about how pregnancy itself affects symptoms of schizophrenia. It is likely that women who are usually maintained on medication to stabilise their condition may stop treatment when they discover they are pregnant because of fears about potential teratogenicity; this is probably why the prevalence of prescriptions of antipsychotics in women with schizophrenia may be lower for the second and third trimesters of pregnancy compared with the first (Toh et al. 2013). What is not clear is the extent to which relapse occurs in pregnant women who continue with medication compared with those who do not.

Pregnant women with schizophrenia are at increased risk of obstetric complications, including pre-eclampsia, poor fetal growth, preterm birth, low birth weight, low Apgar score, congenital defects, still births, and subsequent neonatal deaths and sudden infant death syndrome (Dalman et al. 1999; Bennedsen et al. 2001b; Howard et al. 2003; Howard 2005; Jablensky et al. 2005; Webb et al. 2005; Webb et al. 2006; Matevosyan 2011). Many risk factors for obstetric complications are also more frequent in women with schizophrenia, such as smoking (Howard et al. 2003; Goodwin et al. 2007), alcohol and substance misuse (Menezes et al. 1996), financial difficulties (Howard et al. 2001), domestic violence (Trevillion et al. 2012), nutritional deficiencies (McColl et al. 2013), obesity and diabetes (Howard and Croker 2012), and decreased access to antenatal care (Howard 2005). Smoking is the leading preventable cause of fetal morbidity and mortality in high income countries and is associated with an increased risk of pre-eclampsia, miscarriage, congenital malformations, low birth weight, prematurity, stillbirths, sudden infant death syndrome, and physical and mental disorders in childhood (Royal College of Physicians 2010). Women with mental disorders are more likely to be smoking at conception, at antenatal booking, and up until delivery (Shah and Howard 2006; Goodwin et al. 2007) and to find it more difficult to stop smoking (Webb et al. 2010) even if they accept referral to smoking cessation services (Howard et al. 2013). Women with severe mental disorders are particularly likely to smoke heavily and be more addicted to nicotine (Aubin et al. 2012) and when pregnant are less likely to be asked about smoking than women from the general population (Howard et al. 2003).

Similarly, other health and social care needs of women with a diagnosis of schizophrenia may not be detected by professionals, but are likely to affect health during pregnancy (Howard and Hunt 2008; Wan et al. 2008a; Webb et al. 2010). However, even after adjusting for risk factors such as smoking and socio-economic status, maternal schizophrenia appears to predict poorer obstetric and perinatal outcomes (Matevosyan 2011). In addition, women who are chronically unwell may develop psychotic denial of pregnancy, particularly if there has been previous loss of custody of a child (Miller 1990). This can lead to refusal of antenatal care or failure to recognise labour, with consequent unassisted delivery (Jenkins et al. 2011). It is therefore of paramount importance that women with a diagnosis of schizophrenia should be provided with optimal psychiatric, as well as antenatal, care.

In the postpartum, there is an increased risk of relapse of psychosis—a Danish population-based register study found a relative risk of 5 for hospital admissions in women with a diagnosis of schizophrenia within the first month following delivery (Munk-Olsen et al. 2006). This represents a far lower risk than that for postpartum women with bipolar disorder (see Chap. 8). This increased risk of relapse persists throughout the first year postpartum, probably because of a number of factors associated with new motherhood, including sleep deprivation and the stress of looking after an infant, potentially with social services supervision (Howard et al. 2004a). Other risk factors include affective symptoms, recent active symptoms, hospitalisation during pregnancy, and severe illness history, including long admissions (McNeil 1987; Kumar et al. 1995; Harlow et al. 2007). In addition to risk of relapse of psychosis, mothers with a diagnosis of schizophrenia may also be more likely to be depressed postnatally than controls (Howard et al. 2004b).

In general, infanticide and suicide are rare. They are also rare in women with a diagnosis of schizophrenia (Flynn et al. 2007). The UK Confidential Enquiry into Maternal Death has consistently reported low rates of suicide during pregnancy for all women, but an increased risk of suicide in the first year postpartum for women with psychosis, although this is more common in women with severe affective disorders than schizophrenia (Cantwell et al. 2011). A study of the homicide of infants in England and Wales between 1996 and 2001 showed that 24 % (17 out of 112) had symptoms of mental illness at the time of the offence, mostly depression, and only four perpetrators were women with a lifetime diagnosis of schizophrenia (Flynn et al. 2007).

9.3   Summary of the Evidence for Treatment Improving the Condition in the Perinatal Period

There has been little research into interventions for schizophrenia in the perinatal period and no high-quality studies of antipsychotic medication in pregnancy (Webb et al. 2004). There is weak evidence from a small before and after study of 20 women with schizophrenia treated with antipsychotics that non-drug-related support, such as liaison with maternity care staff and consent for partner to carry out child care, contributed to improvements in mental state (Nishizawa et al. 2007). We, therefore, rely on other sources of evidence for practice guidelines when considering how to care for women with a diagnosis of schizophrenia in the perinatal period.

9.4   Risk of Not Treating Schizophrenia in Pregnancy (for Mother, Pregnancy, and Fetus)

As discussed above, it is unclear to what extent prophylactic antipsychotic medication will reduce risk of relapse of schizophrenia during pregnancy. Data for relapse rates in schizophrenia in non-pregnant populations suggest that rehospitalisation rates and relapse rates are significantly increased following discontinuation of antipsychotic medication in women and men, and risk associated with discontinuation of antipsychotics may be especially increased in the first years after illness onset (Robinson et al. 1999; Morken et al. 2008). Acute and untreated psychosis is well recognised to be associated with psychological distress and behavioural disturbance that may put the mother and fetus at risk and affect the ability of a mother to care for her infant should acute relapse persist postpartum. Acute psychosis is associated with significant activation of the hypothalamic–pituitary–

adrenal axis (Abel et al. 1996). These and other physiological changes associated with acute illness could also affect fetal development through changes in feto-placental integrity and fetal central nervous system development (Cohen and Rosenbaum 1998). Acute illness may also increase the risk of suicide and/or infanticide, although the risk is less in mothers with schizophrenia than in mothers with affective disorders (Flynn et al. 2007). Importantly, reinstatement of treatment for an acute episode following discontinuation often requires higher doses of medication compared with maintenance treatment, exposing the fetus to higher doses of drug.

Social withdrawal, delusional thinking, and inappropriate behaviour can impair daily living (Howard 2005), mother–infant interaction, and consistent caregiving behaviour (Wan et al. 2007; Wan et al. 2008a, b). However, there is some evidence that reducing the symptoms of severe mental illness in the mother can improve mother–child relations (Kahng et al. 2008), so if women are treated during pregnancy and the postpartum period, they may avoid the high levels of social services intervention, supervision, and custody loss reported in many studies of mothers with schizophrenia (Howard et al. 2004a, b).

9.5 Maternal–Fetal Exposure to Psychotropic Medications as a Contemporary Problem

Pregnant women and fetuses are more likely than ever to be exposed to antipsychotic medications and perhaps to the newer second-generation agents in particular. Drugs such as clozapine, olanzapine, risperidone, and quetiapine are increasingly used in women of reproductive age for a range of psychiatric and behavioural disorders other than schizophrenia (Buchanan et al. 2010). Reproductive safety data remain surprisingly incomplete and guideline recommendations lend limited support to clinical risk–benefit analyses (Howard 2005; McKenna et al. 2005; NICE 2007) (Abel 2013). This is a problem not least because the gold standard randomised controlled trial is considered unethical for assessing psychotropic medication use during pregnancy while available observational studies are generally underpowered with biased samples and therefore remain unfit for this purpose in a rapidly changing prescribing landscape (Abel 2013).

In a UK population approaching 66 million, 3–4,000 births per year are likely to be exposed to antipsychotics or other psychotropic medications. This chapter provides a critical summary of current knowledge about the potential risks of fetal antipsychotic drug exposure and proposes how future observational studies might fill crucial gaps in the evidence to deliver workable new clinical guidance in an evidence-poor arena.

Most incident cases of severe mental illness (schizophrenia, related disorders, and bipolar disorder) in women occur during the reproductive years and most are treated with continuous psychotropic pharmacotherapy. In the last few decades, some key changes in care, including deinstitutionalisation and the use of newer agents with fewer effects on fertility, mean that women treated with antipsychotics are increasingly likely to become pregnant, while the broadening use of newer "atypical" antipsychotics for other more common mental disorders among women of childbearing age is also expanding. Psychotropic medications are therefore increasingly likely to be prescribed to mothers during pregnancy (Newport et al. 2007). It is surprising then that the reproductive safety data for these agents remain so incomplete, and guideline recommendations lend limited support to women, their partners, and their treating clinicians in difficult clinical risk–benefit analyses (NICE 2007). Recent reports conclude that prospective studies are needed which can access unbiased and reliable (i.e. large enough) samples of ill mothers exposed to psychotropic medication that they can take account of key characteristics (e.g. maternal psychiatric diagnosis, smoking, pre-pregnancy weight, and polypharmacy) in the estimation of risk.

9.6 Antipsychotics

Antipsychotic drugs will be considered under the two classes commonly referred to as first (FGA) and second-generation antipsychotic (SGA) drugs. It is generally believed that studies are limited for SGAs, but that there is a wealth of information for FGAs. In fact, most of the information on adverse drug effects has been slowly accumulated through spontaneous reports or through reports accumulated by pharmaceutical companies of adverse effects. By their very nature, these data are biased, unrepresentative, and unreliable. For both antipsychotic drug classes, studies examining the key outcomes that we shall consider (congenital malformations, pregnancy and maternal outcomes, and developmental outcomes) remain limited in number and size and, as a result, yield inconsistent findings overall (Table 9.1).

9.6.1 Congenital Malformations

First-Generation Antipsychotics

In 1960, Sobel reported that women with a psychotic illness were twice as likely as women in the general population to have a pregnancy resulting in congenital malformation or death, irrespective of chlorpromazine use in pregnancy (Sobel 1961). Currently, it is uncertain whether or not antipsychotics as a group lead to increases in congenital anomalies above the general population rate of 2–4 % (http://www.statisticsgov.uk) ONS Congenital Anomaly Statistics, England and Wales (Series MB3, No.23, 2008; EUROCAT classification of congenital malformations http://www.eurocat-network.eu/content/EUROCAT-Guard-1.3-Chapeter-3.3-Jan2012.pdf). Older studies have not found an association between birth defects and maternal nonorganic psychosis (McNeil et al. 1992) or maternal postpartum psychosis (Paffenbarger et al. 1961). Theoretically, offspring of mothers with major mental illness should indeed develop more neural tube defects because of higher rates of maternal obesity and reduced serum folate levels related to poor diet (McColl et al. 2013). In a relatively small population sample from

Table 9.1 Risks of adverse outcomes following antipsychotic (AP) exposure in pregnancy

Study	Outcome	Prenatal exposure	n	Findings
Boden et al (2012)	GDM Prematurity SGA	All APs 1st trimester	507 exposed	2× increased risk 60 % increased risk >2 fold increased risk (but likely confounded)
Reis and Kallen (2008)	Severe CMs GDM LSCS Prematurity SGA LGA Prematurity	All APs 1st trimester	576 exposed	50 % increased risk 2× increased risk No increased risk 70 % increased risk 50 % increased risk No increased risk No increased risk
Newham et al. (2008)	SGA LGA	All APs 1st trimester	70 exposed	No increased risk Increased risk for atypicals but v small numbers ($n = 5$)
Newport et al (2007)	LBW Hypoxia	Atypical APs	41 exposed	No significant increase risk
McKenna et al (2005)	CMs Spontaneous Abortion Prematurity Pregnancy complications LBW	Atypical APs	151 exposed	No significant increase
Lin et al (2010)	Prematurity LBW SGA/LGA Prematurity	All APs 1st trimester Compared to women with SCZ on NO APs	242 exposed SCZ only	two fold increase typical antipsychotics only No increased risk No increased risk No increased risk

LBW low birth weight, *SGA or LGA* small or large for gestational age, *GDM* gestational diabetes mellitus, *CMs* congenital malformations, *APs* antipsychotics, *SCZ* schizophrenia

Western Australia, Jablensky and colleagues reported no increased risk of overall birth defects associated with maternal schizophrenia; they did however report an increase in cardiovascular defects and other defects such as minor physical anomalies (Jablensky et al. 2005). The most robust attempts to answer this question come from Scandinavian population-based samples. Bennedsen reported a small increase in the risk of birth defects in children of mothers with schizophrenia using Danish register data (Bennedsen et al. 2001b). Webb et al. observed a markedly elevated risk of fatal birth defects with maternal schizophrenia (RR 2.34), but not with paternal schizophrenia (Webb et al. 2008). While increased rates of birth defects in the children of women with psychosis may imply a role for maternal genetic factors, environmental effects exclusive to mother such as smoking or drug exposure become more likely. None of the studies discussed above have been able to take maternal exposure to medication into account, but the size and lipophilicity of psychotropic and especially antipsychotic medications increase the likelihood that they will cross the placenta (Pinkofsky 1995) and this bioavailability makes them potential candidates as teratogens.

Meta-analysis of older, mainly prospective cohort studies, reports small but significant excess of congenital malformations in infants exposed to phenothiazine ($n = 2,591$) compared with unexposed infants of well mothers ($n = 71,746$) (OR 1.21, 1.01–1.45) (Altshuler et al. 1996). Over the decades, changing antenatal and obstetric care means that the rate of some key outcomes in the background population has also changed so that estimates from more recent cohorts are likely to be more reliable.

Using a 10 year cohort of births (1995–2005) from Swedish national registers, Reis and Kallen report that maternal antipsychotic use *overall* was associated with a moderate excess of congenital malformation compared to well population controls, but the increase was only marginally significant (OR 1.45, 0.99–1.41) (Reis and Kallen 2008). Here, the excess was largely accounted for by cardiovascular anomalies (atrial or ventricular septal defects). Results adjusted for concomitant antiepileptic use, but not for antidepressant use, were also associated with small increases in cardiovascular anomaly (Reis and Kallen 2010). A review to July 2008 (Gentile 2010) also concludes that risk of limb anomalies cannot be excluded with typical antipsychotics (i.e. haloperidol) exposure.

Second-Generation Antipsychotics

Although primarily used to treat schizophrenia and psychotic disorders, newer "second-generation" antipsychotics (SGAs) now treat a spectrum of disorders, including major depression, bipolar disorder, repeated self-harm, PTSD, and other anxiety disorders (McKenna et al. 2005). Far less data have accumulated for newer agents: olanzapine, risperidone, quetiapine, aripiprazole, amisulpride, and clozapine. Again, most data on reproductive safety for these compounds are limited to manufacturers' case series and spontaneous reports. Among reports of olanzapine-exposed pregnancies from the manufacturer, no increase in risk of major malformations is reported. In 523 clozapine-exposed pregnancies, 22 "unspecified malformations" were reported (4.2 %) while in 151 quetiapine-exposed pregnancies, 8 infants had congenital anomalies (5.2 %). Eight malformations were reported in infants born to 250 women taking risperidone (3.2 %); however, pregnancy outcomes were unknown in many of these cases reported to the manufacturer (McKenna et al. 2005). Taken together, these reports do not suggest an increase in major malformation above that seen in the general population, nor do they indicate any specific pattern of abnormalities among second-generation drug-exposed infants. This information does not suggest particular concerns for SGA use in early pregnancy, but again conclusions can only be provisional.

Individual Antipsychotics

Most women exposed to first-generation antipsychotics (FGAs) have been prescribed these medications for hyperemesis gravidarum rather than for mental illness. This represents a potentially important (if not contemporary) control group which might allow distinction between effects of maternal illness from maternal medication. However, for hyperemesis, FGAs tended to be used in much lower doses, and intermittently, limited the benefit of using this as a comparison group. Restricting cases from relatively unbiased population samples, over 200 cases have been reported for olanzapine, haloperidol, or fluphenazine; 100–200 cases for risperidone or flupenthixol and less than 100 for all other antipsychotics, including chlorpromazine, clozapine, sulpiride, trifluoperazine, and quetiapine (Barnes 2011). Taken together these, albeit limited data, and the considerable number of years that many compounds have been available, do not suggest antipsychotic drugs are major teratogens. However, a recent review (Gentile 2010) concluded that risk of limb anomalies associated with early in utero exposure to haloperidol and penfluridol cannot be excluded, and no conclusions can be drawn about the teratogenicity of fluphenazine, thioridazine, and promethazine. To date, there are very few reported first trimester exposures to aripiprazole and one child was born with major congenital anomalies. Little or no published information is currently available for sertindole, amisulpride, and zotepine.

9.6.2 Pregnancy and Maternal Outcomes

The term "obstetric complications" (OCs) refers to a very large set of, in the main, rare obstetric events, ranging from the enigmatic "delivered by an untrained person" (Sacker et al. 1995) to a more clearly defined notion of prematurity or premature labour (Dalman et al. 1999). Even the latter variable can be unclear: some studies do not distinguish between delivery before 37 weeks and 33 weeks, despite rather different risk distributions associated with the two. Some have attempted to get around the problem of rarity of exposure to OCs by grouping together disparate complications. One of the most popular groupings has been "hypoxic–ischaemic-related" events (Zornberg et al. 2000; Cannon et al. 2002). Despite a lack of evidence, categories such as these assume common casual mechanisms for the various OCs within the group. For example "hypoxia" may include events leading to chronic fetal hypoxia (e.g. maternal anaemia, pre-eclampsia, maternal smoking), which may be quite different from those leading to acute fetal hypoxia (e.g. apnoea at birth related to poor Apgar scores, strangulation by prolapse of cord, meconium inhalation, prematurity), and may have quite different sequelae in terms of brain development and risk of subsequent neurodevelopmental outcome. This problem affects both studies which measure OCs as well as those which adjust for OCs as potential confounders of other associations. Furthermore, apart from the risk of obscuring differences, pooling OCs fails to provide sufficient additional information compared to analysis of single complications (Bennedsen et al. 2001a).

Taking such considerations into account, population samples from Australia and Scandinavia have reported varying results for the risk of OCs in women with severe maternal mental illness. An earlier study in Denmark reported an adjusted excess risk of 1.57 for low birth weight and 1.34 for small for gestational age (Bennedsen et al. 1999). In Western Australia, women with a diagnosis of schizophrenia or major affective disorder had raised risk of placental abnormalities and antepartum haemorrhage (Jablensky et al. 2005). Using a similar methodology in a later study, Bennedsen et al. reported no excess OCs for Danish women with schizophrenia (Bennedsen et al. 2001b). Ellman et al. explored whether any adverse outcomes were related to a shared genetic liability in the mother to OC risk and schizophrenia by studying first-degree relatives of mothers with a schizophrenia diagnosis; they found no excess OCs in first-degree relatives compared to controls with no family history of schizophrenia (Ellman et al. 2007). None of these studies was able to assess OC risks associated with exposure to medication. Only more recent linked databases from Sweden have specifically attempted to address this question; of note, findings in these recent reports tend to support the earlier studies and the crude risks are of similar magnitude.

First-Generation Antipsychotics

Reis and Kallen (2008) examined births between 1995 and 2005 from the Swedish Medical Births register. Excess risk of premature delivery (OR 1.73, 1.31–2.29), low birth weight (OR 1.67, 1.21–2.29), and a trend for increased risk of small for gestational age (OR 1.46, 0.99–2.15) was reported for pregnancies exposed to any antipsychotic ($n = 576$) compared to well, unexposed population controls. Boden et al. (2012) examined a slightly different Swedish dataset: the Prescribed Drug Registry. Over a 4-year period (2005–2009), they found that infants exposed to antipsychotics ($n = 507$) overall had higher risk of small for gestational age (OR 2.11, 1.29–3.47) and gestational diabetes (OR 2.78, 1.64–4.70). Risk was further divided into being born small for gestational age for birth length (OR 2.29, 1.41–3.73) and small for gestational age for head circumference (OR 2.19, 1.33–3.62). However, none of these risks remained significant after adjusting for maternal factors, such as smoking.

In a similar era cohort, Lin et al. report on Taiwanese schizophrenia mothers ($n = 242$) prescribed any antipsychotic who had given birth between 2001 and 2003 (Lin et al. 2010). They only found excess risk of prematurity (OR 2.46, 1.50–4.11), and only in mothers receiving *FGAs*, but no excess risk of low birth weight, small, or large for gestational age with early pregnancy antipsychotic exposure overall. No other outcomes were assessed.

A far smaller study in the UK (Newham et al. 2008) reports that infants exposed to FGAs ($n = 45$) and SGAs ($n = 25$) compared to unexposed controls had no significant risk of small for gestational age. Significantly more small-for-gestational-age infants were exposed to typical drugs than the reference group; this difference disappeared after exclusion of mothers exposed to other "weight-altering" drugs. Finally, a review of studies to July 2008 (Gentile 2010) concluded that risk of perinatal complications (ranging from withdrawal symptoms to instability of body temperature) is associated with late in utero exposure to haloperidol and phenothiazine, such as chlorpromazine.

Second-Generation Antipsychotics

McKenna et al. (2005) conclude that women exposed to SGAs have significantly higher rates of low birth weight infants than controls (10 % vs. 2 %), whereas two subsequent studies reported excess of large-for-gestational-age infants: Newham et al. (2008) report increase in infant birth weight and large for gestational age based on only five cases exposed to either clozapine or olanzapine, but excluding cases with gestational diabetes; Bodén et al. (2012) report increased risk of gestational diabetes (OR 2.39, 1.12–5.13) and small for gestational age (OR for 2.42, 1.24–4.70) after early exposure to olanzapine and clozapine as a group. They examine risk of anabolic fetal growth with olanzapine and clozapine as a group, but do not find a significant effect. This latest study has the largest number of cases of women exposed to olanzapine or clozapine ($n = 169$) to date. No studies have been able to look separately at clozapine or other agents, such as olanzapine, quetiapine, or risperidone. This is important because not only are these drugs becoming the most prescribed antipsychotics in the UK (http://www.ic.nhs.uk/statistics-and-data-collections/primary-care/prescriptons/precription-cost-analysis-england-2010), but also because recent examination of placental passage (umbilical cord: maternal plasma concentration) of antipsychotics shows olanzapine had highest passage (mean 72.1 %, SD = 42.0 %) and, also, higher rates of either low birth weight and/or perinatal complications than other antipsychotics (Newport et al. 2007).

Finally, it is worth noting that to date, no studies have examined drug adherence, or time to, or risk of, relapse in mothers with a diagnosis of schizophrenia or related disorder who discontinue antipsychotic medication in pregnancy in powerful enough datasets. Furthermore, outcomes increasingly noted as relevant by service users, such as quality of life, are missing from most older, larger population register datasets.

9.6.3   Neonatal Risks

There is a remarkable absence of systematic studies of neonatal reaction following pregnancy exposure to antipsychotics. Several cases of neonatal extrapyramidal syndrome have been reported following exposure to first-generation antipsychotics (Gentile 2010), but there are no other consistent patterns of adverse effects in the literature.

9.6.4   Developmental and Longer Term Outcomes

Neurocognitive and Intellectual Disability

Over 40 years ago, Barbara Fish published her seminal paper on developmental delay and neurological deviation in so-called "high-risk" children of women with schizophrenia (Fish 1977). Since then, many have reported delays in neurological and motor development, generalised cognitive deficits and learning difficulties, as well as poorer performance than controls on specific neurocognitive tasks in these children. For excellent reviews, see (Goodman 1984; Asarnow 1988; Cornblatt and Obuchowski 1997; Niemi et al. 2003; Wan et al. 2008a). However, effects of fetal antipsychotic exposure on cognitive, psychopathological, or developmental outcomes have not been taken into consideration. This is particularly important because much of the so-called "high-risk" literature *does* show evidence of poorer cognitive, social, and clinical outcomes (Wan et al. 2008a). For example, Niemi et al. (2003) report on 145 children of mothers with psychosis and found them significantly more likely to have a severe academic problem (15 %) than controls (8 %). Impairments are more consistently reported in specific cognitive domains, such as verbal ability, executive functioning, and processing speed (Wan et al. 2008a).

In the older studies, when mothers *could* have been exposed to typical antipsychotics, deficits reported in infancy and early childhood may have poor predictive value and have disappeared later in childhood (Sameroff et al. 1987). Meanwhile, two reviews of the older literature fail to find differences in behavioural functioning or IQ up to 5 years (Thiels 1987; Altshuler et al. 1996). One contemporary study by Morgan et al., including mothers likely to have been exposed to atypical agents, found children of mothers with schizophrenia, bipolar disorder, and unipolar depression up to three times more likely to have intellectual disability as comparison children (Morgan et al. 2009). Morgan suggested that multivariate analysis indicated both genetic and environmental risks acted independently.

Much evidence implies substantial familiality *across* outcomes/disorders, i.e. greater rates of intellectual disability in families with schizophrenia (Heston 1966; Modrzewska 1980; Alaghband-Rad et al. 1998), and vice versa (Gustavson et al. 1986), as well as increased rates of multiply affected families in people with co-occurring intellectual disability and schizophrenia compared to those with schizophrenia only or intellectual disability only (Penrose 1938; Doody et al. 1998). Similarly, neurocognitive impairment in unaffected schizophrenia relatives (Gur et al. 2007) suggests a genetic component to neurocognitive outcomes. However, environmental risks factors, including obstetric complications, are also strongly implicated in the aetiology of both neurocognitive impairments and intellectual disability (Leonard and Wen 2002), including autism (Glasson et al. 2004; Abel et al. 2013).

Psychiatric Outcomes

In the general population, it is likely that multiple genes of small effect contribute to risk of developing serious mental illness, including schizophrenia, and that a range of environmental risk factors interact with this genetic susceptibility (Abel 2004). Children of women with schizophrenia have an eight- to tenfold higher risk of developing the disorder compared to the general population (Gottesman et al. 1987), with the risk in a monozygotic co-twin increased to about 50-fold (Gottesman and Erlenmeyer-Kimling 2001). A recent Danish register study reported that the cumulative incidence by age 52 of schizophrenia in children where one parent had a psychiatric inpatient or outpatient admission for schizophrenia was 7.0 % (Gottesman et al. 2010). If both parents had schizophrenia admissions, the cumulative incidence of schizophrenia in children was 27.3 %, rising to 39.2 % for schizophrenia and related disorders (schizotypal and delusional disorder) and 67.5 % for any psychiatric diagnosis. These population data for schizophrenia consider presence of illness by recording primarily inpatient admissions only. While this is likely to represent a good approximation of risk for schizophrenia (nearly all sufferers are admitted at some point), it provides a poorer representation of risk for less severe, more common psychiatric outcomes.

None of the literature discussed in this section accounts for fetal psychotropic exposure, and much cannot account for unmeasured family influences and confounders. In the Rochester high-risk sample of children of women with schizophrenia, low socio-economic status, and maternal illness chronicity were more important predictors of early outcomes of children to age 4 years than maternal diagnosis per se (Sameroff et al. 1987). This suggests that fetal antipsychotic exposure becomes less likely as a powerful explanatory variable in the generation of risk the more distal and the more complex the behavioural outcomes become. However, unlikely it may be that a drug causes intellectual disability, interactions which prove "risky-for-neurodevelopment" occurring between genetic predisposition and drug exposure are not only conceivable, but also increasingly plausible.

The very limited availability of data on potential longer term neurobehavioural sequelae of fetal exposure to antipsychotics is not difficult to understand. Long-term follow-up is expensive and challenging. It is hard to account for many postnatal risk factors also likely to be associated with being born to a mother with symptoms severe enough to warrant psychotropic agents during pregnancy (Abel and Morgan 2011). However, given the evidence suggesting a range of poorer adverse outcomes for these families, more translational research is needed to delineate modifiable risk factors so that appropriate interventions can be developed and implemented for both mother and child across the developmental life course, commencing in the antenatal period.

9.7   Management Recommendations

The pregnancies of women with a diagnosis of schizophrenia are high risk. As such, identifiable risk factors ideally should be addressed as far as possible before conception. But many of these women are likely to be sexually active and less likely to use contraception or be able to negotiate condom use than well women in the community (Abel and Rees 2010). Reproductive health planning should therefore be a part of the routine care for all women with serious mental illness of reproductive age (Abel et al. 2011). Interventions for the illness and for co-morbid problems such as smoking, obesity, and nutritional deficiencies need tailoring for individual patients; this means time for trials off medications and, as women are at greatest risk (compared to men) of developing metabolic syndrome and morbid obesity with second-generation antipsychotics (Goff et al. 2005), mental health teams need to consider the possibility of pregnancy when planning treatments for young women of reproductive potential. Intensive support is also needed to prepare for smoking cessation, diet and exercise management programmes, etc. These are best delivered before pregnancy with family planning advice. Preconception counselling, at a time when women are not acutely ill and have capacity to make decisions, should also include a discussion of the risks and benefits of taking medication compared with not taking medication so that women with their families can make informed collaborative decisions.

Lack of reproductive and pregnancy planning means that most women with schizophrenia are likely to become pregnant while taking medications. This means that maternity and mental health professionals need to be aware of the increased risk of adverse obstetric and psychosocial outcomes so that they can ensure delivery of optimal care. For example, women with a diagnosis of schizophrenia are more likely than healthy women to have a partner with a psychiatric illness or to have no partner and few or no social supports (Abel et al. 2005). Helping women to engage with antenatal care may be an important way to offer support and guidance and may improve antenatal clinic attendance. Optimal care also needs to identify and address risk factors such as domestic violence and smoking, and comprehensive care is likely to need coordination by a named health professional and modification of maternal care pathways (NICE 2010).

Many women with a diagnosis of schizophrenia and related (non-affective) psychoses are likely to relapse if medication is stopped; women with severe illnesses and recent long hospitalisations will be at particularly high risk. The consequences of an acute episode of illness—child protection proceedings for the unborn child, behavioural disturbance, and/or self-neglect that may put the woman and the fetus at risk, and adverse obstetric and fetal outcomes—are potentially devastating. Women who are likely to relapse will need antipsychotic medication throughout their pregnancies and into the postpartum period, and decisions around medication will often focus on *which* medication to take and *what monitoring* is needed, e.g. increased monitoring of glucose metabolism during pregnancy (SIGN 2012). Switching and/or withdrawal of medication may itself lead to relapse, particularly if an untried medication is started because of its putative lower risk. We would therefore recommend that where possible changes in medication are avoided if the woman is already on medication that keeps her well. Of note, clozapine will usually have been prescribed for treatment resistant illness and should be continued, as stopping may lead to a severe psychotic relapse.

In addition to medication, management should address other risk factors for adverse outcomes such as smoking and substance misuse, and providing psychosocial interventions that will reduce stressors and enhance support for the whole family. This should include consistent support through the perinatal period, monitoring for early relapse indicators which can be quickly treated, and interventions that will help the woman prepare for motherhood, as well as active involvement of other members of the family to help with child care in the postnatal period. Careful multidisciplinary planning with women and relevant others offers women with a diagnosis of schizophrenia the opportunity to minimise harms and to maximise the very many benefits and joys associated with new motherhood.

References

Abel KM. Foetal origins of schizophrenia: testable hypotheses of genetic and environmental influences. Br J Psychiatry. 2004;184:383–5.

Abel KM. Fetal antipsychotic exposure in a changing landscape: seeing the future. Br J Psychiatry. 2013;202:1–3.

Abel KM, Morgan VA. Mental illness, women, mothers and their children. Psychiatric epidemiology. Oxford: Wiley-Blackwell; 2011. p. 483–514.

Abel KM, Rees S. The reproductive and sexual health of women service users: what's the fuss? Adv Psychiatr Treat. 2010;16:279–89.

Abel KM, O'Keane V, Murray RM. Enhancement of the prolactin response to D-fenfluramine challenge in drug-naive schizophrenia. Br J Psychiatry. 1996;168:57–60.

Abel KM, Webb RT, Salmon MP, Wan MW, Appleby L. Prevalence and predictors of parenting outcomes in a cohort of mothers with schizophrenia admitted for joint mother and baby psychiatric care in England. J Clin Psychiatry. 2005;66(6):781–9. quiz 808–789.

Abel KM, Evans DT, Davies R. 2011. eLearning: Sexual, reproductive and mental health. 2013, from http://www.scie.org.uk/publications/elearning/sexualhealth/index.asp

Abel KM, Dalman C, Svensson AC, Susser E, Dal H, Idring S, et al. Deviant fetal growth and autism spectrum disorder. Am J Psychiatry. 2013;170:391–8.

Alaghband-Rad J, Kumra S, Lenane MC, Jacobsen LK, Brown AS, Susser E, et al. Early-onset schizophrenia: mental retardation in siblings. J Am Acad Child Adolesc Psychiatry. 1998;37(2):137–8.

Altshuler LL, Cohen L, Szuba MP, Burt VK, Gitlin M, Mintz J. Pharmacologic management of psychiatric illness during pregnancy: dilemmas and guidelines. Am J Psychiatry. 1996;153(5):592–606.

Alvarez-Jimenez M, Priede A, Hetrick SE, Bendall S, Killackey E, Parker AG, et al. Risk factors for relapse following treatment for first episode psychosis: a systematic review and meta-analysis of longitudinal studies. Schizophr Res. 2012;139:116–28.

Asarnow JR. Children at risk for schizophrenia: converging lines of evidence. Schizophr Bull. 1988;14(4):613–31.

Aubin HJ, Rollema H, Svensson TH, Winterer G. Smoking, quitting, and psychiatric disease: a review. Neurosci Biobehav Rev. 2012;36(1):271–84.

Barnes TR. Evidence-based guidelines for the pharmacological treatment of schizophrenia: recommendations from the British Association for Psychopharmacology. J Psychopharmacol. 2011;25(5):567–620.

Bennedsen BE, Mortensen PB, Olesen AV, Henriksen TB. Preterm birth and intra-uterine growth retardation among children of women with schizophrenia. Br J Psychiatry. 1999;175:239–45.

Bennedsen BE, Mortensen PB, Olesen AV, Henriksen TB, Frydenberg M. Obstetric complications in women with schizophrenia. Schizophr Res. 2001a;47:167–75.

Bennedsen BE, Mortensen PB, Olesen AV, Henriksen TB. Congenital malformations, stillbirths, and infant deaths among children of women with schizophrenia. Arch Gen Psychiatry. 2001b;58(7):674–9.

Bodén R, Lundgren M, Brandt L, Reutfors J, Kieler H. Antipsychotics during pregnancy: relation to fetal and maternal metabolic effects. Arch Gen Psychiatry. 2012;69(7):715–21.

Buchanan RW, Kreyenbuhl J, Kelly DL, Noel JM, Boggs DL, Fischer BA, et al. The 2009 schizophrenia PORT psychopharmacological treatment recommendations and summary statements. Schizophr Bull. 2010;36(1):71–93.

Buckley PF, Miller BJ, Lehrer DS, Castle DJ. Psychiatric comorbidities and schizophrenia. Schizophr Bull. 2009;35:383–402.

Cannon TD, van Erp TG, Rosso IM, Huttunen M, Lönnqvist J, Pirkola T, et al. Fetal hypoxia and structural brain abnormalities in schizophrenic patients, their siblings, and controls. Arch Gen Psychiatry. 2002;59(1):35–41.

Cantwell R, Clutton-Brock T, Cooper G, Dawson A, Drife J, Garrod D, et al. Saving Mothers' lives: reviewing maternal deaths to make motherhood safer, 2006–2008. The eighth report of the confidential enquiries into maternal deaths in the United Kingdom. BJOG. 2011;118 Suppl 1:1–203.

Cohen LS, Rosenbaum JF. Psychotropic drug use during pregnancy: weighing the risks. J Clin Psychiatry. 1998;59:18–28.

Cornblatt B, Obuchowski M. Update of high-risk research: 1987-1997. Int Rev Psychiatry. 1997;9:437–47.

Dalman C, Allebeck P, Cullberg J, Grunewald C, Köster M. Obstetric complications and the risk of schizophrenia: a longitudinal study of a national birth cohort. Arch Gen Psychiatry. 1999;56:234–40.

Dolman C, Jones I, Howard LM. Pre-conception to parenting: a systematic review and meta-synthesis of the qualitative literature on motherhood for women with severe mental illness. Arch Womens Ment Health. 2013;16(3):173–96.

Doody GA, Johnstone EC, Sanderson TL, Owens DG, Muir WJ. 'Pfropfschizophrenie' revisited. Schizophrenia in people with mild learning disability. Br J Psychiatry. 1998;173:145–53.

Ellman LM, Huttunen M, Lönnqvist J, Cannon TD. The effects of genetic liability for schizophrenia and maternal smoking during pregnancy on obstetric complications. Schizophr Res. 2007;93:229–36.

Emsley R, Rabinowitz J, Medori R, Early Psychosis Global Working Group. Remission in early psychosis: rates, predictors, and clinical and functional outcome correlates. Schizophr Res. 2007;89:129–39.

Fish B. Neurobiologic antecedents of schizophrenia in children. Arch Gen Psychiatry. 1977;34:1297–313.

Flynn SM, Shaw JJ, Abel KM. Homicide of infants: a cross-sectional study. J Clin Psychiatry. 2007;66(10):1501–9.

Gentile S. Antipsychotic therapy during early and late pregnancy. A systematic review. Schizophr Bull. 2010;36:518–44.

Glasson EJ, Bower C, Petterson B, de Klerk N, Chaney G, Hallmayer JF. Perinatal factors and the development of autism: a population study. Arch Gen Psychiatry. 2004;61(6):618–27.

Goff DC, Sullivan LM, McEvoy JP, Meyer JM, Nasrallah HA, Daumit GL, et al. A comparison of ten-year cardiac risk estimates in schizophrenia patients from the CATIE study and matched controls. Schizophr Res. 2005;80(1):45–53.

Goodman SH. Children of disturbed parents: the interface between research and intervention. Am J Community Psychol. 1984;12(6):663–87.

Goodwin RD, Keyes K, Simuro N. Mental disorders and nicotine dependence among pregnant women in the united states. Obstet Gynecol. 2007;109(4):875–83.

Gottesman II, Erlenmeyer-Kimling L. Family and twin strategies as a head start in defining prodromes and endophenotypes for hypothetical early-interventions in schizophrenia. Schizophr Res. 2001;51:93–102.

Gottesman II, McGuffin P, Farmer AE. Clinical genetics as clues to the "real" genetics of schizophrenia (a decade of modest gains while playing for time). Schizophr Bull. 1987;13:23–44.

Gottesman II, Laursen TM, Bertelsen A, Mortensen PB. Severe mental disorders in offspring with 2 psychiatrically ill parents. Arch Gen Psychiatry. 2010;67(3):252–7.

Gur RE, Calkins ME, Gur RC, Horan WP, Nuechterlein KH, Seidman LJ, et al. The consortium on the genetics of schizophrenia: neurocognitive endophenotypes. Schizophr Bull. 2007;33 (1):49–68.

Gustavson KH, Modrzewska K, Wetterberg L. Mental retardation in a North Swedish isolate. Clin Genet. 1986;30:374–80.

Harlow BL, Vitonis AF, Sparen P, Cnattingius S, Joffe H, Hultman CM. Incidence of hospitalization for postpartum psychotic and bipolar episodes in women with and without prior prepregnancy or prenatal psychiatric hospitalizations. Arch Gen Psychiatry. 2007;64(1):42–8.

Heston L. Psychiatric disorders in foster home reared children of schizophrenic mothers. Br J Psychiatry. 1966;112:819–25.

Howard LM. Fertility and pregnancy in women with psychotic disorders. Eur J Obstet Gynecol Reprod Biol. 2005;119(1):3–10.

Howard LM, Croker H. Obesity and mental health. In: Gilman M, Poston LE, editors. Maternal obesity. Cambridge: Cambridge University Press; 2012.

Howard LM, Hunt K. The needs of mothers with severe mental illness: a comparison of assessmentts of needs by staff and patients. Arch Womens Ment Health. 2008;11(2):131–6.

Howard LM, Kumar R, Thornicroft G. Psychosocial characteristics and needs of mothers with psychotic disorders. Br J Psychiatry. 2001;178:427–32.

Howard LM, Kumar C, Leese M, Thornicroft G. The general fertility rate in women with psychotic disorders. Am J Psychiatry. 2002;159(6):991–7.

Howard LM, Goss C, Leese M, Thornicroft G. Medical outcome of pregnancy in women with psychotic disorders and their infants in the first year after birth. Br J Psychiatry. 2003;182:63–7.

Howard LM, Thornicroft G, Salmon M, Appleby L. Predictors of parenting outcome in women with psychotic disorders discharged from mother and baby units. Acta Psychiatr Scand. 2004a;110(5):347–55.

Howard LM, Goss C, Leese M, Appleby L, Thornicroft G. The psychosocial outcome of pregnancy in women with psychotic disorders. Schizophr Res. 2004b;71(1):49–60.

Howard LM, Bekele D, Rowe M, Demilew J, Bewley S, et al. Smoking cessation in pregnant women with mental disorders: a cohort and nested qualitative study. Br J Obstet Gynaecol. 2013;120(3):362–70.

Jablensky AV, Morgan V, Zubrick SR, Bower C, Yellachich LA. Pregnancy, delivery, and neonatal complications in a population cohort of women with schizophrenia and major affective disorders. Am J Psychiatry. 2005;162:79–91.

Jenkins A, Millar S, Robins J. Denial of pregnancy: a literature review and discussion of ethical and legal issues. J R Soc Med. 2011;104(7):286–91.

Jones C, Hacker D, Meaden A, Cormac I, Irving CB. WITHDRAWN: cognitive behaviour therapy versus other psychosocial treatments for schizophrenia. Cochrane Database Syst Rev. 2011;(4):CD000524.

Kahng SK, Oyserman D, Bybee D, Mowbray C. Mothers with serious mental illness: when symptoms decline does parenting improve? J Fam Psychol. 2008;22(1):162–6.

Kumar R, Marks M, Platz C, Yoshida K. Clinical survey of a psychiatric mother and baby unit: characteristics of 100 consecutive admissions. J Affect Disord. 1995;33:11–22.

Leonard H, Wen X. The epidemiology of mental retardation: challenges and opportunities in the new millennium. Ment Retard Dev Disabil Res Rev. 2002;8:117–34.

Leucht S, Corves C, Arbter D, Engel RR, Li C, Davis JM. Second-generation versus first-generation antipsychotic drugs for schizophrenia: a meta-analysis. Lancet. 2009;373(9657):31–41.

Leucht S, Tardy M, Komossa K, Heres S, Kissling W, Salanti G, et al. Antipsychotic drugs versus placebo for relapse prevention in schizophrenia: a systematic review and meta-analysis. Lancet. 2012;379(9831):2063–71.

Lin HC, Chen IJ, Chen YH, Lee HC, Wu FJ. Maternal schizophrenia and pregnancy outcome: does the use of antipsychotics make a difference? Schizophr Res. 2010;116(1):55–60.

Matevosyan NR. Pregnancy and postpartum specifics in women with schizophrenia: a meta-study. Arch Gynecol Obstet. 2011;283:141–7.

McColl H, Dhillon M, Howard LM. A systematic review of the nutritional status of pregnant women with severe mental illness. Arch Womens Ment Health. 2013;16(1):39–46.

McGrath J, Saha S, Welham J, El Saadi O, MacCauley C, Chant D. A systematic review of the incidence of schizophrenia: the distribution of rates and the influence of sex, urbanicity, migrant status and methodology. BMC Med. 2004;2:13.

McKenna K, Koren G, Tetelbaum M, Wilton L, Shakir S, Diav-Citrin O, et al. Pregnancy outcome of women using atypical antipsychotic drugs: a prospective comparative study. J Clin Psychiatry. 2005;66(4):444–9.

McNeil TF. A prospective study of postpartum psychoses in a high-risk group: 2. Relationships to demographic and psychiatric history charateristics. Acta Psychiatr Scand. 1987;75:35–43.

McNeil TF, Kaij L, Malmquist-Larsson A. Women with nonorganic psychosis: mental disturbance during pregnancy. Acta Psychiatr Scand. 1984;70:27–39.

McNeil TF, Blennow G, Lundberg L. Congenital malformations and structural developmental anomalies in groups at high risk for psychosis. Am J Psychiatry. 1992;149:57–61.

Menezes PR, Johnson S, Thornicroft G, Marshall J, Prosser D, Bebbington P, et al. Drug and alcohol problems among individuals with severe mental illness in south London. Br J Psychiatry. 1996;168(5):612–9.

Miller LJ. Psychotic denial of pregnancy: phenomenology and clinical management. Hosp Community Psychiatry. 1990;41:1233–7.

Miller LJ, Finnerty M. Sexuality, pregnancy, and childbearing among women with schizophrenia-spectrum disorders. JAMA. 1996;296:2582–9.

Modrzewska K. The offspring of schizophrenic parents in a North Swedish isolate. Clin Genet. 1980;17:191–201.

Morgan D, Kirkbride H, Hewitt K, Said B, Walsh AL. Assessing the risk from emerging infections. Epidemiol Infect. 2009;137(11):1521–30.

Morken G, Widen JH, Grawe RW. Non-adherence to antipsychotic medication, relapse and rehospitalisation in recent-onset schizophrenia. BMC Psychiatry. 2008;8:32.

Munk-Olsen T, Laursen TM, Pedersen CB, Mors O, Mortensen PB. New parents and mental disorders: a population-based register study. JAMA. 2006;296(21):2582–9.

Newham JJ, Thomas SH, MacRitchie K, McElhatton PR, McAllister-Williams RH. Birth weight of infants after maternal exposure to typical and atypical antipsychotics: prospective comparison study. Br J Psychiatry. 2008;192:333–7.

Newport DJ, Calamaras MR, DeVane CL, Donovan J, Beach AJ, Winn S, et al. Atypical anipsychotic administration during late pregnancy: placental passage and obstetrical outcomes. Am J Psychiatry. 2007;164:1214–20.

NICE. Antenatal and Postnatal Mental Health guidelines: Clinical guidelines CG45. N. I. f. H. a. C. E. London: British Psychological Society and the Royal College of Psychiatrists; 2007.

NICE. Pregnancy and complex social factors. NICE Clinical Guideline 110. N. I. f. H. a. C. E. NICE. London: NICE, National Institute for Health and Clinical Excellence; 2010.

Niemi LT, Suvisaari JM, Tuulio-Henriksson A, Lönnqvist JK. Childhood developmental abnormalities in schizophrenia: evidence from high-risk studies. Schizophr Res. 2003;60:239–58.

Nishizawa O, Sakumoto K, Hiramatsu K, Kondo T. Effectiveness of comprehensive supports for schizophrenic women during pregnancy and puerperium: preliminary study. Psychiatry Clin Neurosci. 2007;61(6):665–71.

Jr Paffenbarger RS, Steinmetz CH, Pooler BG, Hyde RT. The picture puzzle of the postpartum psychoses. J Chronic Dis. 1961;13:161–73.

Penrose LS. A clinical and genetic study of 1280 cases of mental defect. Medical Research Council 1938: Special Report Number 229. London: H. M. Stationary Office; 1938.

Pharoah F, Mari J, Rathbone J, Wong W. Family intervention for schizophrenia. Cochrane Database of Systematic Reviews 2010;(12):CD000088.

Pinkofsky HB. Psychosis during pregnancy: treatment considerations. Ann Clin Psychiatry. 1995;9:175–9.

Reis M, Kallen B. Maternal use of antipsychotics in early pregnancy and delivery outcome. J Clin Psychopharmacol. 2008;28(3):279–88.

Reis M, Kallen B. Delivery outcome after maternal use of anidepssant drugs in pregnancy: an update using Swedish data. Psychol Med. 2010;40:1723–33.

Robinson D, Woerner MG, Alvir JM, Bilder R, Goldman R, Geisler S, et al. Predictors of relapse following response from a first episode of schizophrenia or schizoaffective disorder. Arch Gen Psychiatry. 1999;56:241–7.

Royal College of Physicians. Passive smoking and children: A report of the Tobacco Advisory Group of the Royal College of Physicians, Royal College of Physicians; 2010.

Sacker A, Done DJ, Crow TJ, Golding J. Antecedents of schizophrenia and affective illness. Obstetric complications. Br J Psychiatry. 1995;166:734–41.

Sameroff A, Seifer R, Zax M, Barocas R. Early indicators of developmental risk: Rochester Longitudinal Study. Schizophr Bull. 1987;13(3):383–94.

Shah N, Howard LM. Screening for smoking and substance misuse in pregnant women with mental illness. Psychiatr Bull. 2006;30:3.

SIGN. Scottish Intercollegiate Guidelines Network. Management of Perinatal Mood Disorders; 2012.

Sobel DE. Infant mortality and malformations in children of schizophrenic women. Psychiatr Q. 1961;35:60–4.

Thiels C. Pharmacotherapy of psychiatric disorder in pregnancy and during breastfeeding: a review. Pharmacopsychiatry. 1987;20(4):133–46.

Toh S, Li Q, Cheetham TC, Cooper WO, Davis RL, Dublin S, et al. Prevalence and trends in the use of antipsychotic medications during pregnancy in the U.S., 2001-2007: a population-based study of 585,615 deliveries. Arch Womens Ment Health. 2013;16(2):149–57.

Trevillion K, Oram S, Feder G, Howard LM. Experiences of domestic violence and mental disorders: a systematic review and meta-analysis. PLoS One. 2012;7(12):e51740.

Vigod SN, Seeman MV, Ray JG, Anderson GM, Dennis CL, Grigoriadis S, et al. Temporal trends in general and age-specific fertility rates among women with schizophrenia(1996-2009): a population-based study in Ontario, Canada. Schizophr Res. 2012;139(1–3):169–75.

Wan MW, Salmon MP, Riordan DM, Appleby L, Webb R, Abel KM. What predicts poor mother-infant interaction in schizophrenia? Psychol Med. 2007;37(4):537–46.

Wan MW, Abel KM, Green J. The transmission of risk to children from mothers with schizophrenia: a developmental psychopathology model. Clin Psychol Rev. 2008a;28(4):613–37.

Wan MW, Moulton S, Abel KM. A review of mother-child relational interventions and their usefulness for mothers with schizophrenia. Arch Womens Ment Health. 2008b;11(3):171–9.

Webb RT, Howard L, Abel KM. Antipsychotic drugs for non-affective psychosis during pregnancy and postpartum. Cochrane Database of Systematic Reviews. 2004;(2):CD004411.

Webb RT, Abel KM, Pickles AR, Appleby L. Mortality in offspring of parents with psychotic disorders: a critical review and meta-analysis. Am J Psychiatry. 2005;162(6):1045–56.

Webb RT, Abel KM, Pickles AR, Appleby L, King-Hele SA, Mortensen PB. Mortality risk among offspring of psychiatric inpatients: a population-based follow-up to early adulthood. Am J Psychiatry. 2006;163(12):2170–7.

Webb RT, Pickles AR, King-Hele SA, Appleby L, Mortensen PB, Abel KM. Parental mental illness and fatal birth defects in a national birth cohort. Psychol Med. 2008;38(10):1495–503.

Webb RT, Wicks S, Dalman C, Pickles AR, Appleby L, Mortensen PB, et al. Influence of environmental factors in higher risk of sudden infant death syndrome linked with parental mental illness. Arch Gen Psychiatry. 2010;67(1):69–77.

Wiersma D, Nienhuis FJ, Slooff CJ, Giel R. Natural course of schizophrenic disorders: a 15-year follow up of a Dutch incidence cohort. Schizophr Bull. 1998;24:75–85.

Wiersma D, Wanderling J, Dragomirecka E, Ganev K, Harrison G, An Der Heiden W, et al. Social disability inschizophrenia: its development and prediction over 15 years in incidence cohorts in six European centres. Psychol Med. 2000;30:1155–67.

Wildgust HJ, Beary M. Are there modifiable risk factors which will reduce the excess mortality in schizophrenia? J Psychopharmacol. 2010;24(4 Suppl):37–50.

Wykes T, Huddy V, Cellard C, McGurk SR, Czobor P. A meta-analysis of cognitive remediation for schizophrenia: methodology and effect sizes. Am J Psychiatry. 2011;168(5):472–85.

Zornberg GL, Buka SL, Tsuang MT. PUB. Am J Psychiatry. 2000;157:196–202.

Postpartum Psychosis

10

Veerle Bergink and Steven A. Kushner

Abstract

Postpartum psychosis is a severe and potentially life-threatening disorder that warrants acute clinical intervention. The initial clinical evaluation for postpartum psychosis requires a thorough medical and psychiatric history, physical and neurological examination, and comprehensive laboratory analysis to exclude known organic causes for acute psychosis. Unfortunately, little is known about what interventions are most effective, as research has been very limited and no randomized trials have been performed. Antipsychotic medication, lithium, and ECT have been described in case series and are frequently used in clinical practice as treatment options for postpartum psychosis.

Prevention of postpartum psychosis is a major challenge for mental health practitioners and obstetricians. Recently, we have proposed distinct clinical treatment algorithms for women with bipolar disorder versus women with a history of psychosis limited to the postpartum period. In bipolar women, prophylaxis during pregnancy appears critically important for maintaining mood stability during pregnancy and postpartum. In contrast, we recommend initiating prophylactic treatment immediately postpartum in women with a history of psychosis limited to the postpartum period. Considering together the available phenomenological, epidemiological, and treatment outcome data, we believe that postpartum psychosis should not be considered as a primary psychotic disorder as its name might otherwise suggest, but rather as a diagnostically independent entity within the group of bipolar affective disorders.

Keywords

Bipolar disorder • Mood stabilizers • Postpartum psychosis • Pregnancy

V. Bergink (✉) • S.A. Kushner
Erasmus Medical Center, Department of Psychiatry, 's Gravendijkwal 230, 3000 CA Rotterdam, The Netherlands
e-mail: v.bergink@erasmusmc.nl

10.1   Epidemiology, Phenomenology and Diagnosis

After childbirth, women are vulnerable to the onset of serious psychiatric symptomatology. Women are approximately 22 times more likely to experience the onset of a manic or psychotic episode in the first month postpartum than at any other time in their lives. Postpartum psychosis is the most severe form of childbirth-related psychiatric illness. The prevalence of postpartum psychosis in the general population is estimated as 1–2 per 1,000 childbirths (Munk-Olsen et al. 2006).

In the majority of cases, the onset is rapid and within 2 weeks postpartum. The early symptoms include insomnia, mood fluctuation, and sometimes obsessive concerns regarding the newborn, followed by more severe symptoms such as delusions, hallucinations, disorganized behavior, and serious mood symptoms. The occurrence of these severe mood symptoms such as mania, depression, or a mixed state is very prominent in postpartum psychosis. Affective phenomenology seems to be a hallmark of the disease and is more prevalent in postpartum psychosis compared to non-postpartum psychosis. Apart from its prominent affective symptoms, postpartum psychosis is also notable for its curious delirium-like appearance. Women with postpartum psychosis sometimes exhibit atypical cognitive symptoms such as disorientation, confusion, perplexity, misrecognition of people, derealization, and depersonalization. Of note, there is a relatively low incidence of schizophrenia-like symptoms, such as "Schneiderian first-rank symptoms" (Spinelli 2009; Sit et al. 2006; Brockington et al. 1981). Together, given that postpartum psychosis is generally considered a mood disorder and not a primary psychotic disorder, the term postpartum *psychosis* is therefore somewhat misleading.

By far, the most important risk factors of postpartum psychosis are a history of bipolar disorder or a previous episode of postpartum psychosis. In either case, the risk of postpartum psychosis is estimated as 25–50 % following every (subsequent) delivery. A family history of postpartum psychosis or bipolar disorder is also a well-known risk factor. Several family studies have consistently reported familial aggregation of psychiatric (particularly affective) disorders in first-degree relatives of women with postpartum psychosis (Jones and Craddock 2007). Previous studies have suggested a number of demographic and clinical variables that may be associated with postpartum psychosis, such as primiparity and complications during delivery (Blackmore et al. 2006). Indeed, primiparity has been repeatedly observed as a significant covariate in modeling the risk factors for postpartum psychosis. However, a recent large population-based study in primiparous mothers without previous psychiatric hospitalization found no significant influence of delivery complications on the risk of postpartum psychosis (Valdimarsdottir et al. 2009). Furthermore, no significant evidence has ever implicated psychosocial factors.

Postpartum psychosis must be clearly differentiated from postpartum depression (Table 10.1). In particular, postpartum depression refers to a non-psychotic depressive episode that affects approximately 10 % of mothers after childbirth. Women with postpartum depression experience symptoms of misery, apathy, irritability, social isolation, anxiety, failure to cope, and guilt, which are likely to have an

Table 10.1 Mood symptoms and syndromes during the postpartum period

	Estimated incidence	Onset	Frequent symptoms	Management
Maternity "blues"	50 %	3–5 days postpartum	Emotional lability, moodswings, anxiety	Self-limited, emotional support
Postpartum depression	10 %	Variable window: during pregnancy up to 1 year postpartum	Low mood, feelings of guilt, impaired feelings of bonding with the child	Psychotherapy, antidepressant medication, mother–baby therapy
Postpartum psychosis[a]	0.1–0.2 %	Within 4 weeks postpartum (usually within 2 weeks)	Agitation, irritablility, euphoric mood, depression, delusions, hallucinations, confusion, cognitive symptoms	Hospitalization, medical workup, lithium, antipsychotics, ECT

[a]Including postpartum mania and postpartum depression with psychotic features

impact on a mother's relationship with her child. Like non-puerperal depression, this disease entity is highly heterogeneous: psychosocial risk factors, such as a poor social background, lack of support, and stressful life events, factor prominently in the risk and clinical manifestations. Postpartum depression has a markedly different onset from postpartum psychosis. The onset of postpartum depression is highly variable: often with symptoms during pregnancy (in almost half of the cases), as well as episodes of depression with their onset throughout the entire first year postpartum.

Although an early postpartum onset is typical for postpartum psychosis, prodromal symptoms of postpartum psychosis are sometimes difficult to distinguish from the normal, physiological maternity blues. About half of recently delivered mothers experience the maternity blues between day 3 and 5 postpartum. This term refers to the brief occurrence of dysphoria, irritability, and mood swings. In contrast to postpartum psychosis, the duration of maternity blues ranges from a few hours to a few days, and for which the more severe symptoms that define postpartum psychosis are entirely absent (Table 10.1).

Understandably, most studies and scientific reviews have focused on postpartum blues and depression. The relatively low incidence, the clinical severity, and diagnostic uncertainty regarding the proper classification of postpartum psychosis have all contributed to the paucity of research.

10.2 Diagnostic Classification of Postpartum Psychosis: A Brief History

One of the initial case reports of postpartum psychosis arose from the autobiographical work of Margery Kempe who delivered her first baby in the UK in 1393 (Staley and Kemp 2000). In brief, she described that she became gravely ill after delivery and called for a priest. The priest began to censure her before she could divulge her sins, and then left. Fearing eternal damnation, she fell into a delusional state, where she described seeing devils around her. Because she tried to throw herself out of the window and tried to bite through the veins in her wrist, her husband chained her in a storeroom. After 6 months, she saw Jesus sitting at her bedside; the effect was miraculous as she was suddenly sane. Later case reports from Germany, France, and the UK describe similar cases: women with an acute onset of severe affective psychosis immediately postpartum. Importantly, some of these case reports described women with multiple postpartum episodes but none outside the postpartum period, which suggested the existence of a specific postpartum disease. Over time, several names have been given to this postpartum disease, such as "mania lacteal", "amentia", "puerperal insanity", "puerperal psychosis", "puerperal mania", "dreamlike delirium", and finally "postpartum psychosis". Since the eighteenth century, postpartum psychosis has been widely appreciated as a severe disease, requiring acute intervention (Brockington 1996).

The first treatments described were cutting of hair, applying ice packs to the head, and/or application of leeches. In the nineteenth century, physicians focused on the control of excitement, guarding against suicide, and supportive management pending an expected spontaneous remission. Remarkably, current treatments of postpartum psychosis do not have a substantially improved empirical basis than the treatments over the last centuries (Doucet et al. 2010). Furthermore, in the second half of the twentieth century, the diagnostic category of "postpartum psychosis" was abolished: the prevailing view from experts in the field has been that postpartum psychoses are not specific and fall mainly within the bipolar spectrum.

Childbirth is considered a general stressor, which can trigger an attack of any kind of psychiatric illness. Accordingly, the widely used American psychiatric classification system (DSM-IV and DSM-V: Diagnostic Statistic Manual of Disease) does not have a specific category for postpartum psychosis.

Meanwhile in the UK, the British psychiatric classification system ICD-10 (International Classification of Disease) contains a specific section entitled "mental and behavioral disorders associated with the puerperium". Notably, however, the addendum to this section encourages a very cautious use of this category:

> Most experts in this field are of the opinion that a clinical picture of puerperal psychosis is so rarely (if ever) reliably distinguishable from affective disorder or schizophrenia that a special category is not justified. Any psychiatrist who is of the minority opinion that special postpartum psychoses do indeed exist may use this category, but should be aware of its real purpose.

Despite these serious warnings, and while the term "postpartum psychosis" is officially excommunicated, there is an undiminished interest from researchers to understand this phenomenon. In particular, over the last decades clinical research has focused intensely on the strong link with bipolar disorder.

10.3   Postpartum Psychosis and Bipolar Disorder

Women with a diagnosed bipolar disorder are at very high risk (25–50 %) for affective psychosis in the weeks following delivery (Viguera et al. 2011). Cross-sectional symptomatology, family history, and the longitudinal illness course all support the notion of a strong link to bipolar disorder. First, most studies have shown a preponderance of manic symptoms in postpartum psychosis. Further, family studies of patients with postpartum psychosis have consistently found the risk for bipolar disorder to be higher than the risk within the general population. Lastly, a widely held estimate is that after an incipient postpartum affective psychosis, a woman has between 35 and 65 % chance of developing a bipolar disorder (Chaudron and Pies 2003).

Although bipolar disorder is certainly an important risk factor for postpartum psychosis, a large proportion of postpartum psychosis patients have no history of prior manic or psychotic episodes (Oates 2003; Boyce and Barriball 2010). In our research, we have particularly focused on this group: patients with first-onset psychosis postpartum. First-onset postpartum psychosis has markedly different characteristics compared to postpartum psychosis in bipolar patients. Postpartum psychosis patients demonstrate a significantly delayed postpartum onset compared to postpartum relapses in bipolar patients. Further, and in contrast to bipolar patients, obstetric complications are not a risk factor for patients with psychosis limited to the postpartum period. Finally, with clinical treatment an overwhelming majority of patients experience a complete symptom remission within 3 months postpartum. Together, our data contribute to the emerging consensus that women with a history of psychosis limited to the postpartum period might have a distinct variant of bipolar disorder (Bergink et al. 2011b).

10.4   Treatment

Postpartum psychosis is a psychiatric emergency that requires immediate medical attention and psychiatric referral. Inpatient psychiatric treatment is essential to ensure the safety of mother and baby. Within the UK, national guidelines (NICE) recommend that all women requiring postpartum admission are admitted with their infants to specialist Mother and Baby Units (MBU). There is some evidence that admission to an MBU is associated with improved satisfaction with care and reduced time to recovery.

The initial clinical evaluation for postpartum psychosis requires a thorough history, physical and neurological examination, and laboratory analysis to exclude known organic causes for acute psychosis. There are case reports on misdiagnosis of postpartum psychosis revealing a late-onset urea cycle disorder, paraneoplastic encephalitis, citrullinemia type I, and primary hypoparathyroidism. Differential diagnosis should further include infectious diseases, eclampsia, autoimmune diseases, metabolic diseases, vitamin deficiencies, stroke, and drug-induced psychosis (Sit et al. 2006). Therefore, tests should include a complete blood count, electrolytes, blood urea nitrogen, creatinine, calcium, liver function tests, thyroid function, and glucose. With proper indication, head CT or MRI, vitamins B1, B12, and folate, urinalysis, and urine drug screen should also be performed.

We showed that autoimmune thyroid disease is much more prevalent in women with first-onset postpartum psychosis (19 %) than in postpartum women from the general population (5 %). Furthermore, clinical thyroid failure occurs significantly faster and in a greater percentage of patients with postpartum psychosis. Therefore, screening for TPO antibodies, TSH, and fT4 is warranted in patients with postpartum psychosis (Bergink et al. 2011a).

Lastly, and perhaps most importantly, for any mother who presents with a postpartum mood disorder, the clinician must inquire about thoughts of harming herself or the infant. Delusional thoughts about harm to the infant or herself in postpartum psychosis are ego-syntonic and associated with psychotic belief. The urge to act on psychotic beliefs, combined with loss of reality testing, can quickly and easily lead to dangerous life-threatening situations.

10.5 Pharmacotherapy

Little is known about what interventions are most effective for patients with postpartum psychosis, as research has been very limited and no randomized trials have been performed. In total, only 21 treatment studies of postpartum psychosis can be found in the recent literature (Doucet et al. 2010). Sample sizes are very small: the majority is case reports describing a single patient and very few studies included more than ten patients.

The effects of hormones, propranolol, antipsychotics, lithium, and ECT were examined. Three studies conducted by the same group have found beneficial effects of estrogen (Ahokas et al. 2000). The potential beneficial use of progesterone and hormonal replacement therapy has been described through case reports (Boyce and Barriball 2010). Other case reports have provided support for propranolol (a beta-adrenergic blocker used to treat hypertension) as a treatment option for postpartum psychosis (Steiner et al. 1973).

Lithium and antipsychotic medication are commonly used in the treatment of postpartum psychosis. In our prospective cohort study, we report on the duration of episode while 51 patients received naturalistic treatment using the sequential addition of benzodiazepines, antipsychotics, and finally lithium. Our treatment algorithm was based on our clinical experience, guided by the larger literature for treatment of bipolar patients. Specifically, all patients were initially treated with benzodiazepines. For those patients without a marked improvement on benzodiazepine monotherapy, antipsychotic medication was initiated within the first week of admission. After 2 weeks of combination antipsychotic/benzodiazepine treatment, adjunctive lithium was initiated in those patients without a significant clinical response.

In our cohort, 47 of 51 patients achieved full remission prior to discharge. The median duration of episode, defined as onset (median day 8) until full remission of all affective, cognitive, and psychotic symptoms, was 40 days (Bergink et al. 2011b).

In earlier studies, lithium was found to be effective in one case study where it was used as monotherapy (Lichtenberg et al. 1988), and in two studies where it was used as adjunctive therapy (Silbermann et al. 1975; Targum et al. 1979). The effects of antipsychotics have been described in four case reports, for which treatment was reportedly successful on chlorpromazine, clozapine, and pimozide (Doucet et al. 2010).

A few studies have explored the influence of ECT in the treatment of PP (Focht and Kellner 2012). In one case study, treatment with chlorpromazine was ineffective, while ECT treatment led to remission (Stanworth 1982). Similarly, a case series of five women with treatment refractory PP described positive treatment outcomes with ECT (Forray and Ostroff 2007). Furthermore, a retrospective study compared the clinical responses to ECT of women with postpartum psychosis versus non-postpartum psychosis. Notably, the postpartum group was found to have greater clinical improvement following ECT compared to the non-postpartum group (Reed et al. 1999). Finally in a recent study, 34 women received successful ECT treatment and ECT was proposed as first-line treatment option (Babu et al. 2013).

Unfortunately, few treatment recommendations are available in the literature regarding the treatment of postpartum depression with psychotic features. According to DSM-IV criteria, postpartum depression with psychotic features does not constitute a bipolar depression. However, based on our clinical experience, we have followed the view that early-onset postpartum depression is likely to have a bipolar diathesis, particularly if psychotic features are present. Therefore, we followed the guidelines for treatment of bipolar II depression in patients with the acute onset of depression with psychotic features during the postpartum period, even in the absence of hypomanic symptoms immediately postpartum or of a history of hypomania (Bergink, Koorengevel 2010).

Of our patients ($n = 7$) diagnosed with a major depressive episode with psychotic features and an onset of symptoms within 4 weeks of the postpartum period, six women were treated with lithium and antipsychotics and one woman refused treatment. Except for one woman, all patients with depression had a complete remission with the combination of lithium and antipsychotics. The one patient who did not respond to treatment with lithium and antipsychotics received ECT, and her depression subsequently remitted (Bergink, Koorengevel 2010).

We do not know what would have happened if we had treated these seven women with antidepressants, but in our opinion antidepressant treatment could have put these patients at an unacceptable risk for exacerbation of symptoms. Similar to Sharma et al. (Sharma 2006); Sharma et al. 2009), we also have the clinical experience that antidepressants should be used cautiously in the postpartum period. Over the last 4 years, eight postpartum patients were referred to our clinic as a result of a very unstable illness course (manic and psychotic symptoms) after treatment with antidepressants in the absence of mood stabilization.

10.6   Mother–Infant Bonding

Interrupted development of a secure mother–infant bond can lead to long-term problems in a child's emotional, cognitive, and behavioral development (Murray et al. 2010). Importantly, severe postpartum psychiatric disorders, such as postpartum psychosis, represent a major challenge to maintaining the integrity of mother–infant bonding while symptoms persist. Two small studies have confirmed a deleterious influence of postpartum psychosis on mother–child bonding during the acute phase of the illness (Chandra et al. 2006; Hornstein et al. 2007). Remarkably, however, a recent study from our group demonstrated that women with a postpartum psychosis, in contrast to postpartum depression, experience few difficulties in establishing a healthy bond with their child after discharge from the hospital (Noorlander et al. 2008). Therefore, a more comprehensive series of studies is required to define optimal treatment algorithms for specific postpartum psychiatric disorders based upon empirical evidence and long-term outcomes.

10.7   Prevention of Subsequent Episodes

The strongest predictors for postpartum psychosis are a history of bipolar disorder and/or postpartum psychosis (Munk-Olsen et al. 2009; Doucet et al. 2010; Chaudron and Pies 2003). Consequently, guiding women at high risk for psychosis through pregnancy and the postpartum period is a major challenge for mental health practitioners and obstetricians (Cohen 2007; Viguera et al. 2002; Yonkers et al. 2004; Galbally et al. 2010), for which safe and effective relapse prevention would be the optimal strategy.

Six studies have assessed the efficacy of various prophylactic treatments for prevention of postpartum psychosis in bipolar patients: lithium (three studies) (Stewart et al. 1991; Cohen et al. 1995; Austin 1992), estrogen, valproate, and olanzapine (Kumar et al. 2003; Wisner et al. 2004; Sharma et al. 2006). In all 3 studies using lithium, bipolar women receiving prophylactic treatment had significantly lower rates of postpartum psychosis. In contrast, both estrogen and valproate failed to demonstrate significant prophylactic benefits. Olanzapine prophylaxis was equivocal and therefore warrants further investigation. Notably, a major limitation of these studies was that they included both women who initiated prophylaxis during pregnancy and postpartum, without differentiating between these groups. However, the timing of onset for pharmacological prophylaxis is of paramount clinical importance given that the benefits of prophylaxis during pregnancy need to be carefully weighed against the risks for the fetus (Burt, et al. 2010).

In our recent work, we evaluated the outcome of lithium prophylaxis during pregnancy, compared to immediately postpartum, in 70 women at high risk for postpartum psychosis using standardized clinical guidelines (Bergink et al. 2012). Specifically, we have investigated relapse rates both during pregnancy and in the postpartum period for 41 women with bipolar disorder and 29 women with a history of postpartum psychosis. Women with postpartum psychosis, compared to those with bipolar disorder, had a substantial difference in their clinical outcomes and prophylaxis requirements.

Notably, all women with a history of psychosis limited to the postpartum period were stable throughout their entire pregnancy despite using no prophylactic medication. In contrast, women with bipolar disorder had high rates of relapse during pregnancy. Furthermore, initiation of prophylaxis using either lithium or antipsychotics immediately postpartum in women with a history of psychosis limited to the postpartum period was highly effective for preventing postpartum relapse. In contrast, the efficacy of postpartum prophylaxis in women with bipolar disorder was much lower. During the postpartum period, relapse was highest in women with bipolar disorder who experienced mood episodes during pregnancy.

Therefore, we have proposed distinct clinical treatment algorithms for women with bipolar disorder versus women with a history of psychosis limited to the postpartum period. In bipolar women, prophylaxis during pregnancy appears critically important for maintaining mood stability during pregnancy and to minimize the high risk of postpartum relapse. In contrast, we recommend initiating prophylactic treatment immediately postpartum in women with a history of psychosis limited to the postpartum period, offering an important clinical advantage by avoiding in utero fetal exposure to prophylactic medication.

Disclosure None of the authors report a competing interest.

References

Ahokas A, Aito M, Rimon R. Positive treatment effect of estradiol in postpartum psychosis: a pilot study. J Clin Psychiatry. 2000;61(3):166–9.

Austin MP. Puerperal affective psychosis: is there a case for lithium prophylaxis? Br J Psychiatry. 1992;161:692–4.

Babu GN, Thippeswamy H, Chandra PS. Use of electroconvulsive therapy (ECT) in postpartum psychosis—a naturalistic prospective study. Arch Womens Ment Health. 2013;16(3):247–51. doi:10.1007/s00737-013-0342-2.

Bergink V, Koorengevel KM. Postpartum depression with psychotic features. Am J Psychiatry. 2010;167(4):476–7; author reply 477. doi:10.1176/appi.ajp.2009.09111655. 167/4/476-a [pii]

Bergink V, Kushner SA, Pop V, Kuijpens H, Lambregtse-van den Berg MP, Drexhage RC, et al. Prevalence of autoimmune thyroid dysfunction in postpartum psychosis. Br J Psychiatry. 2011a;198(4):264–8. doi:10.1192/bjp.bp.110.082990.

Bergink V, den Berg MP L, Koorengevel KM, Kupka R, Kushner SA. First-onset psychosis occurring in the postpartum period: a prospective cohort study. J Clin Psychiatry. 2011b;72 (11):1531–7. doi:10.4088/JCP.10m06648.

Bergink V, Bouvy PF, Vervoort JS, Koorengevel KM, Steegers EA, Kushner SA. Prevention of postpartum psychosis and mania in women at high risk. Am J Psychiatry. 2012;169(6):609–15. doi:10.1176/appi.ajp.2012.11071047.

Blackmore ER, Jones I, Doshi M, Haque S, Holder R, Brockington I, et al. Obstetric variables associated with bipolar affective puerperal psychosis. Br J Psychiatry. 2006;188:32–6. doi:10.1192/bjp.188.1.32. 188/1/32 [pii].

Boyce P, Barriball E. Puerperal psychosis. Arch Womens Ment Health. 2010;13(1):45–7. doi:10.1007/s00737-009-0117-y.

Brockington I. Motherhood and mental health. Oxford: Oxford University Press; 1996.

Brockington IF, Cernik KF, Schofield EM, Downing AR, Francis AF, Keelan C. Puerperal psychosis. Phenomena and diagnosis. Arch Gen Psychiatry. 1981;38(7):829–33.

Burt VK, Bernstein C, Rosenstein WS, Altshuler LL. Bipolar disorder and pregnancy: maintaining psychiatric stability in the real world of obstetric and psychiatric complications. Am J Psychiatry. 2010;167(8):892–7. doi:10.1176/appi.ajp.2009.09081248. 167/8/892 [pii].

Chandra PS, Bhargavaraman RP, Raghunandan VN, Shaligram D. Delusions related to infant and their association with mother-infant interactions in postpartum psychotic disorders. Arch Womens Ment Health. 2006;9(5):285–8. doi:10.1007/s00737-006-0147-7.

Chaudron LH, Pies RW. The relationship between postpartum psychosis and bipolar disorder: a review. J Clin Psychiatry. 2003;64(11):1284–92.

Cohen LS. Treatment of bipolar disorder during pregnancy. J Clin Psychiatry. 2007;68 Suppl 9:4–9.

Cohen LS, Sichel DA, Robertson LM, Heckscher E, Rosenbaum JF. Postpartum prophylaxis for women with bipolar disorder. Am J Psychiatry. 1995;152(11):1641–5.

Doucet S, Jones I, Letourneau N, Dennis CL, Blackmore ER. Interventions for the prevention and treatment of postpartum psychosis: a systematic review. Arch Womens Ment Health. 2010. doi:10.1007/s00737-010-0199-6.

Focht A, Kellner CH. Electroconvulsive therapy (ECT) in the treatment of postpartum psychosis. J ECT. 2012;28(1):31–3. doi:10.1097/YCT.0b013e3182315aa8.

Forray A, Ostroff RB. The use of electroconvulsive therapy in postpartum affective disorders. J ECT. 2007;23(3):188–93. doi:10.1097/yct.0b013e318074e4b1. 00124509-200709000-00014 [pii].

Galbally M, Snellen M, Walker S, Permezel M. Management of antipsychotic and mood stabilizer medication in pregnancy: recommendations for antenatal care. Aust N Z J Psychiatry. 2010;44 (2):99–108. doi:10.3109/00048670903487217.

Hornstein C, Trautmann-Villalba P, Hohm E, Rave E, Wortmann-Fleischer S, Schwarz M. Interactional therapy program for mothers with postpartum mental disorders. First results of a pilot project. Nervenarzt. 2007;78(6):679–84.

Jones I, Craddock N. Searching for the puerperal trigger: molecular genetic studies of bipolar affective puerperal psychosis. Psychopharmacol Bull. 2007;40(2):115–28.

Kumar C, McIvor RJ, Davies T, Brown N, Papadopoulos A, Wieck A, et al. Estrogen administration does not reduce the rate of recurrence of affective psychosis after childbirth. J Clin Psychiatry. 2003;64(2):112–8.

Lichtenberg P, Navon R, Wertman E, Dasberg H, Lerer B. Post-partum psychosis in adult GM2 gangliosidosis. A case report. Br J Psychiatry. 1988;153:387–9.

Munk-Olsen T, Laursen TM, Pedersen CB, Mors O, Mortensen PB. New parents and mental disorders: a population-based register study. JAMA. 2006;296(21):2582–9. doi:10.1001/jama. 296.21.2582. 296/21/2582 [pii].

Munk-Olsen T, Laursen TM, Mendelson T, Pedersen CB, Mors O, Mortensen PB. Risks and predictors of readmission for a mental disorder during the postpartum period. Arch Gen Psychiatry. 2009;66(2):189–95. doi:10.1001/archgenpsychiatry.2008.528. 66/2/189 [pii].

Murray L, Arteche A, Fearon P, Halligan S, Croudace T, Cooper P. The effects of maternal postnatal depression and child sex on academic performance at age 16 years: a developmental approach. J Child Psychol Psychiatry. 2010;51(10):1150–9. doi:10.1111/j.1469-7610.2010. 02259.x.

Noorlander Y, Bergink V, van den Berg MP. Perceived and observed mother-child interaction at time of hospitalization and release in postpartum depression and psychosis. Arch Womens Ment Health. 2008;11(1):49–56. doi:10.1007/s00737-008-0217-0.

Oates M. Perinatal psychiatric disorders: a leading cause of maternal morbidity and mortality. Br Med Bull. 2003;67:219–29.

Reed P, Sermin N, Appleby L, Faragher B. A comparison of clinical response to electroconvulsive therapy in puerperal and non-puerperal psychoses. J Affect Disord. 1999;54(3):255–60. S0165-0327(99)00012-9 [pii].

Sharma V. A cautionary note on the use of antidepressants in postpartum depression. Bipolar Disord. 2006;8(4):411–4. doi:10.1111/j.1399-5618.2006.00336.x. BDI336 [pii].

Sharma V, Smith A, Mazmanian D. Olanzapine in the prevention of postpartum psychosis and mood episodes in bipolar disorder. Bipolar Disord. 2006;8(4):400–4. doi:10.1111/j.1399-5618. 2006.00335.x. BDI335 [pii].

Sharma V, Burt VK, Ritchie HL. Bipolar II postpartum depression: detection, diagnosis, and treatment. Am J Psychiatry. 2009;166(11):1217–21. doi:10.1176/appi.ajp.2009.08121902. 166/11/1217 [pii].

Silbermann RM, Beenen F, de Jong H. Clinical treatment of post partum delirium with perfenazine and lithium carbonate. Psychiatr Clin (Basel). 1975;8(6):314–26.

Sit D, Rothschild AJ, Wisner KL. A review of postpartum psychosis. J Womens Health (Larchmt). 2006;15(4):352–68. doi:10.1089/jwh.2006.15.352.

Spinelli MG. Postpartum psychosis: detection of risk and management. Am J Psychiatry. 2009;166 (4):405–8. doi:10.1176/appi.ajp.2008.08121899. 166/4/405 [pii].

Staley L, Kemp M. The book of Margery Kemp. New York, NY: W.W. Norton; 2000.

Stanworth HM. After-care of puerperal psychosis in the community. Nurs Times. 1982;78 (22):922–5.

Steiner M, Latz A, Blum I, Atsmon A, Wijsenbeek H. Propranolol versus chlorpromazine in the treatment of psychoses associated with childbearing. Psychiatr Neurol Neurochir. 1973;76 (6):421–6.

Stewart DE, Klompenhouwer JL, Kendell RE, van Hulst AM. Prophylactic lithium in puerperal psychosis. The experience of three centres. Br J Psychiatry. 1991;158:393–7.

Targum SD, Davenport YB, Webster MJ. Postpartum mania in bipolar manic-depressive patients withdrawn from lithium carbonate. J Nerv Ment Dis. 1979;167(9):572–4.

Valdimarsdottir U, Hultman CM, Harlow B, Cnattingius S, Sparen P. Psychotic illness in first-time mothers with no previous psychiatric hospitalizations: a population-based study. PLoS Med. 2009;6(2):e13. doi:10.1371/journal.pmed.1000013. 06-PLME-RA-0854 [pii].

Viguera AC, Cohen LS, Bouffard S, Whitfield TH, Baldessarini RJ. Reproductive decisions by women with bipolar disorder after prepregnancy psychiatric consultation. Am J Psychiatry. 2002;159(12):2102–4.

Viguera AC, Tondo L, Koukopoulos AE, Reginaldi D, Lepri B, Baldessarini RJ. Episodes of mood disorders in 2,252 pregnancies and postpartum periods. Am J Psychiatry. 2011;168(11):1179–85. doi:10.1176/appi.ajp.2011.11010148. appi.ajp.2011.11010148 [pii].

Wisner KL, Hanusa BH, Peindl KS, Perel JM. Prevention of postpartum episodes in women with bipolar disorder. Biol Psychiatry. 2004;56(8):592–6. doi:10.1016/j.biopsych.2004.07.022. S0006-3223(04)00856-X [pii].

Yonkers KA, Wisner KL, Stowe Z, Leibenluft E, Cohen L, Miller L, et al. Management of bipolar disorder during pregnancy and the postpartum period. Am J Psychiatry. 2004;161(4):608–20.

Borderline Personality Disorder and the Eating Disorders in the Perinatal Period

11

Gaynor Blankley, Josephine Power, and Andrew Chanen

Abstract

Borderline Personality Disorder and the Eating Disorders are severe disorders that are associated with significant psychiatric and physical co-morbidity. Yet, there is limited research to draw upon regarding the natural history and risks associated with these disorders across pregnancy and the postnatal period. The risks to the mother and the infant of these conditions and their treatments require careful consideration and patients require individualised clinical care.

Keywords

Borderline Personality Disorder • Eating disorders • Perinatal • Psychopharmacological management

11.1 Borderline Personality Disorder

11.1.1 Brief Overview of Borderline Personality Disorder

Borderline Personality Disorder (BPD) is a severe mental disorder that is characterised by a pervasive pattern of impulsivity, emotional instability, interpersonal dysfunction, and disturbed self-image (Leichsenring et al. 2011), affecting 0.7–2.7 % of the general adult population (Coid et al. 2006; Trull et al. 2010), 9.3–22.5 % of psychiatric outpatients, and in some settings over 40 % of inpatients (Zimmerman et al. 2008). The outcome for BPD in American adults is now reliably

G. Blankley (✉) • J. Power
Mercy Hospital for Women, Heidelberg, Australia
e-mail: gblankley@mercy.com.au

A. Chanen
Orygen Youth Health Research Centre, Centre for Youth Mental Health, The University of Melbourne, Melbourne, Australia

Orygen Youth Health Clinical Program, Northwestern Mental Health, Melbourne, Australia

M. Galbally et al. (eds.), *Psychopharmacology and Pregnancy*,
DOI 10.1007/978-3-642-54562-7_11, © Springer-Verlag Berlin Heidelberg 2014

characterised by attenuation of diagnostic criteria over time, with severe and continuing functional disability across a broad range of domains that is comparable to, or greater than, that associated with many mental state disorders (Gunderson et al. 2011; Zanarini et al. 2010). Patients with BPD also have continuing high rates of co-occurring conditions (Zanarini et al. 2004a), health service utilisation (Zanarini et al. 2004b; Horz et al 2010; Sansone et al. 2011), and a suicide rate of around 8 % (Pompili et al. 2005). Although effective interventions exist for adults with BPD (e.g. Bateman and Fonagy 2009; Giesen-Bloo et al. 2006; Linehan et al. 2006), the overall outcomes from such interventions are modest and their availability is limited.

BPD appears to arise from the interaction of biological and environmental risk and protective factors, but the developmental pathways remain unclear. Findings from prospective longitudinal studies of community samples and studies of young people with borderline pathology suggest a variety of genetic, neurobiological, psychopathological, and environmental risk factors (Chanen and Kaess 2012). However, these risk factors are common to other mental disorders and are generally not specific for BPD (Chanen and McCutcheon 2013).

Temperamental and mental state abnormalities that resemble aspects of the BPD phenotype emerge in childhood and adolescence and presage the BPD syndrome in adolescence or adulthood (Chanen and McCutcheon 2013). However, it is usually first identifiable during adolescence to early adulthood, which corresponds to the years when women are most fertile (De Genna et al. 2012).

11.1.2 Natural History of BPD in the Perinatal Period

Individuals with BPD are more likely to experience exacerbation of symptoms at times of interpersonal stress (Zanarini et al. 1997). Given that pregnancy and early parenthood are times of transition and for many a developmental crises (Cohen and Slade 2000), it could be expected that women with BPD might be more vulnerable to an exacerbation of mental health issues during these times. However, there are few studies that describe or quantify the mental health, obstetric, and early infant outcomes for women with this diagnosis across pregnancy and the postpartum period. There is some evidence that women with BPD might be less likely to have used contraception and to have teenage and unplanned pregnancies (Chen et al. 2007; De Genna et al. 2011, 2012) and sexually transmitted infections (Chanen et al. 2007): factors that might contribute to an exacerbation of symptoms in the perinatal period.

Developmental trauma, including childhood sexual abuse, is common among women with BPD (Zanarini et al. 1997), and childbirth and parenting may reactivate past traumas for this group of women, such that they might be unable to focus and think about their new baby and its experiences and needs (Newman 2008). Shame and guilt-proneness is generally high among women with BPD (Rusch et al. 2007). These women frequently describe feelings such as anxiety, shame, ambivalence, loss of identity, depression, anger, and emptiness in the perinatal period and might struggle with their parenting, feel less satisfied, experience higher levels of parenting stress, and have difficulty with affect regulation and recognition of their infant's cues (Newman and Stevenson 2005; Newman et al. 2007).

Currently there is only one guideline published for the management of BPD in the perinatal period (Government of South Australia, Maternity Care Guidelines 2006), which is based on clinical opinion, with no data available on the evaluation of its implementation. Issues described included the need to be aware of the risks for both mother and foetus, frequent requests for early delivery and issues associated with polypharmacy. However, the guidelines are for the management of patients with BPD as they access care within the maternity care setting and are not comprehensive guidelines for the management of BPD in the perinatal period.

11.1.3 Summary of Evidence for Treatment Improving the Course and Outcome of BPD

The most recently published national guidelines for BPD are the Clinical Practice Guidelines for the Management of BPD, developed by the Australian Government's National Health and Medical Research Council (NHMRC) (National Health and Medical Research Council 2012). This systematic literature review supports interventions for people with BPD and found that the characteristics of effective treatments involved treatment that was founded on an explicit theory of BPD, delivered by an appropriately trained and supervised therapist regularly over a planned treatment course, whilst attending to the patient's emotional state and focused on achieving change and the relationship between the clinician and the patient. It was further recommended that pharmacotherapy should not be routinely added to psychological interventions. They concluded that there is insufficient evidence to support that any one specific treatment has advantages over another in improving the outcomes for patients with BPD in the long term and that further research is required to clarify this.

11.1.4 Risks of Not Treating BPD

Whist there is evidence that a diagnosis of BPD carries significant risks for physical and psychiatric co-morbidity, including Substance Use Disorders (Zanarini et al. 2004b), risk of impulsive and risk taking behaviour, deliberate self-harm, suicide attempts, and suicide, all of which have known risks for mothers and infants across the perinatal period, there is no evidence currently that this diagnosis carries specific risks for the pregnancy or the foetus. However, there are risks associated with *treating* BPD, including the risks of polypharmacy, which in pregnancy would expose the unborn infant unnecessarily to medications that are unlikely to be helpful to the mother.

11.1.5 Specific Pharmacological Treatment Options for BPD

Whilst there is no specific pharmacological treatment for BPD, polypharmacy is common (Zanarini et al. 2004a, b). The NH&MRC (2012) reviewed the evidence basis for the pharmacological treatments for BPD including a meta-analysis of RCTs for pharmacotherapy versus placebo. They found the studies to be difficult to interpret because of the small sample sizes and the different outcome measures across studies. They concluded that pharmacotherapy did not alter the course or outcome of BPD. Furthermore, they determined that specific recommendations could not be made about the use of a particular medication to target specific symptoms when less than 3 RCTs were available for the meta-analysis.

They found that SSRIs may have some effect on mood symptoms, but that they also needed to be prescribed with caution because overall they were less efficacious in treating depression in patients with BPD and they have potentially harmful side effects such as an increase in suicidal ideation, especially in patients under 25 years of age. Lithium was reviewed in four studies with findings that it had some benefits for mood symptoms and anger. Sodium valproate was found to help with mood symptoms, anger, aggression, and impulsivity, and lamotrigine and topiramate were found to have some benefits for impulsivity, mood lability, and anger. Antipsychotic medications were found to have been prescribed for cognitive and perceptual abnormalities, dysphoria, anxiety, anger, and depressive symptoms. Olanzapine was found to provide some benefits for the management of hostility, irritability, general psychopathology, and general functioning. Ariprazole was found in one study to be beneficial for anger, hostility, irritability, anxiety, depression, and interpersonal functioning, and quetiapine has been reported to provide benefits for affective symptoms and impulsivity.

However, it must be stressed that the findings from these studies are insufficient to recommend the routine or common use of psychotropic medications in BPD. Moreover, many of the agents studied pose significant risks to the developing foetus. The findings must be replicated before any of these medications are adopted and prescribed as 'mainstay' treatments.

The NHMRC (2012) recommendations are summarised below.

1. Medication should not be used as the primary therapy for BPD.
2. Time limited use of medication can be considered as an adjunct to a structured psychological therapy for specific symptoms.
3. Caution should be taken when prescribing medications as they may be lethal and there is a high risk of suicide in patients with BPD.
4. Caution should be taken if prescribing medication in patients with associated substance abuse.
5. Before prescribing: ensure that the medication is not being used in place of more appropriate interventions, that the psychological role of prescribing

(continued)

(including the impact it may have on the therapeutic relationship) is considered, and that single medication is recommended and polypharmacy avoided wherever possible. Once these risks have been considered, and collaboration established between all health-care providers, it needs to be determined whom the prescriber will be.

6. If medications are used in crises they should be withdrawn as soon as the crisis is resolved.

There is no evidence available to support the prescribing of benzodiazepines to patients with BPD, and as a class they are associated with issues of abuse and dependence, and in pregnancy they should be prescribed sparingly.

Prescribing for BPD in pregnancy

Given the lack of data to support the effectiveness of pharmacological treatments in patients with BPD clinicians should have an even higher threshold for prescribing during pregnancy and wherever possible avoided. There is insufficient evidence available to develop concise prescribing guidelines for patients with BPD. In addition, prescribing medication may result in a missed opportunity to engage the patient in an effective structured psychosocial treatment plan. If a decision is made to prescribe medications during pregnancy the risks of individual medications, both known and unknown, including teratogenic risks, risks during pregnancy, delivery and the postpartum period, risks for the newborn, and longer term risks for neurobehavioral development should be clearly discussed with the patient and documented.

11.1.6 Management Recommendations for BPD in the Perinatal Period

Management of BPD requires structured psychosocial interventions that are based upon a theory of BPD and delivered by appropriately trained and supervised clinical staff. This might occur intermittently or on a continuous basis, depending upon the patient's needs. During the perinatal period, it is appropriate to follow recommendations of the NH&MRC's recent guidelines (2012). Wherever possible management should include:

Preconception: Sexual and Reproductive Health

Sexual and reproductive health should be a focus of management for all women of childbearing age with BPD. As already noted, impulsivity may result in unsafe sex and unplanned pregnancies, many of which may remain undiagnosed well into the first trimester (Chanen et al. 2007; De Genna et al. 2011, 2012; Chen et al. 2007; Henshaw and Protti 2010). Thus, it is ideal for female patients in their reproductive years to be referred to their general practitioner or family planning clinic for consultation regarding the management of their sexual and reproductive health and the risks associated with unplanned or planned pregnancy. Consideration should be given to a second opinion from a specialist perinatal psychiatrist when psychotropic medications are prescribed in pregnancy. Specific liaison with the patient's general practitioner or gynaecologist about the patient's anxieties accessing health care may be required.

If a woman with a pre-existing diagnosis of BPD is planning a pregnancy, then a discussion about the impact of pregnancy and parenting on her mental health and the impact that treatments may have on her unborn infant should be undertaken. Management options and their associated risks and benefits should also be discussed. Wherever possible, the partner/father of the baby should be involved in discussions.

Pregnancy may be the first time a patient presents for mental health assessment and therefore assessment and management may only begin at this time.

Management During Pregnancy

A comprehensive clinical assessment, diagnosis, and formulation including co-morbid psychiatric diagnoses, co-existing medical and obstetric conditions, assessment of the foetus, and the relationship developing between the mother and her infant should be undertaken during pregnancy. Management planning should include an understanding of the effect of pregnancy and parenting on the woman's mental illness and its treatment and the impact that the illness and its treatment will have on the pregnancy, foetus, and neonate. The particular physical, psychological, social, and relationship changes associated with pregnancy need to be considered (Galbally et al. 2013). Particular attention should be paid to how anxiety, 'affective storms', impulsivity, suicidality, idealisation, and/or devaluation of the unborn infant as well as staff, family, and friends caring for her may affect maternal and infant care and how this can be best managed. The antenatal period may provide a good opportunity, and possibly an incentive, to provide supportive psychoeducation and preparatory psychotherapy for parenthood.

In more severe BPD, multiple health providers and agencies may be involved in patient care and there is a risk that there may be a lack of coordination between care providers. Staff may experience difficulties caring for patients with BPD, including powerful countertransference feelings, which might affect care decisions. It is recommended that a management plan be developed in collaboration with the patient and as many health professionals as possible, relevant to the patient's care and that particular attention be paid to communication among these professionals.

The following specific issues as they arise within the obstetric care setting may require attention:

1. Identify particular sources of distress for the patient being triggered by pregnancy (e.g. shame, ambivalence, feelings of dependence, relationship issues, family of origin issues, re-arousal of memories of developmental trauma, and fears about giving birth).
2. Provide education about the need for appropriate antenatal care whilst encouraging engagement and consider whether assertive outreach is necessary for this to occur (e.g. by a case manager or community midwife) and that specific monitoring recommendations are adhered to.
3. Identify and list the names and contact details of those involved in the patient's care and their management role. Encourage communication between maternity and mental health-care providers and provide education about BPD to all professionals involved.
4. If medication is to be prescribed during pregnancy follow the principles described above.
5. Clarify safety plans including the specifics of who is to be contacted and strategies that are helpful at times of crisis.
6. Consider the safest mode of delivery for mother and infant including who will be in attendance at delivery.
7. Recommend an antenatal paediatric consultation where it is clinically relevant.
8. Recommend a referral to social work for planning around accommodation, income, and parenting support services, etc.
9. Develop a perinatal mental health-care plan as described that includes recommendations for the mother and her infant.

As pregnancy progresses, management plans should be reviewed, updated (in collaboration with the patient), and circulated to all relevant clinicians and kept in the patient's obstetric file.

Throughout pregnancy, attention also needs to be given to the developing foetus. Specific issues include:

1. Risks to the unborn infant associated with the presence of co-morbid illness and medications prescribed need to be considered and the monitoring requirements recommended for the medications prescribed should be adhered to.
2. Consideration should be given to the developing mother–infant relationship, in particular the mother's capacity to consider the needs of her unborn infant and what psychiatric and psychosocial interventions may be required antenatally and postnatally.
3. Recommendations about appropriate parenting supports, including the possibility of making an unborn infant protective notification if required.
4. Referral to a paediatrician antenatally should be recommended where indicated clinically.

Longer term treatment options, as outlined in the NHMRC guidelines, should also be discussed with the patient, and wherever possible, liaison between health-care providers involved in the patients' longer term care and those involved in perinatal care should occur.

11.2 Eating Disorders

11.2.1 Brief Overview of the Key Features of the Eating Disorders

Eating disorders (EDs) are severe psychiatric illnesses that are most common in women of childbearing age. Anorexia nervosa (AN) and bulimia nervosa (BN) are the two eating disorders specified in the DSM-IV; however, the most common diagnosis in clinical and community samples is the residual category 'eating disorder not otherwise specified' (EDNOS) (Smink et al. 2012). EDNOS is a poorly defined group in the DSM-IV that includes partial syndromes of AN and/or BN, purging disorder, and binge eating disorder (BED). The DSM-V contains a revised ED section with broadening of existing criteria and includes BED as a separate diagnosis (APA 2013), but hitherto research has been hampered by a lack of clear or consensus criteria. All EDs have serious physical, emotional, psychological, and social sequelae that greatly impact on pregnancy, transition to motherhood, and parenting.

AN mostly affects young women with 40 % of incident cases being girls aged 15–19 (Smink et al. 2012). It has a prevalence of 1.9–4.3 % depending on the population studied and criteria used (Wade et al. 2006). It is characterised by an intense fear of weight gain, disordered body image, and refusal to maintain normal weight through rigorous exercise, restricted eating, and sometimes bingeing and purging. Amenorrhea, either primary or secondary, may be present as a consequence of starvation and hormonal imbalance.

Psychiatric co-morbidities are common in AN, with depression present in 65 %, social phobia in 34 %, and OCD in 26 %. Medical co-morbidities are almost ubiquitous, with every major organ system potentially affected. AN has the highest rate of mortality among all mental disorders (Harris and Barraclough 1998) with a crude mortality rate of 0.51 % per year. In one study, one in five deaths was due to suicide (Arcelus et al. 2011). The natural history is of recovery in a third of patients, chronic relapsing and remitting illness in another third, and severe illness leading to premature death for the remainder.

BN has a mean age of onset at 17 years (Hoek and van Hoeken 2003) and a point prevalence of 1 % in young females (Keski-Rahkonen et al. 2009). It is characterised by episodes of binge eating during which there is a sense of loss of control over the amount and type of food eaten. Binges are typically followed by feelings of self-loathing, guilt, and disgust, with consequent frantic compensatory behaviour to reduce the amount of weight gained by purging or using laxatives, diuretics, or enemas. Despite this, weight may be normal. Psychiatric co-morbidities are common with substance abuse and depression being found most frequently. The medical consequences include hormonal, oral, and gastrointestinal complications and electrolyte imbalances that may lead to cardiac arrhythmias and potentially death. Relapse–remission is the most common pattern of illness, but overall the prognosis is better than for AN. Remission rates of 74 % have been quoted, but this same sample showed 42 % relapse over the study period (Grilo et al. 2007).

Point prevalence of EDNOS is difficult to establish as there has been no consistent criteria for clinical diagnosis and research. BED, in which sufferers engage in binges with associated abnormal attitudes to food (APA 2013), has a lifetime prevalence of up to 10 % (Machado et al. 2007). Patients are usually obese, which leads to a range of other medical problems such as metabolic syndrome and cardiovascular disease. Studies suggest that it has a similar relapsing–remitting course to BN (Grilo et al. 2007).

11.2.2 Natural History of Eating Disorders in the Perinatal Period

Despite the significance of EDs in women of childbearing age, there has been limited research interest until recently. Early studies suggested that women with ED rarely became pregnant due to nutritional deficiency and hormone imbalance (Weinfeld et al. 1977). However, despite common menstrual irregularities, it would appear that fertility rates do not differ significantly from the general population (Kohmura et al. 1986; Bulik et al. 1999; Crow et al. 2002). In addition, women with AN may be more likely to have unplanned pregnancies (Bulik et al. 2010), potentially due to poor contraceptive advice based on the assumption of infertility. BN also appears to have little impact on later fertility (Crow et al. 2002). Studies are lacking in BED and fertility, but obesity is associated with reduced ability to conceive.

Most studies in this area are limited by being based on retrospective reports from clinical samples. The Norwegian Mother and Child Cohort Study is a large prospective population-based birth cohort study of 10,000 women (Bulik et al. 2007). It found that 0.1 % pregnant women met broad criteria for AN prior to pregnancy, 0.7 % reported BN, and 3.5 % reported BED. Rates of remission during pregnancy varied: 35 % BN remitted (higher in purging subtype) and 39 % BED with no data available for AN. Other studies have found remission of ED symptoms during pregnancy (Lacey and Smith 1987; Morgan et al. 1999), but only 23 % remain well postpartum and preoccupation with weight may recur acutely. Some women may deteriorate in comparison with pre-pregnancy symptoms (Morgan et al. 1999).

There is an increased rate of anxiety and depression in women with ED who become pregnant and fear of weight gain may lead to increased symptoms in pregnancy. When ED symptoms continue during pregnancy there is a higher risk of complications at all stages and into the postpartum period (Abraham 1998; Conti et al. 1998). A history of BN, active or not, raises the risk of hyperemesis, small head circumference, and SGA (Kouba et al. 2005), and active BN has been associated with lower birth weight, low Apgars, breech presentation, congenital malformations, smaller head circumference, miscarriage, gestational diabetes, and postpartum depression (Lacey and Smith 1987; Kouba et al. 2005; Mitchell et al. 1991; Franko et al. 2001; Morgan et al. 2006). Women with AN have higher rates of miscarriage and caesarean delivery (Bulik et al. 1999; Franko et al. 2001; Mitchell et al. 1991). Low pre-pregnancy weight and poor weight gain in pregnancy are associated with adverse outcomes such as stillbirth, IUGR, low Apgars, and breech presentation (Arbuckle and Sherman 1989; Wen et al. 1990), as well as congenital malformations such as cleft lip and palate. Intra-uterine growth retardation (IUGR) is itself associated with significant sequelae for the infant; in the short term there is a greater risk of neonatal asphyxia and neonatal adaptive problems such as meconium aspiration, pulmonary hypertension, failure of glucose regulation, and temperature instability necessitating increased medical attention and intervention (Rosenberg 2008). As the infant develops, there is an increased incidence of chronic lung disease, necrotising enterocolitis, and retinopathy with ongoing failure to thrive. Further-reaching consequences are still being investigated, but links have been established with IUGR and breast cancer risk and cardiovascular disease in adulthood (Kok et al. 1998; Michels et al. 1996; Rich-Edwards et al. 1997).

Women with BED and consequent obesity are at higher risk of miscarriage, thromboembolism, and pre-eclampsia (Yu et al. 2006). Obesity in pregnancy is a risk factor for gestational diabetes (Metzger et al. 2007). This in turn increases the risk of an infant being large for gestational age that has been linked to metabolic syndrome in childhood and future obesity (Boney et al. 2005). There is elevated perinatal mortality (Yu et al. 2006). Specific studies in this area are lacking.

Postpartum, the risk of depression is greater in women with ED (Abraham 1998). Even without depression, the physical disruption of ED symptoms may affect capacity to parent and interact with the infant. Ongoing ED symptoms may also increase the likelihood of marital instability and conflict, which further compromises the well-being of the child.

11.2.3 Summary of Evidence of Treatment Improving Eating Disorders

The 2006 APA guidelines recommend a combined approach including nutritional rehabilitation and psychological support for the management of AN and state that prescribing SSRIs to patients offers no advantage. For patients with severe resistance to weight gain the atypical antipsychotics may be useful for those with severe obsessional thinking and pro-motility agents may be useful for the treatment of abdominal pain and bloating. The SSRIs are recommended for the treatment of BN and BED.

Psychological interventions for EDs have been recommended for AN, BN, and EDNOS with Cognitive Behaviour Therapy (CBT) focusing on cognitive distortions and negative thinking patterns around body image and Interpersonal

Therapy (IPT) focusing on addressing interpersonal issues that are associated with ED symptoms rather than the symptoms themselves.

Yager et al. (2012) reviewed 342 articles that related to the evidence available supporting the key recommendations of the APA 2006 guidelines for the treatment of eating disorders. They found that there were few randomised controlled trials (RCTs) and that the studies available suffered from a range of methodological issues, such as small sample sizes, recruitment and retention issues, and poorly defined predictors of recovery across the different studies. However, their review supported hospital-based treatment in order to provide either tube feeding or nutritional rehabilitation in severely underweight patients with AN, but not in normal weight patients.

Whilst the theoretical underpinnings for psychological interventions appear sound, Yager et al. (2012) found that the research on psychotherapy for individuals with EDs was limited, with the methodology and outcome measures of studies being variable. They found some evidence that CBT and IPT are efficacious in the treatment of BN and that 'guided self-help' was more effective than being on a 'wait list' for treatment. Overall, they concluded that larger studies with more robust methodologies are required to substantiate evidence for the efficacy of psychotherapeutic treatments commonly prescribed.

11.2.4 Risks of Not Treating Eating Disorders in Pregnancy

Pregnancy is a time of great nutritional and metabolic strain on a woman's body, as well as a period of potentially intense emotional upheaval. With compromise of physical or emotional reserves, there may be serious consequences for both mother and infant if EDs are left untreated.

During pregnancy, the developing foetus derives all nutrition from the mother. If stores of energy in the form of carbohydrates, protein, and fat are inadequate, or reserves of vitamins and minerals are low, they will be drained to support the growing foetus. Without adequate nutritional replacement, malnutrition is a real risk and this in turn may lead to physical illness in the mother.

The required weight gain in pregnancy can be extremely threatening for women who have been preoccupied with their weight and this may lead to avoidance of medical and obstetric care. Some women may be able to view the weight gain as a necessary sacrifice, but others can enter a crisis of their eating symptoms or develop serious mood disorder symptoms.

Women with untreated AN tend to have low weight gain during pregnancy and are at higher risk of having a baby with IUGR and its consequences. If purging is ongoing, the risks of dehydration, electrolyte imbalance, and cardiac arrhythmias are exacerbated during pregnancy. Those women who are overweight are at increased risk of elevated blood pressure and gestational diabetes.

In the postpartum period, untreated ED symptoms may escalate in response to the physical changes of pregnancy or as a means of coping with loss of control and other difficulties faced during the transition to motherhood. These symptoms can be a distraction for the mother and reduce her availability and responsiveness to her infant. This may lead to a failure of the attachment and bonding process, with potentially disastrous, long-lasting effects. Furthermore, women with a history of ED are more likely to experience difficulties in feeding their babies (Park et al. 2003).

11.2.5 Specific Pharmacological Treatment Options for the Management of Eating Disorders

Flament et al. (2012) reviewed the evidence for the efficacy and safety of pharmacological agents prescribed to treat EDs. They found that no single medication is indicated for the treatment of AN, although antipsychotics, antidepressants, mood stabilisers, gastric motility agents, appetite stimulants, and bi-phosphonates have all been prescribed. Their review found that high doses of the antidepressant fluoxetine (60 mg) were effective in relapse prevention in weight-restored patients with AN in 50 % of studies. Olanzapine was found to demonstrate an adjunctive effect for the treatment of underweight patients with an increase in weight gain and a decrease in obsessive ruminations about body size.

Tricyclic antidepressants (TCAs), mono-amine oxidase inhibitors (MAOIs), and SSRIs have been trialled for treating BN, all with positive results in the reduction of symptoms of bingeing and purging as well as ruminating about body image. However, given the potential toxicity of MAOIs and TCAs, the SSRIs are recommended as first line treatment.

The mood stabiliser's and naltrexone have also been trialled for the treatment of AN and BN. However, given the potential for toxicity in patients who are already physically vulnerable, they are not recommended as part of treatment.

Eight RCTs were identified in which the SSRIs have been trialled for BED, with findings that they all resulted in a decrease in the frequency of bingeing.

Overall, there is insufficient evidence to provide the basis for developing prescribing guidelines for patients with EDs during the perinatal period. Prescribing needs to be considered in the context of each individual patient's clinical presentation and with a clear understanding between clinician and patient of the goals of the medication and the risks to her if that medication is not prescribed. The specific risks of these medications, with respect to any increased risk of malformation, pregnancy and obstetric risks, neonatal risks, and longer term risks must also be considered. Monitoring recommendations have been described in previous chapters.

11.2.6 Management Recommendations for the Eating Disorders during the Perinatal Period

All the eating disorders require long-term psychiatric and medical care. AN is characterised by marked denial of the illness and noncompliance with treatment

(McKnight and Park 2010), an issue that requires consideration during the perinatal period because of the additional risks of untreated illness on infant development. Management during the perinatal period should focus on encouraging appropriate weight gain/maintenance, monitoring for the particular medical, psychological, obstetric, and foetal growth and development issues that may emerge during this time. A multidisciplinary team approach is ideal, and wherever possible, consent should be obtained from the woman to enable close communication between herself, her partner/family (as appropriate), and all professionals involved in her care.

Preconception: Reproductive and Sexual Health

Women with EDs may have menstrual irregularities and may assume that they cannot conceive which can lead to inadequate use of contraception and the risk of an unplanned pregnancy. Thus a referral to the patient's GP or a family planning clinic should be considered in order to discuss reproductive health.

Pre conception planning should include:

1. A full discussion about the impact that the eating disorder may have on fertility and conception, early pregnancy loss, foetal growth, and development throughout pregnancy as well as the risks of deterioration in maternal physical and mental health as a result of the pregnancy.
2. Enquiry about substance use such as smoking and alcohol, as well as the use of drugs such as laxatives, diuretics, and appetite suppressants. Specific education about risks of use during pregnancy should be provided.
3. Specific education about body changes, weight gain, and cravings that may occur in pregnancy and the importance of healthy eating in order to enable the baby to grow and develop.
4. A full discussion about the medical and obstetric care, and monitoring that is recommended throughout pregnancy, to ensure optimal outcomes for mother and infant.
5. A referral to a dietician for pre-pregnancy education about the nutritional requirements required across pregnancy and the postpartum period with the aim of helping the woman gain a better understanding of her dietary requirements and to make specific plans for how to ensure her nutritional needs can be met and give her a sense of control over her situation. In addition, the nutritional and dietary supplements, especially zinc, folic acid, calcium, and protein that may be required preconception should be discussed.

Pregnancy

Whether pregnancy is the first time the patient presents for psychiatric assessment and management, or the patient is already engaged in active treatment, a comprehensive clinical assessment, diagnosis, and formulation including co-morbid psychiatric diagnoses, co-existing medical and obstetrical conditions, assessment of her unborn infant, and the relationship developing between the mother and her infant are essential.

Throughout pregnancy and the early postpartum period the severity of the ED should be monitored and liaison between the treating psychiatric, medical, and obstetric teams is essential in order to ensure that adequate monitoring of maternal and infant physical health occurs and that appropriate treatment can begin if required. Developing a management plan, together with the patient, which includes both short- and long-term management goals and plans, is recommended.

Specific issues that may require focus during the perinatal period include:

(a) Identifying particular sources of distress for the patient being triggered by pregnancy. In particular issues around weight gain in pregnancy and changes in body shape.
(b) Aiming to normalise weight gain in pregnancy and framing weight gain as 'healthy growth of the baby'. Monitoring of weight gain as the pregnancy progresses.
(c) Providing education about the need for good antenatal care (ANC). Consideration may be given to assertive outreach (e.g. by a case manager or community midwife) to ensure ANC occurs.
(d) Regular surveillance of electrolytes if required.
(e) Clarifying crisis plans for medical, obstetric, or psychiatric emergencies.
(f) Specific recommendations about medications to be prescribed as already noted above.
(g) Close monitoring of foetal growth and development across pregnancy.
(h) Having a low threshold for maternal admission if there is either:
  1. Evidence of deterioration in the patient's own health or
  2. Evidence that the growth and development of the unborn infant is compromised. (The aim of admission is to ensure that active treatment of maternal physical and mental health can occur whilst close monitoring of foetal growth and development across the second and third trimesters can take place. The choice of the setting for admission will depend on the particular resources available within the location that the mother lives and may be to either an obstetric unit that has a psychiatric liaison service, or a specialist eating disorders unit with close obstetric liaison. Involuntary treatment of the mother may be considered, in order to care for her and her unborn infant, if she is unable to consent to treatment).
(i) An antenatal paediatrics referral to discuss any issues relating to co-morbid conditions or biological treatments that may impact on the newborn infant should be recommended.

(continued)

(j) A perinatal mental health-care plan should be written and included in the patient's obstetric file detailing specific management recommendations and the clinicians involved in the patient's care. Consent should be obtained from the woman to have the plan circulated to all relevant treating clinicians involved in her care and the names, contact details, and their role in the patient's management should be included. Regular communication between all clinicians involved in her care during pregnancy is ideal, in order to optimise outcomes for mother and infant. When clinically indicated, the plan should be reviewed (in collaboration with the patient) and updated.

(k) Consideration be given to protective concerns in some cases, and recommendations about appropriate parenting supports may be required.

(l) Throughout pregnancy and prior to discharge from the obstetric care setting, longer term treatment recommendation and goals should be discussed and referral and liaison with long-term clinicians undertaken.

Early Postpartum

Postnatal monitoring and support are essential as there is a risk of relapse of EDs postnatally. Continued consultation with a dietician, physician, and psychiatrist is recommended to ensure that education and advice around healthy eating and nutrition can be ongoing and that maternal physical and mental health can be monitored and early treatment (including physical investigations) initiated if required. Drugs such as laxatives, diuretics, and appetite suppressants may be used in an effort to lose weight quickly without realising the effect on the infant if breastfeeding.

Additional support and planning, particularly around the developing mother–infant relationship and breastfeeding, and admission to an inpatient mother baby unit to support this should be considered. There should be a low threshold for early referral to a paediatrician for infant assessment and monitoring throughout development.

References

Abraham S. Disordered eating and pregnancy, part 1. Eur Eat Disord Rev. 1998;9:1–4.

American Psychiatric Association. Diagnostic and statistical manual of mental disorders. 5th ed. Arlington, VA: American Psychiatric Publishing; 2013.

Arcelus J, Mitchell AJ, Wales J, Nielsen S. Mortality rates in patients with anorexia nervosa and other eating disorders. A meta-analysis of 36 studies. Arch Gen Psychiatry. 2011;68(7):724–31.

Arbuckle TE, Sherman GJ. Comparison of the risk factors for preterm delivery and intrauterine growth retardation. Paediatr Perinat Epidemiol. 1989;3:115–29.

Bateman A, Fonagy P. Randomized controlled trial of outpatient mentalization-based treatment versus structured clinical management for borderline personality disorder. Am J Psychiatry. 2009;166(12):1355–64.

Boney CM, Verma A, Tucker R, Vohr BR. Metabolic syndrome in childhood: associations with birth weight, maternal obesity, and gestational diabetes mellitus. Pediatrics. 2005;115:290–6.

Bulik C, Sullivan P, Fear J, Pickering A, Dawn A, McCullin M. Fertility and reproduction in women with a history of anorexia nervosa: a controlled study. J Clin Psychiatry. 1999;60:130–5.

Bulik CM, von Holle A, Hamer R, Berg CK, Torgersen L, Magnus P, et al. Patterns of remission, continuation, and incidence of broadly defined eating disorders during early pregnancy in the Norwegian Mother and Child Cohort Study. Psychol Med. 2007;37(8):1109–18.

Bulik CM, Hoffman ER, Von Holle A, Torgersen L, Stoltenberg C, Reichborn-Kjennerud T. Unplanned pregnancy in women with anorexia nervosa. Obstet Gynecol. 2010;116 (5):1136–40.

Chanen A, Jovev M, Jackson HJ. Adaptive functioning and psychiatric symptoms in adolescents with borderline personality disorder. J Clin Psychiatry. 2007;68(2):297–306.

Chanen AM, Kaess M. Developmental pathways toward borderline personality disorder. Curr Psychiatry Rep. 2012;14(1):45–53.

Chanen AM, McCutcheon LK. Prevention and early intervention for borderline personality disorder: current status and recent evidence. Br J Psychiatry. 2013;202(S54):s24–9.

Chen EY, Brown MZ, Lo TY, Linehan MM. Sexually transmitted disease rates and high-risk sexual behaviours in borderline personality disorder versus borderline personality disorder with substance use disorder. J Nerv Ment Dis. 2007;195:125–9.

Cohen LJ, Slade A. The psychology and psychopathology of pregnancy: reorganization and transformation. In: Jr. Zeanah CH, editor. Handbook of infant mental health. 2nd ed. New York, NY: Guildford; 2000.

Coid J, Yang M, Tyrer P, Roberts A, Ullrich S. Prevalence and correlates of personality disorder in Great Britain. Br J Psychiatry. 2006;188:423–31.

Conti J, Abraham S, Taylor A. Eating behavior and pregnancy outcome. J Psychosom Res. 1998;44:465–77.

Crow S, Thuras P, Keel PK, Mitchell JE. Long-term menstrual and reproductive function in patients with bulimia nervosa. Am J Psychiatry. 2002;159:1048–50.

De Genna NM, Feske U, Angiolieri T, Gold MA. Race and sexually transmitted diseases in women with and without borderline personality disorder. J Womens Health. 2011;20:333–40.

De Genna N, Feske U, Larkby C, Angilieri T, Gold M. Pregnancies, abortions and births among women with and without borderline personality disorder. Women's Health Isuues. 2012;22–4: e371–7.

Flament MF, Bissada H, Spettigue W. Evidence-based pharmacotherapy of eating disorders. J Neuropsychopharmacol. 2012;15:189–207.

Franko D, Blais M, Becker A, Delinsky S, Greenwood DN, Flores AT, et al. Pregnancy complications and neonatal outcomes in women with eating disorders. Am J Psychiatry. 2001;158:1461–6.

Galbally M, Blankley G, Power J, Snellen M. Perinatal mental health services: What are they and why do we need them? Australas Psychiatry. 2013;21(2):165–70.

Giesen-Bloo J, van Dyck R, Spinhoven P, van Tilburg W, Dirksen C, van Asselt T, et al. Outpatient psychotherapy for borderline personality disorder: randomized trial of schema-focused therapy vs transference-focused psychotherapy. Arch Gen Psychiatry. 2006;63(6):649–58.

Grilo CM, Pagano ME, Skodol AE, Sanislow CA, McGlashan TH, Gunderson JG, et al. Natural course of bulimia nervosa and eating disorder not otherwise specified: 5-year prospective study of remissions, relapses, and the effects of personality disorder psychopathology. J Clin Psychiatry. 2007;68(5):738–46.

Government of South Australia. Personality Disorders in Pregnancy, Ch 146. South Australian Perinatal Practice Guidelines. Maternity care in South Australia; 2006.

Gunderson JG, Stout RL, McGlashan TH, Shea MT, Morey LC, Grilo CM, et al. Ten-year course of borderline personality disorder: psychopathology and function from the collaborative longitudinal personality disorders study. Arch Gen Psychiatry. 2011;68(8):827–37.

Harris EC, Barraclough B. Excess mortality of mental disorder. Br J Psychiatry. 1998;173:11–53.

Henshaw C, Protti O. Addressing the Sexual and reproductive health needs of women who use mental health services. Adv Psychiatr Treat. 2010;16:272–8.

Hoek HW, van Hoeken D. Review of the prevalence and incidence of eating disorders. Int J Eat Disord. 2003;34(4):383–96.

Horz S, Zanarini MC, Frankenburg FR, Reich DB, Fitzmaurice G. Ten-year use of mental health services by patients with borderline personality disorder and with other axis II disorders. Psychiatr Serv. 2010;61(6):612–6.

Keski-Rahkonen A, Hoek HW, Linna MS, Raevuori A, Sihvola E, Bulik CM, et al. Incidence and outcomes of bulimia nervosa: a nationwide population-based study. Psychol Med. 2009;39 (5):823–31.

Kohmura H, Miyake A, Aono T, Tanizawa O. Recovery of reproductive function in patients with anorexia nervosa: a 10-year follow-up study. Eur J Obstet Gynecol Reprod Biol. 1986; 22:293–6.

Kok JH, den Ouden LA, Verloove-Vanhorick SP, Brand R. Outcome of very preterm small for gestational age infants: the first nine years of life. Br J Obstet Gynaecol. 1998;105:162–8.

Kouba S, Hallstrom T, Lindholm C, Hirschberg A. Pregnancy and neonatal outcomes in women with eating disorders. Obstet Gynecol. 2005;105:255–60.

Lacey J, Smith G. Bulimia nervosa: the impact of pregnancy on mother and baby. Br J Psychiatry. 1987;50:777–81.

Leichsenring F, Leibing E, Kruse J, New AS, Leweke F. Borderline personality disorder. Lancet. 2011;377(9759):74–84.

Linehan MM, Comtois KA, Murray AM, Brown MZ, Gallop RJ, Heard HL, et al. Two-year randomized controlled trial and follow-up of dialectical behavior therapy vs therapy by experts for suicidal behaviors and borderline personality disorder. Arch Gen Psychiatry. 2006;63 (7):57–766.

Machado PP, Machado BC, Gonçalves S, Hoek HW. The prevalence of eating disorders not otherwise specified. Int J Eat Disord. 2007;40(3):212–7.

McKnight RF, Park RJ. Atypical antipsychotics and anorexia nervosa: a review. Eur Eat Disord Rev. 2010;18(1):10–21.

Metzger BE, Buchanan TA, Coustan DR, de Leiva A, Dunger DB, Hadden DR, et al. Summary and recommendations of the fifth international workshop-conference on gestational diabetes mellitus. Diabetes Care. 2007;30:S251–60.

Michels KB, Trichopoulos D, Robins JM, Rosner BA, Manson JE, Hunter DJ, et al. Birthweight as a risk factor for breast cancer. Lancet. 1996;348:1542–6.

Mitchell JE, Seim HC, Glotter D, Soll EA, Pyle RL. A retrospective study of pregnancy in bulimia nervosa. Int J Eat Disord. 1991;10:209–14.

Morgan J, Lacey J, Sedgwick P. Impact of pregnancy on bulimia nervosa. Br J Psychiatry. 1999;174:135–40.

Morgan JF, Lacey JH, Chung E. Risk of postnatal depression, miscarriage and preterm birth in bulimia nervosa: Retrospective controlled study. Psychosom Med. 2006;68:487–92.

National Health and Medical Research Council. Clinical practice guideline for the management of borderline personality disorder. Melbourne: National Health and Medical Research Council; 2012.

Newman L, Stevenson C. Parenting and borderline personality disorder: ghosts in the nursery. Clin Child Psychol Psychiatry. 2005;10:385–90.

Newman L, Stevenson CS, Bergman LR, Boyce P. Borderline personality disorder, mother–infant interaction and parenting perceptions: preliminary findings. Aust N Z J Psychiatry. 2007;41 (7):598–605.

Newman L. Trauma and ghosts in the nursery: parenting and borderline personality disorder. In: Sved-Williams A, Cowling V, editors. Infants of parents with mental illness: developmental, clinical, cultural and personal perspectives. Bowen Hills: Australian Academic; 2008. p. 212–27.

Park R, Senior R, Stein A. The offspring of mothers with eating disorders. Eur Child Adolesc Psychiatry. 2003;12:110–9.

Pompili M, Girardi P, Ruberto A, Tatarelli R. Suicide in borderline personality disorder: a meta-analysis. Nord J Psychiatry. 2005;59(5):319–24.

Rich-Edwards JW, Stampfer MJ, Manson JE, Rosner B, Hankinson SE, Colditz GA, et al. Birth weight and risk of cardiovascular disease in a cohort of women followed up since 1976. Br Med J. 1997;315:396–400.

Rosenberg A. The IUGR newborn. Semin Perinatol. 2008;32(3):219–24.

Rusch N, Lieb K, Gottler I, Hermann C, Schramm E, Richter H, et al. Shame and implicit self-concept in women with borderline personality disorder. Am J Psychiatry. 2007;164(3):500–8.

Sansone RA, Farukhi S, Wiederman MW. Utilization of primary care physicians in borderline personality. Gen Hosp Psychiatry. 2011;33(4):343–6.

Smink FE, van Hoeken D, Hoek HW. Epidemiology of eating disorders: incidence, prevalence and mortality rates. Curr Psychiatry Rep. 2012;14(4):406–14.

Trull TJ, Jahng S, Tomko RL, Wood PK, Sher KJ. Revised NESARC personality disorder diagnoses: gender, prevalence, and comorbidity with substance dependence disorders. J Pers Disord. 2010;24(4):412–26.

Wade TD, Bergin JL, Tiggemann M, Bulik CM, Fairburn CG. Prevalence and long-term course of lifetime eating disorders in an adult Australian twin cohort. Aust N Z J Psychiatry. 2006;40 (2):121–8.

Wen SW, Goldenberg RL, Cutter GR, Hoffman HJ, Cliver SP. Intrauterine growth retardation and preterm delivery: prenatal risk factors in an indigent population. Am J Obstet Gynecol. 1990;162(1):213–8.

Weinfeld R, Dubay M, Burchell R, Mellerick J, Kennedy A. Pregnancy associated with anorexia and starvation. Am J Obstet Gynecol. 1977;15:698–9.

Yager J, Devlin MJ, Halmi KA, Herzog DB, Mitchell III JE, Powers P, Zerbe KJ. Guideline watch (August 2012): Practice guideline for the treatment of patients with eating disorders. 3rd ed. Washington, DC: American Psychiatric Association (APA); 2006. 128 p [765 references].

Yu CKH, Teoh TG, Robinson S. Review article: obesity in pregnancy. Br J Obstet Gynaecol. 2006;113:1117–25.

Zanarini MC, Williams AA, Lewis RE, Reich RB, Vera SC, Marino MF, et al. Reported pathological childhood experiences associated with the development of borderline personality disorder. Am J Psychiatry. 1997;54:1101–6.

Zanarini MC, Frankenburg J, Hennen J, Silk KR. Mental Health service utilization by borderline personality disorder patients and Axis II comparison subjects followed prospectively for 6 years. J Clin Psychiatry. 2004a;65(1):28–36.

Zanarini MC, Frankenburg FR, Hennen J, Reich DB, Silk KR. Axis I comorbidity in patients with borderline personality disorder: 6-year follow-up and prediction of time to remission. Am J Psychiatry. 2004b;161(11):2108–14.

Zanarini MC, Frankenburg FR, Reich DB, Fitzmaurice G. The 10-year course of psychosocial functioning among patients with borderline personality disorder and axis II comparison subjects. Acta Psychiatr Scand. 2010;122(2):103–9.

Zimmerman M, Chelminski I, Young D. The frequency of personality disorders in psychiatric patients. Psychiatr Clin North Am. 2008;31(3):405–20.

Management of Substance Abuse in Pregnancy: Maternal and Neonatal Aspects

12

Laura Brandt, Anna K. Leifheit, Loretta P. Finnegan, and Gabriele Fischer

Abstract

In Europe, the USA and Australia the prevalence of smoking during pregnancy ranges between 10 and 27 %. Drinking alcohol is reported by 8.5–19.5 % of pregnant women, with a potentially significant number of unreported cases. Additionally, there are as many as 60,000–100,000 pregnant women using illicit drugs per year, with a high percentage of poly-drug users. Substance-dependent women have a high incidence of co-morbid psychiatric disorders, with DSM-IV axis I affective and post-traumatic stress as well as axis II personality disorders being the most frequent co-morbidities. Due to serious consequences of licit and illicit substance use during pregnancy as well as undetected/untreated psychiatric co-morbidities, the primary focus must be on adequate diagnostic assessment. Treatment, tailored individually to the kind of substance dependence and under consideration of evidence-based treatment options available as early as possible during pregnancy, leads to better pregnancy outcomes and fewer birth complications. Neonates born to mothers who are chronic illicit drug users or provided maternal medication-assisted treatment frequently develop a Neonatal Abstinence Syndrome (NAS). Pharmacological NAS treatment should be provided based on principles of accurate assessment and diagnosis, with non-pharmacological measures such as rooming-in being vital supportive

L. Brandt (✉) • A.K. Leifheit
Center for Public Health, Medical University of Vienna, Vienna, Austria
e-mail: laura.brandt@meduniwien.ac.at; anna.leifheit@meduniwien.ac.at

L.P. Finnegan
Finnegan Consulting, LLC, Avalon, NJ, USA

Office of Research on Women's Health, National Institutes of Health, Bethesda, MD, USA
e-mail: finnegal337@aol.com

G. Fischer
Department of Psychiatry and Psychotherapy & Center for Public Health,
Medical University of Vienna, Vienna, Austria
e-mail: gabriele.fischer@meduniwien.ac.at

M. Galbally et al. (eds.), *Psychopharmacology and Pregnancy*,
DOI 10.1007/978-3-642-54562-7_12, © Springer-Verlag Berlin Heidelberg 2014

interventions. The economic burden of substance dependence during pregnancy and related follow-up costs are significant. To lower societal costs and increase the quality of life of both mothers and children, international treatment standards, building on previous recommendations, must be established and implemented.

Keywords

Substance use disorder • Pregnancy • Neonatal abstinence syndrome • Opioids • Psychiatric co-morbidity • Costs • Treatment

12.1   Substance Abuse/Dependence in Pregnant Women

Since the childbearing ages encompass the years of 15–44, many young women who are misusing substances will become pregnant and deliver a drug-exposed newborn. The stigma of substance use and pregnancy are a combination that is difficult for young women. The result may be avoidance of prenatal care and substance abuse treatment. A healthy mother and baby are more probable when prenatal care is elected providing recognition and treatment of any medical or obstetric complications that may arise during pregnancy. Good prenatal care by physicians knowledgeable in treating high-risk pregnancies can stabilise the pregnant woman and provide appropriate measures for the health of the foetus and newborn. Certain medical conditions in the pregnant woman can influence the infant's outcome. For example, infection in the mother may cause neonatal infection with pneumonia; hypertension in the mother influences foetal growth; sexually transmitted diseases in the mother can cause infection in the infant; pre-eclampsia in the mother can cause growth restriction, preterm birth or foetal death in the infant; placental abruption or insufficiency in the mother can cause foetal distress, growth restriction or foetal death of the infant; and preterm delivery in the mother will result in an immature low-birth-weight infant who may suffer respiratory distress or intracranial haemorrhage with the potential of long-term developmental problems and disabilities.

Pregnant substance misusing young women may have psychiatric illnesses, histories of physical and/or sexual abuse, family dysfunction and low frustration tolerance coupled with a chaotic lifestyle. These issues predispose the newborn to the potential for serious outcomes including ineffective/poor parenting, failure to thrive, child neglect, child abuse, abandonment and death.

Within the delivery of the necessary services that should be provided to pregnant substance misusing young women, a comprehensive, multidisciplinary approach must be utilised in order to normalise the medical and psychological status of the mother and to ensure a better outcome for the newborn and child.

12.1.1 Prevalence of Substance Use Among Pregnant Women

Many epidemiological studies highlight that smoking tobacco, alcohol consumption and illicit substance abuse are increasing in women of childbearing age (De Santis et al. 2011). Even though consequences of licit drug use during pregnancy can be just as or even more severe than those of illicit drug use, prevalence rates are listed separately. Illicit drug use has special characteristics such as higher stigmatisation and legal consequences that influence the willingness to report use and seek help. Especially for Europe, data on the prevalence of substance use among pregnant women are often derived from isolated studies using various methodologies, and findings are not readily comparable (European Monitoring Centre for Drugs and Drug Addiction 2012). Thus, results have to be considered with caution and cannot simply be generalised.

For Europe, it has been estimated that 10–27 % of pregnant women smoke during pregnancy (European Medicine Agency 2007), whereas in the USA the prevalence was reported as 17.3 % (National Survey on Drug Use and Health 2007). US pregnant women were more likely to have smoked cigarettes during their first trimester (22.9 %) compared to second (14.3 %) and third (15.3 %) trimester (National Survey on Drug Use and Health 2007). According to estimates by the Australian Institute of Health and Welfare 11 % of women smoke during pregnancy. However, the proportion decreases to 7.7 % after women become aware of their pregnancy (National Drug Strategy Household Survey Report 2011).

The 2005 Comparative Risk Assessment Study reported that the pattern of pregnant women's drinking in Europe is similar to estimates for the USA (Alcohol Consumption, Alcohol Dependence and Attributable Burden of Disease in Europe 2012). In the USA 8.5 % of pregnant women reported current alcohol use, 2.7 % binge drinking and 0.3 % heavy drinking (National Survey on Drug Use and Health 2012). In Australia, 47.3 % of pregnant women drank alcohol prior to the knowledge of their pregnancy and 19.5 % despite knowledge of their pregnancy. The drinking rate, despite knowledge of pregnancy, increases with age and socio-economic status. The majority (over 90 %) of those aged 25 and younger who were drinking prior to knowledge of pregnancy stopped drinking when they became aware of their pregnancy, but only half of those over 36 years of age stopped (National Drug Strategy Household Survey Report 2011).

There is little information on the prevalence of prescription drug use, especially the *types of drugs* prescribed to pregnant women. Daw et al. (2011) reviewed literature describing patterns of prescription drug use during pregnancy including mainly European studies (12 out of 17). They reported the lowest rates of prescription drug use for Northern European countries ranging from 44.2 to 57 % and the highest rates for the Netherlands (69.2 %), Germany (85.2 %) and France (93 %), excluding vitamins and minerals. However, the authors did not include information on particular therapeutic class. For a German sample of women who gave birth between 2000 and 2001 ($n = 41,293$), a prevalence of 0.2 % for antidepressant and 0.1 % sedative (benzodiazepines and barbiturates) prescription drug use during pregnancy was reported (Egen-Lappe and Hasford 2004). Based on data of the prospective, population-based Avon Longitudinal Study of Parents and Children (ALSPAC) 39.6 % of pregnant women with a delivery between 1991 and 1992 in Southwest England self-reported analgesic use during pregnancy (Headley et al. 2004). Andrade et al. (2004) provide information on the prevalence of prescription drug use among pregnant women in the USA. Among women who delivered in a hospital between 1996 and 2000 ($n = 129{,}616$) 2.8 % were prescribed antidepressants (1st trimester: 2.2 %, 2nd: 1.3 %, 3rd: 1.4 %), 1.3 % sedative hypnotics (1st trimester: 0.5 %, 2nd: 0.3 %, 3rd: 0.7 %) and 14.2 % opioid and non-opioid analgesics (1st trimester: 6.1 %, 2nd: 5.6 %, 3rd: 5.6 %). Information on prescription drug use among Australian pregnant women is limited and based on small sample sizes. Henry and Crowther (2000) reported a prevalence of 97.1 % total (including "over the counter" medication), 2.1 % antidepressant and 50 % analgesic prescription drug use during the first trimester among 140 women delivering at the Women's and Children's Hospital in Adelaide in 1999.

The number of European pregnant women using illicit drugs each year is estimated at 60,000 (Gyarmathy et al. 2009). In the USA the use of illicit drugs during pregnancy is known to affect over 100,000 women annually (Benningfield et al. 2010). The National Survey on Drug Use and Health (2013) showed that 5.9 % of US pregnant women aged 15–44 were current illicit substance users based on data averaged across 2011 and 2012, compared to 10.7 % of women in this age group who were not pregnant. For Australia, a prevalence rate of 8 % for illicit substance use among pregnant and breastfeeding women was reported (O'Donnell et al. 2009).

Each year there are as many as 30,000 pregnant women using opioids in Europe (Gyarmathy et al. 2009). For the USA in 2009, the rate of mothers being dependent on, or using opioids at the time of delivery, was 5.6 per 1,000 hospital life births, reflecting an almost fourfold increase compared to 2000 (1.19 per 1,000 hospital 130 births; Patrick et al. 2012). Australian data on opiate use during pregnancy are sparse and mainly reported within the illicit drug category and not listed separately. The prevalence of heroin use increased from 4 % in 1992 to 8 % in 1998 and declined to 2 % in 2001 (O'Donnell et al. 2009). However, it needs to be noted that 2001 is the year of the so-called Australian "heroin shortage" (Degenhardt et al. 2006). A more recent study examining obstetric and perinatal outcomes for women with a drug-related hospital admission during pregnancy in New South Wales (1998–2002) found 1974 records with an opioid ICD-10 diagnosis in a sample of 416,834 women (0.47 %; Burns et al. 2006).

As for the prevalence of cocaine use there are significant differences between countries due to vastly different drug markets. A European multi-centre and multi-modal project illustrated the diverse picture of cocaine use in Europe (Haasen et al. 2004). The 12-month prevalence rate shows an increase from 1990 to 2000/2001 in all studied countries but Sweden. Lifetime prevalence rates show a wide range with the lowest rates in Sweden (1.0 %) and the highest in the UK with 5.6 %. However, not even the highest rates reach anywhere near US rates with a far greater cocaine availability at a higher purity and lower price compared to Europe and

Australia (United Nations Office on Drug and Crime 2013). Therefore, the prevalence rates of females aged 18–25 having used cocaine in the past month are higher in the USA with 5.5 % (Department of Health and Human Services 2006) compared to 2.3 % of females aged 20–29 in Australia (Australian Institute of Health and Welfare 2004–2005). For European pregnant women, a prevalence rate of 3.1 % based on meconium analysis is reported from the "Meconium Project" located in Barcelona, Spain. However, the study sample is not representative for the population of European pregnant women since it included mainly women with a low socio-economic status (Pichini et al. 2005). For the USA, the last national survey data were reported in 1992 with an estimated 1.1 % of women using cocaine during pregnancy (US National Institutes of Health 1992). A more recent study, analysing data from the nationally representative epidemiologic 2002 and 2003 National Survey on Drug Use and Health, found that only 0.3 % of pregnant women compared to 1.0 % of non-pregnant women of childbearing age used cocaine (Havens et al. 2009). For Australia, a study examining the consequences of drug use in Western Australian women found only four women reporting cocaine use during pregnancy in a sample of 911 pregnant women (Werler et al. 2003).

In substance use disorder (SUD), frequently, more than one licit or illicit substance is abused. For example, more than 90 % of opioid-dependent women smoke cigarettes (Fischer 2007). Thus, poly-substance use further complicates the adequate study of epidemiology and outcomes of SUD in pregnancy. In the UK, as an example for Europe, 17,856 pregnant women were screened for illicit drug use. Of the 168 (0.9 %) women who were identified to use illicit drugs during pregnancy, 61.3 % showed illicit poly-substance use and almost all women (97 %) used multiple drugs if alcohol and tobacco were included (Goel et al. 2011). In the USA, poly-substance use during pregnancy was reported in 6.1 % of the cases (defined as using at least two drugs including alcohol, cigarettes, marijuana, prescription analgesics, tranquilisers, sedatives, stimulants, cocaine, crack, heroin and methamphetamine; Havens et al. 2009). In South Australia, 89,080 women were screened for substance use in pregnancy and of the 707 (0.9 %) women reporting substance use, 18.8 % showed poly-substance use (including alcohol but not tobacco; Kennare et al. 2005).

In Table 12.1 all prevalence data on substance use in pregnancy for Europe, the USA and Australia are summarised. It is important to note that the table just serves as an overview and results are not readily comparable since methodologies and sample sizes of included studies differ significantly.

12.1.2 Psychiatric Co-morbidity

The Epidemiologic Catchment Area study (ECA; Regier et al. 1993), the National Comorbidity Study (NCS; Kessler et al. 1994) and the National Epidemiologic Survey on Alcohol and Related Conditions (NESARC; Conway et al. 2006) are the most widely cited US studies on co-morbidity between SUD and psychiatric disorders. In the ECA an estimated 72 % of individuals with SUD had at least

Table 12.1 Prevalence of substance use during pregnancy (EU, USA, Australia)

	Europe	USA	Australia
Nicotine (% of women smoking during pregnancy)	10–27 % European Medicines Agency (2007)	17.3 % National Survey on Drug Use and Health (2007)	11 % National Drug Household Survey Report (2011)
Alcohol (% of pregnant women)	Pattern of drinking was similar to estimates for the US	8.5 % alcohol use 2.7 % binge drinking 0.3 % heavy drinking	19.5 % alcohol use
	Comparative Risk Assessment Study (2005)	National Survey on Drug Use and Health (2012)	National Drug Household Survey Report (2011)
Prescription drugs			
% of pregnant women using any prescription drug	44.2–93 % Daw et al. (2011)	–	97.1 % Henry and Crowther (2000)
% of pregnant women using antidepressants	0.2 % Egen-Lappe and Hasford (2004)	2.8 % Andrade et al. (2004)	2.1 % Henry and Crowther (2000)
% of pregnant women using sedatives	0.1 % Egen-Lappe and Hasford (2004)	1.3 % Andrade et al. (2004)	–
% of pregnant women using analgesics	39.6 % Headley et al. (2004)	14.2 % Andrade et al. (2004)	50 % Henry and Crowther (2000)
Illicit drugs			
Pregnant women using illicit substances per year (*n*)	60.000 Gyarmathy et al. (2009)	100.000 Benningfield et al. (2010)	–
% of pregnant women being illicit substance users	0.9 % Goel et al. (2011)	5.9 % National Survey on Drug Use and Health (2013)	8 % O'Donnell et al. (2009)
Opioids			
Pregnant women using opioids per year (*n*)	30.000 Gyarmathy (2009)	23.130[a] Patrick et al. (2012)	–
% of pregnant women using opioids	–	0.56 % Patrick et al. (2012)	0.47 % Burns et al. (2006)
Cocaine (% of pregnant women being cocaine users)	3.1 % Pichini et al. (2005)	0.3 % Havens et al. (2009)	0.4 % Werler et al. (2003)
Polysubstance use (% of pregnant women using ≥2 substances)	0.9 % (licit + illicit) 0.57 % (illicit) Goel et al. (2011)	6.1 % (licit + illicit) – Havens et al. (2009)	0.15 % (alcohol + illicit) Kennare et al. (2005)

[a] Own calculations based on a total number of births in 2009 of 4,130,665 (Martin et al. 2011)

Table 12.2 Lifetime odds ratios of mood and anxiety disorders associated with substance use disorders (women compared to men; Conway et al. 2006)

	Major depression		Mania			Any anxiety disorder	
	Women	Men	Women	Men		Women	Men
Any drug use disorder	3.6	3.4	6.7	5.6		2.9	3.0
Abuse	2.6	2.3	4.0[a]	2.6		2.2	1.9
Dependence	6.5	5.6	10.7	10.8		5.0	6.1
Opioid use disorder	6.0	4.9	9.5[a]	5.5		4.2	3.3
Abuse	4.8	4.3	5.7	3.8		3.1	2.2
Dependence	10.3	7.6	19.8	12.4		7.8	10.2
Cocaine use disorder	3.2	2.9	6.2	5.5		2.7	3.0
Abuse	1.9	3.0	3.5	2.8		1.7	2.0
Dependence	6.1	4.8	10.0	11.4		4.8	5.0

[a]Significant gender differences ($p < 0.05$)

one co-morbid psychiatric disorder (Regier et al. 1993). Co-morbidity rates are higher in individuals who are dependent on illicit substances compared to alcohol-dependent individuals, while poly-substance use is associated with the highest rates of psychiatric co-morbidity (Kandel et al. 2001). The NCS found an odds ratio (OR) of 2.4 for co-morbidity between any lifetime psychiatric disorder and alcohol or SUD. Half of the NCS respondents with a lifetime alcohol or SUD also met criteria for at least one lifetime psychiatric disorder, while 50.9 % of the NCS respondents with a lifetime psychiatric disorder also had a history of alcohol or substance abuse or SUD (Kessler 2004).

Conway et al. (2006) present nationally representative data from the NESARC sample on DSM-IV lifetime mood and anxiety disorders and co-morbidity with SUDs. The associations between SUDs and psychiatric disorders for women compared to men are displayed in Table 12.2.

The majority of opioid-dependent women suffers from psychiatric co-morbidities (range between 56 and 73 %), mainly affective disorders, PTSD or personality disorders (Fitzsimons et al. 2007; Martin et al. 2009; Unger et al. 2010). Greenfield et al. (2010) found a 12-month prevalence of 29.7 % for mood and anxiety disorders among women with SUDs, with the most common disorder being major depressive disorder (15.4 %). In a study by Benningfield et al. (2010) 48.6 % of the subjects ($n = 174$ opioid-dependent women) reported symptoms of a mood disorder and 12.6 % suicidal thinking at some point in the past 30 days. The prevalence rate of depression (33 %) was consistent with results by Fitzsimons et al. (2007).

In the special population of pregnant women, depression is of major concern in clinical research, especially postpartum depression. Postpartum depression rates are reported between 10 and 15 % in the general population (Rogers et al. 2013). Postpartum depressive syndromes lead to the risk of suicide and in severe cases infanticide if not appropriately diagnosed and treated. Women with a history of depression before or during pregnancy and adolescents with a history of substance abuse constitute high-risk groups for postpartum depression (Pajulo et al. 2001).

Low income and poor social support are additional risk factors (Clare and Yeh 2012). Mothers of preterm infants are at particular risk for postpartum depression with rates ranging from 14 to 27 % (Rogers et al. 2013). Holbrook and Kaltenbach (2012) analysed in a retrospective chart review 125 pregnant women enrolled in a comprehensive substance abuse treatment program. Almost one-third (30.4 %) of the women screened positive for moderate or severe depression at treatment entry. Nearly half of the sample (43.7 %) exhibited postpartum depression at 6 weeks post-delivery. The demographic variables were not related to the incidence of postnatal depression; only antenatal depression at treatment entry was a significant predictor for postpartum depression. Among opioid-dependent pregnant women, the high rate of unintended pregnancies (between 80 and 90 %; Heil et al. 2011) and socio-economic problems such as unemployment, co-addicted partners, and partner violence (Moore et al. 2011) can increase stress, with a close association between stress and maternal depression (Davis et al. 2007). Clare and Yeh (2012) found that postpartum depression is a challenging diagnosis and difficult to treat.

Selective serotonin reuptake inhibitors (SSRIs) (e.g. *fluoxetine, paroxetine, sertraline, citalopram and fluvoxamine*) are the most frequently used drugs to treat depression both in the general population and in pregnant women, even though SSRIs and pharmacological interventions in pregnancy are poorly studied due to the problem of entering pregnant women in clinical trials (Nature Editorial 2010). The US Food and Drug Administration issued a warning on SSRIs during pregnancy in 2006 as a single study showed a potential risk of persistent pulmonary hypertension of the newborn (PPHN), a rare heart and lung condition. To date, new studies show conflicting findings, questioning if the use of SSRIs during pregnancy can cause PPHN. Thus, the current FDA advice is not to alter the current clinical practice of treating depression during pregnancy, but to report any adverse events involving SSRIs (FDA Drug Safety Communication 2011). This serves as an example that pharmacological treatment during pregnancy always must be based on a sound risk–benefit assessment. It is however evident that a multidisciplinary approach to depression in pregnant women is necessary to prevent potentially life-threatening consequences in mothers and their children (Clare and Yeh 2012). Furthermore, it is a crucial task of drug regulators to ensure that treating physicians are aware of gender differences in drug reactions and dosages (Nature Editorial 2010).

In addition to affective disorders, epidemiological data indicate that 3–59 % of substance-dependent women meet diagnostic criteria for post-traumatic stress disorder (PTSD) (Najavits et al. 1997). According to El-Bassel et al. (2005), 25–57 % of substance-dependent women are traumatised as victims of intimate partner violence (IPV). Stene et al. (2010) found that women exposed to IPV show higher rates of abusing psychotropic substances, even after adjusting for mental distress. They examined psychotropic substance use (hypnotics, anxiolytics and antidepressants) among women exposed to different forms of IPV (physical, sexual, psychological). Physical and/or sexual IPV was related to increased use of hypnotics, anxiolytics and antidepressants. Psychological IPV alone was associated with increased use of anxiolytics and antidepressants. After adjustments for mental distress the association persisted only for use of antidepressants. As for the substances used, many women suffering from PTSD are poly-drug users, but the most common substance involved in abuse is alcohol (Back et al. 2003). Back et al. (2003) examined the differences between women with co-morbid PTSD and cocaine dependence and women with co-morbid PTSD and alcohol dependence. Women in the alcohol/PTSD group showed higher rates of major depression and social phobia as well as stressful life events. In addition, the rate of avoidance and hyperarousal was higher in the alcohol/PTSD group. Women in the cocaine/PTSD group demonstrated greater occupational and social impairment.

Exploration of the association between SUD and personality disorders revealed that opioid dependence often co-occurs with borderline personality disorder (BPD). A literature review found a mean rate of 27 % of patients with any SUD meeting diagnostic criteria for BPD, with the highest rate for opioid abuse/dependence (18.5 %), followed by cocaine (16.8 %) and alcohol abuse/dependence (14.3 %) (Trull et al. 2000). BPD is diagnosed at higher rates among women compared to men in general clinical samples and among women with SUDs. BPD traits such as impulsivity and risk-taking behaviour may be associated with increased risk of unplanned pregnancies at a very young age, frequently resulting in abortions or miscarriage (De Genna et al. 2011). A study by De Genna et al. (2012) showed that women with BPD often become pregnant during the period when BPD symptoms emerge and intensify. These women are at increased risk of teenage and unintended pregnancies.

Another frequent co-morbid personality disorder in SUD patients is the antisocial personality disorder (ASPD). The prevalence of ASPD among injection drug users (IDU) is up to 75 %, but the majority of IDUs with ASPD are men (Havens et al. 2007). The literature suggests that DSM criteria for ASPD may lead to an underestimation of the prevalence of the disorder in women (Dolan and Vollm 2009). ASPD is associated with risk behaviour such as needle sharing and high-risk sexual behaviour. The consequences are significantly increased transmission rates of HIV, hepatitis C and hepatitis B virus. Emotional instability and impulsivity often occur as a consequence of stressful life events such as childbirth. Thus, pregnant substance-dependent women with ASPD constitute a highly vulnerable group in particular need of support (Havens et al. 2007).

In general, substance-dependent women with co-occurring psychiatric symptoms show poorer treatment outcomes with higher rates of illicit substance abuse (Fitzsimons et al. 2007), highlighting the need for early standardised diagnostic assessment and adequate treatment.

12.1.3 Costs

For Europe, substance dependence is the fifth most expensive disorder of the brain (psychiatric and neurologic disorders; Olesen et al. 2012). The European total annual costs of addiction are displayed in Table 12.3 and compared to other

Table 12.3 European
total annual costs of
disorders of the brain
(Olesen et al. 2012)

Disorder	Annual costs in billion € (2010)
Mood disorders	113.4
Psychotic disorders	93.9
Anxiety disorders	74.4
Stroke	64.1
Addiction[a]	65.7

[a]Alcohol and opioid dependence

common disorders of the brain. Total European 2010 costs of disorders of the brain were estimated at €798 billion, with €65.7 billion for addictive disorders alone, composed of 37 % direct health-care costs, 23 % direct non-medical costs and 40 % indirect costs.

In Europe, structured data on (long-term) childcare costs related to mothers' licit and illicit substance use are sparse. Mangham et al. (2009) estimated for the UK costs of early delivery (before the 37th week of gestation), occurring in approximately 15 % of opioid-dependent women, with up to €466.250 per child. In the USA the mean annual costs of health care for children born with foetal alcohol syndrome (FAS) are US$2,842 per child/year. This is US$2,342 more than the annual average costs of care for a child without FAS (US$500). Prevention of FAS in one child would result in savings of US$128,810 in 10 years and US$491,820 in 20 years (Klug and Burd 2003). An investigation measuring trends and costs associated with Neonatal Abstinence Syndrome (NAS) between 2000 and 2009 reported that mean hospital charges per child diagnosed with NAS increased from $39,400 to $53,400 and charges for all other hospital births increased from $6,600 to $9,500 per child (Patrick et al. 2012). The length of hospital stay remained relatively unchanged for NAS during the study period (approximately 16 days) compared with a slightly increased length of stay for all other hospital births of approximately 3 days during the study period. With regard to national estimates, between 2000 and 2009, total hospital charges for NAS are estimated to have increased from $190 million to $720 million adjusted for inflation (Patrick et al. 2012).

12.1.4 Treatment

Treatment as early as possible during pregnancy leads to better pregnancy outcomes and fewer birth complications. Substance-dependent pregnant women are optimally treated in a multi-professional setting with treatment being tailored individually to the kind of substance dependence and under consideration of the evidence-based treatment options available (Metz et al. 2012).

For nicotine dependence, group therapy and cognitive behaviour therapy have shown to be effective in terms of smoking cessation during pregnancy (Windsor et al. 1998). Another psychosocial treatment option, Contingency Management (CM), is based on principles of operant conditioning (i.e. incentives are offered to encourage abstinence) and shows low dropout rates compared with other psychosocial interventions (Dutra et al. 2008). A Cochrane Review reported that CM for pregnant women increases smoking cessation rates significantly compared to other smoking cessation interventions (Lumley et al. 2009). CM interventions also show a positive impact on foetal growth, birth weight and breastfeeding duration (Higgins et al. 2012). Based on these results, pregnant patients with SUD and their offspring could benefit considerably by integration of CM into standard addiction treatment. Contingency Management has been mostly applied in research in the USA and in recent years a growing number of European studies have been published (Winklbaur-Hausknost et al. 2013). As for pharmacological interventions, Brose et al. (2013) examined whether the combination of nicotine replacement therapy (NRT, patch plus a faster acting form) is associated with a higher effect for smoking cessation in pregnancy. Compared with no medication, the use of a combination of nicotine patch and a faster acting form was associated with higher quitting rates, whereas single NRT showed no benefit. However, since NRT is not registered for use in pregnant women it should only be considered under close supervision.

For alcohol, an accurate and early diagnostic assessment not only of addiction, but any consumption during pregnancy, is vital. Alcohol can cause foetal developmental disorders even at the earliest stages of pregnancy while research indicates that binge drinking and regular heavy drinking put a foetus at the greatest risk for Foetal Alcohol Spectrum Disorders (FASD) (US National Institutes of health 1992). Several screening tools for alcohol abuse have been identified and validated for use in prenatal care. The most recently proposed brief and easy to use tool is the T-ACE 3 (Tolerance, Annoyed, Cut down, Eye opener), with high sensitivity and specificity in identifying risk drinking during pregnancy and predicting long-term neurobehavioral outcomes in exposed children. In the treatment of alcohol dependence an appropriate education about consequences of alcohol consumption is recommended (Kraigher et al. 2001). Due to the severe consequences of alcohol consumption on the foetus, abstinence has to be considered a primary goal in pregnant women. In heavy drinking women, detoxification must take place in an inpatient setting under close observation. Concomitant pharmacotherapy should be considered even at early stages of detoxification since elevated stress levels of the mother due to withdrawal pose a significant risk for the foetus. However, a risk–benefit assessment is necessary as pharmacological agents for treating withdrawal symptoms (e.g. benzodiazepines or clomethiazole) are also associated with risks for the foetus. If total abstinence cannot be considered a realistic therapeutic goal, reduction of alcohol intake should be the focus, since any reduction can be beneficial for foetal outcome (Heberlein et al. 2012). Brief interventions (one to three counselling-type sessions providing information and advice to alcohol users), which can be provided by health professionals and nursing staff, have been shown to significantly reduce alcohol consumption during pregnancy (Jones et al. 2013). Brief interventions during pregnancy show the largest effects in women with the highest initial consumption. Furthermore, the effects can be significantly enhanced if the partner is included (Chang et al. 2005).

Opioid maintenance therapy (OMT) is the current standard of care for opioid addiction, with proven efficacy in terms of reducing illegal substance use and increasing treatment retention. The first-line treatment for opioid-dependent pregnant women is OMT with methadone or alternatively with buprenorphine. Winklbaur-Hausknost et al. (2013) compared results of two double-blind, double-dummy, randomised controlled trials on comparison of buprenorphine and methadone [Pilot Study (PS) and European sample of the MOTHER trial (MT)] in opioid-dependent pregnant women. Both groups received vouchers for study attendance and completion of assessments; however, the MT group additionally received a CM intervention following an escalating design for drug-free urine samples. The results demonstrate that earlier treatment enrolment [MT: mean estimated gestational age (EGA) at enrolment week 18.4 vs. PS: mean EGA week 24.3] as well as an escalating incentive structure of CM interventions reduces illicit substance use during pregnancy. The number of opioid- and benzodiazepine-positive urine samples was significantly higher in the PS compared to MT ($p = .03$ and $p < .001$, respectively). Furthermore, the rate of preterm deliveries was increased in the PS (36 %) compared to MT (11 %) and similar results were found for dropout rates, with 10 % in MT compared to 22 % in PS. Even though both results were not significant, they are still clinically relevant, especially since the MT preterm delivery rate was very low and almost equal to general population rates of 5–9 % in most developed countries (Goldenberg et al. 2008). Unger et al. (2011) presented a unique case series investigating OMT with buprenorphine compared to methadone in opioid-dependent pregnant women using a within-subjects design. The results confirm effectiveness in terms of relapse prevention and safety of both medications for all three women and in both pregnancies. Treatment with buprenorphine resulted in a trend towards lower expression of NAS.

The importance of considering site-specific factors was highlighted by a study investigating site differences between MOTHER trial centres (Central Europe, rural US and urban US centres). Women in the urban US sites showed higher concomitant substance consumption and dropout rates compared to other centres and furthermore neonatal outcomes differed between sites (Baewert et al. 2012). Thus, it is important to not only consider medication aspects, but also environmental and cultural features in women's treatment. The final medication decision during pregnancy has to be based on individual benefit ratio decisions, also considering the women's previous experience, acceptance and tolerance of a particular medication to enhance treatment compliance and retention.

Treatment of opioid dependence with state-of-the-art OMT during pregnancy is associated with better pregnancy outcomes and fewer birth complications, representing an important aspect for long-term health-care system costs (Daley et al. 2001). Even though buprenorphine shows more favourable NAS outcomes, women should not be restricted to one medication, but have the choice between buprenorphine and methadone since both have been shown to be effective and safe treatment options (Unger et al. 2011).

12.2   Neonatal Abstinence Syndrome

Although hospitals around the world are experiencing increases in the number of newborns exposed to substances misused by their mothers, identifying the exact number of neonates born following intrauterine chronic exposure to opioids and other addicting agents has always been a challenging task. Contributing to this imprecision are, as demonstrated above, alterations in drug-taking patterns over time, marked variability in drug use patterns between individual hospitals and health-care facilities in an individual city and across countries and the use of many different agents at the same time, both licit and illicit. A study regarding the current extent of maternal drug abuse and its impact on the number of babies with NAS collected information on 7.4 million discharges from 4,121 hospitals in 44 of the 50 states in the USA between 2000 and 2009 (Patrick et al. 2012). Data from this study compared discharges for NAS versus all other hospital births in 2009. NAS was diagnosed at a rate of 3.39 per 1,000 hospital births per year. The investigators also found that newborns with NAS were 19 % more likely than all other hospital births to have low birth weight and 30 % more likely to have respiratory complications and also had feeding difficulties and seizures more often.

12.2.1 Aetiology

Neonates born to mothers who are chronic illicit opioid users or provided maternal medication-assisted treatment, such as methadone or buprenorphine, are frequently born with a passive dependency to those specific agents. However, many factors have been shown to be associated with the variability in the appearance of this syndrome. Because of their low molecular weight and lipid solubility, all of these drugs easily pass through the placenta from the mother to the foetus, which occurs at varying degrees, depending on the properties of the individual drugs. Once the drugs pass across the placenta and accumulate in the foetus, there is an equilibrium established between maternal and foetal blood. Disruption of the trans-placental passage of drugs at birth, when the umbilical cord is cut, terminates the drug supply to the baby with the potential of resulting in the development of symptoms of withdrawal or abstinence. This constellation of symptoms constitutes a multisystem disorder involving the central nervous system, gastrointestinal system, respiratory system and the autonomic nervous system, which is termed the NAS (Finnegan 1986).

NAS presents as a constellation of behavioural and physiological signs and symptoms that are remarkably similar in spite of marked differences in the properties of the causative agents. Drugs involved include opioids such as heroin, methadone, buprenorphine or prescription drugs (*OxyContin, Percodan, Vicodin, Percocet and Dilaudid*). Opioids produce the most dramatic effects of abstinence on both the mother and foetus. Other medications that may cause NAS are the sedative-hypnotics such as benzodiazepines (i.e. diazepam) and barbiturates. These agents have a longer half-life, and withdrawal may not start until after the infant has been discharged from hospital. Seligman et al (2008) studied the maternal variables predicting length of treatment for NAS in methadone-exposed newborns. Later gestational age and concomitant maternal benzodiazepine use were associated with longer treatment. This study demonstrates that maternal poly-drug abuse can increase the severity of NAS. SSRIs, alcohol and nicotine have also been implicated in producing symptoms of NAS (Finnegan 1976; Finnegan and Kandall 2004; Weiner and Finnegan 2011).

A newborn can also develop abstinence symptoms *at birth* if narcotic antagonists are administered in the delivery room. This can be followed by very severe and precipitous symptoms of neonatal abstinence. The type of analgesia and the anaesthesia that the mother receives can also influence the time of onset of NAS. Generally epidural anaesthesia causes fewer problems for the mother and baby (Finnegan and Kandall 2008).

Medications provided for the treatment of opioid dependence in pregnant women (methadone or buprenorphine), although providing many benefits to the maternal–foetal–newborn triad, also have the potential risk of abstinence in the newborn. Between 48 and 94 % of intrauterine opioid-exposed children develop a NAS (Osborn et al. 2010) with a lower incidence in buprenorphine-exposed (47 %) compared to methadone-exposed children (50–81 %; Jones et al. 2010a). Numerous studies have been reported regarding the dose of methadone and its effect on NAS. Some studies found that the greater the dose of methadone, the greater the severity of NAS resulting in physicians lowering the dose in the mother in order to decrease the severity of neonatal symptoms (Arlettaz et al. 2005; Lim et al. 2009; Madden et al. 1977). With inadequate doses of methadone, the women had a significant chance of relapse to heroin use. In contrast, there were an equal number of reports stating that there was *no correlation* between methadone dose and NAS severity (Dryden et al. 2009; Wouldes and Woodward 2010). This debate was settled when Cleary et al. (2010) did a meta-analysis comparing data from 67 studies (29 of which met the criteria for inclusion) to determine if there was a relationship between maternal methadone dose in pregnancy and the occurrence of NAS or the need for medical treatment in severe cases. From their results, they concluded that the severity of the NAS does not appear to differ according to whether mothers are on high- or low-dose methadone maintenance therapy. In addition, evidence-based studies show no association between NAS severity and trimester of methadone initiation, duration and amount of methadone exposure, duration of maternal drug use prior to pregnancy and no apparent relationship between maternal methadone dose (10–100 mg/day) and frequency or severity of abstinence-associated seizures (Berghella et al. 2003; Cleary et al. 2010; Herzlinger et al. 1977; Kaltenbach et al. 2012; Newman and Gevertz 2011).

For buprenorphine, NAS has been reported in varying degrees of severity and incidence. Many of the studies did not control for the use of other drug abuse concomitant with buprenorphine treatment. NAS occurrence was significant in those studies, which included other drug use; however, studies in Austria and the USA showed minimal abstinence symptoms from buprenorphine alone. A well-controlled clinical trial (The MOTHER Study) compared the differences between the occurrence and severity of NAS from methadone and that from buprenorphine

(Jones et al. 2010b). No significant differences between methadone and bupre-norphine were found in overall rates of NAS needing treatment, peak NAS scores and head circumference. There was a reduction of severity of NAS in buprenorphine-exposed neonates defined as the total amount of morphine needed in mg, length of hospital stay and number of days for treatment of NAS. These three items are inter-related in that the more morphine that is needed, the longer the days for treatment and the hospital stay (Jones et al 2010b). In addition, differences were found between centres when categorising the sites as urban or rural American and the Central European site showing less differences between the NAS in buprenorphine versus methadone-exposed babies (Baewert et al. 2012).

Wachman et al. (2013) studied the association of *OPRM1 and COMT* single-nucleotide polymorphisms with length of hospital stay and treatment of NAS in order to determine if there is a link between genetics and the syndrome. Genes tied to addiction in adults may provide future answers for infants with NAS. Certain genes in their common form without variations are associated with a higher risk of opioid addiction in adults. This multi-centre US cohort study (Maine, Massachusetts, Texas & New York) enrolled 86 mother–child pairs exposed to methadone or buprenorphine and analysed their DNA. Infants with variation of the OPRM1 gene were in the hospital 8.5 days less than those without the variation with a higher chance of not needing treatment. With the COMT gene, babies were in the hospital 10.8 fewer days and had less treatment. Concomitant smoking or psychiat-ric drugs (SSRIs) put babies at greater risk for withdrawal symptoms. The eventual goal of this study is to identify the highest risk babies early, attempt to develop treatment strategies that will prevent some of the NAS and try to get the babies home sooner. The US National Institutes of Health is commencing a larger study regarding genes and their influence on NAS severity.

12.2.2 Symptoms

Smoking cigarettes is common in opioid-dependent women and, dependent on the dose, NAS symptoms can be enhanced by this dual addiction in pregnant women (Winklbaur et al. 2009). Infants who have been exposed to heavy nicotine concentrations in utero have been found to be more excitable and hypertonic and demonstrate more stress and abstinence signs (Neonatal Tobacco Syndrome; Law et al. 2003). Symptoms seen in alcohol-exposed babies are present in the first 24 h of life and are especially reported in those with Foetal Alcohol Syndrome features. The newborns exhibit irritability, tremors, seizures, opisthotonus and abdominal distension.

Antidepressants used in depressed pregnant women predispose their newborns to neurobehavioral symptoms. Central Nervous System signs (e.g. irritability, seizures), motor signs (e.g. agitation, tremors, hypertonia), respiratory symptoms (e.g. increased respiratory rate, nasal congestion) and gastrointestinal signs (e.g. emesis, diarrhoea, feeding difficulty), fever and hypoglycaemia may be manifested by infants exposed to SSRIs during the last trimester of pregnancy

(Haddad et al. 2005). The onset of symptoms ranges from several hours to several days after birth and usually resolves by age 2 weeks. Symptoms are more commonly reported with fluoxetine and paroxetine exposure (Lund et al. 2009). A decrease in maternal SSRI use during the third trimester may lower the neonatal risk of developing NAS; however, this needs to be balanced against the harmful effects of depression during pregnancy.

After opioid exposure in utero most infants appear physically and behaviourally normal at birth with symptoms reported to appear shortly after birth and up to 2 weeks of age, but the majority are exhibited within the first 72 h of life (Finnegan 1991; Finnegan and Kandall 2004; Hudak and Tan 2012). Neonatal opioid abstinence is usually apparent within the first 24–72 h of life because most opioids are short-acting and not stored by the foetus in appreciable amounts. Methadone is longer acting and stored in foetal tissues; the occurrence, timing and severity of abstinence signs are therefore more variable. Acute symptoms may persist for several weeks, whereas subacute symptoms may persist for 4 to 6 months (Coyle et al. 2002; Franck and Vilardi 1995).

NAS resulting from opioid exposure in utero is described as a generalised disorder characterized by signs and symptoms of central nervous system hyperirritability, gastrointestinal dysfunction, respiratory and autonomic nervous system symptoms. Descriptions of the four major systems affected are as follows: *central nervous system symptoms* are most prominent in NAS and are those that bring a great deal of attention because of the considerable irritability seen in the babies. Tremors, those occurring when the infant is disturbed and those that occur when sleeping or in a quiet state, are associated with high-pitched cry, increased muscle tone, irritability, increased deep tendon reflexes and an exaggerated Moro reflex. An exaggerated rooting reflex and a voracious appetite manifested as sucking of fists or thumbs are common. When feedings are administered, the infants may have extreme difficulty because of an ineffectual and uncoordinated sucking and swallowing mechanism, all of which are mediated by the mid-brain (Finnegan 1986). Infants demonstrate *gastrointestinal system symptoms* with regurgitation, projectile vomiting and loose stools. Dehydration due to poor intake, coupled with increased losses from the gastrointestinal tract, may cause excessive weight loss, electrolyte imbalance, shock, coma and death. Timely and appropriate pharmacological control of abstinence, as well as provision of extra fluids and calories to offset both clinically apparent and insensible losses, is important in the management of these symptoms (Weinberger et al. 1986). Excessive secretions, nasal stuffiness, rapid respirations sometimes accompanied by chest retractions, intermittent cyanosis and apnea constitute the *respiratory system symptoms* (Finnegan 1980). Infants with acute heroin withdrawal were found to have increased respiratory rates, leading to hypocapnia and an increase in blood pH during the first week of life (Glass et al. 1972). Severe respiratory distress occurs most often when the infant regurgitates, aspirates and develops aspiration pneumonia, which is not often seen in the average NAS. Symptoms related to the *autonomic nervous system* include spontaneous generalised sweating, sneezing, yawning and skin colour changes (mottling). Increases in temperature and shedding of tears by the baby may occur, both of which increase water loss (Behrendt and Green 1972).

Babies exposed to cocaine in utero do not demonstrate typical abstinence symptoms. Neurobehavioral symptoms in cocaine-exposed babies include tremors, lethargy intermittent with irritability, abnormal cry patterns, poor sucking, hypertonia, abnormal sleep patterns and poor interactions with caretakers. These effects have been described by Askin and Diehl-Jones (2001) as neurotoxicity with under-aroused neurobehavioral function, but not a true NAS. Moreover, symptoms of irritability in these infants are difficult to separate in the context of other factors from which they suffer such as prematurity or prenatal exposure to other drugs concomitantly with cocaine such as heroin, alcohol and nicotine (Askin and Diehl-Jones 2001; Bada et al. 2002).

Maturity of the infant is an important issue when considering the onset of NAS. In full-term infants, the NAS onset is earlier, symptoms are more severe, treatment needs are greater and fewer seizures are observed. Preterm babies have a later onset and less severe symptoms (Doberczak et al. 1991; Doberczak et al. 1993). The reduced severity of abstinence in preterm babies could be due to either developmental immaturity of the central nervous system (immaturity of either dendritic ramifications, specific opiate receptors or neurotransmitter function) or reduced total drug exposure due to the shortened gestation.

There is great variability in the expression of abstinence symptoms in different newborns regarding *onset*, *pattern* and *duration* of symptoms. It has been suggested that the rate of decline in the newborns' plasma level of the pharmacological agent from day 1 to 4 of life influences the severity of abstinence symptoms (in these studies the pharmacological agent was methadone; Doberczak et al. 1991; Doberczak et al. 1993; Rosen and Pippenger 1976). Basically, the faster a baby excretes the pharmacological agent, the sooner symptoms will occur and they will be more severe.

If not recognised and not treated, NAS can cause death of the infant from excess fluid losses, high temperatures, seizures, respiratory instability, aspiration of fluid into the lungs or cessation of breathing (Jones et al. 2010b). However, with the current medical knowledge concerning drug abuse in pregnancy and the care of the newborn, no infant mortality should occur as a result of NAS.

12.2.3 Assessment

An assessment tool permits an accurate evaluation of the signs and symptoms and the severity, avoids unnecessary treatment of mildly affected infants and provides a methodology for effective dosing and tapering of medications. A number of scoring tools have been developed and reported in the paediatric literature (Finnegan et al. 1975; Finnegan 1986; Green and Suffet 1981; Lipsitz 1975; Zahorodny et al. 1998). Recommended by the American Academy of Paediatrics for assessment of the baby who may develop NAS as a result of in utero exposure to opioids (Hudak and Tan 2012), the Finnegan Neonatal Abstinence Score is administered by the nursing staff to monitor the newborn for the onset, progression and diminution of NAS.

The Finnegan Neonatal Abstinence Score rates the individual signs and symptoms assigning each a relative weight based on the relationship to newborn morbidity— the higher score of an item relates to more severe morbidity. Due to the undulating pattern of NAS, babies must be scored throughout the day at regular intervals. With severe symptoms, the infant is evaluated more frequently until stabilisation of the NAS occurs (Finnegan 1986). With the available inter-observer reliability manual and DVD for the Finnegan Neonatal Abstinence Score, a clinician should easily be able to assess opioid-exposed infants for the presence of abstinence signs and symptoms, implement appropriate examination techniques required to evaluate NAS, document clinical signs and symptoms of NAS and achieve a 90 % reliability with other examiners using the score. If individuals are properly trained and inter-rater reliability is achieved, the score becomes a valuable objective measure to assess the onset, progression and diminution of symptoms of abstinence (D'Apoliti and Finnegan 2010).

Assessment for other neonatal conditions should also be considered since the symptoms of NAS can mimic such conditions as septicaemia, encephalitis, meningitis, post-anoxic CNS irritation, hypoglycaemia, hypocalcaemia and cerebral haemorrhage, for all of which the infant born to the substance misusing woman is at risk, especially because of maternal infections and preterm birth.

12.2.4 Treatment

Routine prophylactic pharmacological treatment is not recommended for NAS since not all drug-exposed newborns experience abstinence symptoms; however, it is very important to closely observe the newborns for symptoms that may occur over the first 4–5 days of life. Treatment should be provided based on principles of accurate assessment and diagnosis. The diagnosis should be confirmed by maternal history of opioid use and a urine or meconium toxicology screen.

Routinely in hospital, the opioid-exposed baby is usually separated from the mother, admitted for observation in a quiet, dimly lit environment, or more likely to a Neonatal Intensive Care Unit (NICU) and treated for abstinence, if necessary. Separation from the mother and sensory deprivation have not been studied as independent predictors of improvement in NAS; however, separation may contribute to increased abstinence symptoms, decreased maternal attachment and neonatal abandonment. It has been hypothesised that rooming in might promote more effective mothering and might reduce the prevalence and severity of NAS (Velez and Jansson 2008). Abrahams et al. (2007) studied rooming-in compared with standard care for newborns of mothers using methadone or heroin. Two groups were studied: newborns who roomed in with their mothers and those who received traditional care in the NICU. Results of this study revealed that newborns who roomed-in with their mothers were less likely to require treatment for NAS and more likely to be discharged home with their mothers using weight gain as treatment criteria. Later studies also showed that the incidence of treatment for

NAS and the days in hospital were reduced when babies were rooming-in (RI) with their mothers (RI.11 %; NICU.45 %; RI.7 days; NICU.13 days; Hodgson and Abrahams 2012).

Metz et al. (2011) compared maternal and neonatal outcome of women in OMT (buprenorphine or methadone) throughout pregnancy in a randomised double-blind double-dummy clinical trial (CT: daily prenatal visits, assessment of NAS blinded for intrauterine medication exposure and mandatory rooming-in of mother and child after delivery) compared to a group undergoing structured standard protocol (SP: frequency of prenatal visits ranged on average between 2 and 3 per week). Newborns showed significantly better outcomes regarding NAS parameters for buprenorphine in both groups, but a lower total morphine dose administered and shorter length of hospital stay in the CT compared to SP group. These results refer to the benefit of rooming-in with mothers over the total NAS period in CT in addition to the blinded assessment of NAS as the treatment duration was much longer in SD with no significant differences (equivalently low rates) in structured maternal urine toxicology results between the groups.

Provision of supportive interventions, many of which are traditional methods of soothing a newborn infant, is important in the treatment of neonatal abstinence. Some of these supportive interventions include offering a pacifier (Non-Nutritive Sucking), skin to skin contact with the mother, swaddling snugly with hands available for sucking, not overdressing the baby, aspiration of the naso-pharynx, feeding of small amounts frequently (every 2h) if poor feeding persists without overfeeding and finally, positioning baby to right side-lying to reduce aspiration if vomiting or regurgitation is a problem (Weiner and Finnegan 2011). Although there is much that we still need to explore concerning the treatment of NAS, what we do know will provide comfort for the baby and decrease the chances of associated complications such as aspiration pneumonia, dehydration and seizures (Finnegan 1986; Unger et al. 2013). Using supportive care will enhance the baby's ability to feed normally, gain weight and permit adequate sleep (Finnegan and Kandall 2004).

Another issue that has been explored is whether maternal breast feeding can influence neonatal abstinence expression in view of the fact that very small quantities of methadone and buprenorphine have been detected in breast milk samples (McCarthy and Posey 2000). Methadone is detected in breast milk, but at very low levels. The ratio of breast milk to maternal blood plasma concentrations was found to range from 0.05 to 1.2 (McCarthy and Posey 2000; Wojnar-Horton et al. 1997). Buprenorphine is also detected in breast milk with a maternal blood plasma ratio which approximates one. Buprenorphine is not absorbed well by mouth so the infant is exposed to 1/5 to 1/10 of the total amount available in the breast milk. Absorption of buprenorphine from the breast milk is much less than other opioids (Johnson et al. 2001). Therefore, breast feeding in methadone- or buprenorphine-treated mothers who express an interest in doing so is recommended providing that they are HIV negative, are compliant with their treatment plan and do not use other licit or illicit drugs (Gynaecologists ACoOa Committee Opinion

2012; Paediatrics AAo Policy Statement 2005) since it supports mother–child attachment.

Pharmacological treatment is provided according to the severity of the score which monitors the infant's clinical response to medication and the amount necessary to control the symptoms, followed by progressive tapering of the dose. Clinicians should provide an opioid medication in the treatment of NAS using a titration method to increase the dose (in mg/kg) according to severity of the scores. Prompt escalation of dose, with aggressive decreases in dose as symptoms abate, are essential principles. Specific medications generally administered for neonatal abstinence from opioids include *oral morphine or tincture of opium or methadone* according to body weight and score (Osborn et al. 2010). Morphine drops were proven to be superior to other medications (Ebner et al. 2007). Clonidine is used infrequently and is not a first-choice medication. Sublingual administration of buprenorphine has been studied in the treatment of neonatal abstinence and a dose schema has been developed (Anagnostis et al. 2011; Kraft et al. 2011). In the UK 94 % and in the USA 83 % of physicians use morphine or methadone to treat neonatal opioid abstinence (Hudak and Tan 2012). With abstinence syndrome from other substances (e.g. barbiturates, ethanol, sedatives hypnotics), phenobarbital is generally administered.

The development of the infant who has experienced NAS is always of concern. Although many will predict a guarded prognosis for future development of infants who have experienced NAS, it is a transient and treatable condition and, within a stable environment, NAS per se should not influence outcomes. Many wish to implicate the exposure of a particular pharmacological agent, illicit or treatment opioid; however child development is related to multi-factorial issues with the environment in which the child exists and poverty amongst the myriad of influences. Through appropriate *recognition, assessment and treatment* of NAS coupled with good orientation of the future caretaker, we can better assure a nurturing, healthy environment for the child with a good chance of normal developmental outcomes.

Conclusion

This chapter provides an overview of the prevalence, consequences and treatment of substance use and related disorders in pregnant women and their neonates. Due to the lack of comparable structured data from Latin America and Africa these regions could not be included, which poses a limitation.

The data and results described above highlight the complexity of substance dependence during pregnancy. Affected women constitute a highly vulnerable group of patients with multiple psychiatric co-morbidities. Co-morbid disorders need to be recognised and treated adequately, since poor prognosis is expected if treatment fails to address both. Optimally managed substance-dependent pregnant women should receive treatment individually tailored to the kind of substance dependence and psychiatric co-morbidity that is being experienced. Initiation of a standardised diagnostic process and treatment of SUD and co-morbidities as early as possible leads to better pregnancy outcomes. Neonates have to be observed closely since between 48 % and 94 % of intrauterine opioid-exposed children develop a NAS. Collective randomised controlled trials, prospective and retrospective data show a less severe NAS for buprenorphine compared to methadone exposure in utero. However, it is of utmost importance that NAS is not used as criteria for selection of OMT. NAS is an easily identifiable and treatable condition that is only one aspect of the complete risk: Benefit ratio decisions have to be considered individually for every patient when making medication decisions during pregnancy. Pharmacological NAS treatment should be provided based on principles of accurate assessment and diagnosis and successful non-pharmacological measures as rooming-in should be considered for integration into standard clinical care. The most important outcome measure for treatment success is the well-being of both mother and child, which can be achieved by a diversification of treatment (i.e. the option of both buprenorphine or methadone for opioid dependence treatment) as well as special treatment options (e.g. CM) and standards of care resulting in superior maternal and neonatal outcomes. Furthermore, all intervention measures that prolong the pregnancy, prevent preterm delivery and shorten the duration of hospital stay also lead to a decrease in societal costs.

References

Abrahams RR, Kelly SA, Payne S, Thiessen PN, Mackintosh J, Janssen PA. Rooming-in compared with standard care for newborns of mothers using methadone or heroin. Can Fam Physician. 2007;53(10):1722–30.

Administration USFaD. FDA Drug Safety Communication: Selective serotonin reuptake inhibitor (SSRI) antidepressant use during pregnancy and reports of a rare heart and lung condition in newborn babies; 2011.

Alcohol consumption, alcohol dependence and attributable burden of disease in Europe 2012. Available from: http://amphoraproject.net/w2box/data/AMPHORAReports/CAMH_Alcohol_Report_Europe_2012.pdf

Anagnostis EA, Sadaka RE, Sailor LA, Moody DE, Dysart KC, Kraft WK. Formulation of buprenorphine for sublingual use in neonates. J Pediatr Pharmacol Ther. 2011;16(4):281–4.

Andrade SE, Gurwitz JH, Davis RL, Chan KA, Finkelstein JA, Fortman K, et al. Prescription drug use in pregnancy. Am J Obstet Gynecol. 2004;191(2):398–407.

Arlettaz R, Kashiwagi M, Das-Kundu S, Fauchere JC, Lang A, et al. Methadone maintenance program in pregnancy in a Swiss perinatal center (II): neonatal outcome and social resources. Acta Obstet Gynecol Scand. 2005;84(2):145–50.

Askin DF, Diehl-Jones B. Cocaine: effects of in utero exposure on the fetus and neonate. J Perinat Neonatal Nurs. 2001;14(4):83–102.

Australian Institute of Health and Welfare. National Drug Strategy Household Survey: First Results Canberra (AUST): AIHW; 2004–2005.

Back SE, Sonne SC, Killeen T, Dansky BS, Brady KT. Comparative profiles of women with PTSD and comorbid cocaine or alcohol dependence. Am J Drug Alcohol Abuse. 2003;29(1):169–89.

Bada HS, Das A, Bauer CR, Shankaran S, Lester B, Wright LL, et al. Gestational cocaine exposure and intrauterine growth: maternal lifestyle study. Obstet Gynecol. 2002;100(5 Pt 1):916–24.

Baewert A, Jagsch R, Winklbaur B, Kaiser G, Thau K, Unger A, et al. Influence of site differences between urban and rural American and Central European opioid-dependent pregnant women and neonatal outcome characteristics. Eur Addict Res. 2012;18(3):130–9.

Behrendt H, Green M. Nature of the sweating deficit of prematurely born neonates. Observations on babies with the heroin withdrawal syndrome. N Engl J Med. 1972;286(26):1376–9.

Benningfield MM, Arria AM, Kaltenbach K, Heil SH, Stine SM, Coyle MG, et al. Co-occurring psychiatric symptoms are associated with increased psychological, social, and medical impairment in opioid dependent pregnant women. Am J Addict. 2010;19(5):416–21.

Berghella V, Lim PJ, Hill MK, Cherpes J, Chennat J, Kaltenbach K. Maternal methadone dose and neonatal withdrawal. Am J Obstet Gynecol. 2003;189(2):312–7.

Brose LS, McEwen A, West R. Association between nicotine replacement therapy use in pregnancy and smoking cessation. Drug Alcohol Depend. 2013;132(3):660–4.

Burns L, Mattick RP, Cooke M. Use of record linkage to examine alcohol use in pregnancy. Alcohol Clin Exp Res. 2006;30(4):642–8.

Chang G, McNamara TK, Orav EJ, Koby D, Lavigne A, Ludman B, et al. Brief intervention for prenatal alcohol use: a randomized trial. Obstet Gynecol. 2005;105(5 Pt 1):991–8.

Clare CA, Yeh J. Postpartum depression in special populations: a review. Obstet Gynecol Surv. 2012;67(5):313–23.

Cleary BJ, Donnelly J, Strawbridge J, Gallagher PJ, Fahey T, Clarke M, et al. Methadone dose and neonatal abstinence syndrome-systematic review and meta-analysis. Addiction. 2010;105(12):2071–84.

Conway KP, Compton W, Stinson FS, Grant BF. Lifetime comorbidity of DSM-IV mood and anxiety disorders and specific drug use disorders: results from the National Epidemiologic Survey on Alcohol and Related Conditions. J Clin Psychiatry. 2006;67(2):247–57.

Coyle MG, Ferguson A, Lagasse L, Oh W, Lester B. Diluted tincture of opium (DTO) and phenobarbital versus DTO alone for neonatal opiate withdrawal in term infants. J Pediatr. 2002;140(5):561–4.

Daley M, Argeriou M, McCarty D, Callahan Jr JJ, Shepard DS, et al. The impact of substance abuse treatment modality on birth weight and health care expenditures. J Psychoactive Drugs. 2001;33(1):57–66.

D'Apoliti K, Finnegan LP. Assessing signs & symptoms of neonatal abstinence using the Finnegan scoring tool, an Inter-Observer Reliability Program. 2010. Available from: http://www.neoadvances.com

Davis EP, Glynn LM, Schetter CD, Hobel C, Chicz-Demet A, et al. Prenatal exposure to maternal depression and cortisol influences infant temperament. J Am Acad Child Adolesc Psychiatry. 2007;46(6):737–46.

Daw JR, Hanley GE, Greyson DL, Morgan SG. Prescription drug use during pregnancy in developed countries: a systematic review. Pharmacoepidemiol Drug Saf. 2011;20(9):895–902.

Degenhardt L, Day C, Gilmour S, Hall W. The "lessons" of the Australian "heroin shortage". Subst Abuse Treat Prev Policy. 2006;1:11.

De Genna NM, Feske U, Angiolieri T, Gold MA. Race and sexually transmitted diseases in women with and without borderline personality disorder. J Womens Health. 2011;20(3):333–40.

De Genna NM, Feske U, Larkby C, Angiolieri T, Gold MA. Pregnancies, abortions, and births among women with and without borderline personality disorder. Womens Health Issues. 2012;22(4):e371–7.

Department of Health and Human Services. Results from the 2005 National Survey on Drug Use and Health: National Findings. Rockville, MD: DHHS; 2006.

De Santis M, De Luca C, Mappa I, Quattrocchi T, Angelo L, et al. Smoke, alcohol consumption and illicit drug use in an Italian population of pregnant women. Eur J Obstet Gynecol Reprod Biol. 2011;159(1):106–10.

Doberczak TM, Kandall SR, Wilets I. Neonatal opiate abstinence syndrome in term and preterm infants. J Pediatr. 1991;118(6):933–7.

Doberczak TM, Kandall SR, Friedmann P. Relationship between maternal methadone dosage, maternal-neonatal methadone levels, and neonatal withdrawal. Obstet Gynecol. 1993;81(6):936–40.

Dolan M, Vollm B. Antisocial personality disorder and psychopathy in women: a literature review on the reliability and validity of assessment instruments. Int J Law Psychiatry. 2009;32(1):2–9.

Dryden C, Young D, Hepburn M, Mactier H. Maternal methadone use in pregnancy: factors associated with the development of neonatal abstinence syndrome and implications for healthcare resources. Br J Obstet Gynaecol. 2009;116(5):665–71.

Dutra L, Stathopoulou G, Basden SL, Leyro TM, Powers MB, et al. A meta-analytic review of psychosocial interventions for substance use disorders. Am J Psychiatry. 2008;165(2):179–87.

Ebner N, Rohrmeister K, Winklbaur B, Baewert A, Jagsch R, et al. Management of neonatal abstinence syndrome in neonates born to opioid maintained women. Drug Alcohol Depend. 2007;87(2–3):131–8.

Egen-Lappe V, Hasford J. Drug prescription in pregnancy: analysis of a large statutory sickness fund population. Eur J Clin Pharmacol. 2004;60(9):659–66.

El-Bassel N, Gilbert L, Wu E, Go H, Hill J. Relationship between drug abuse and intimate partner violence: a longitudinal study among women receiving methadone. Am J Public Health. 2005;95(3):465–70.

European Medicine Agency. 2007. Available from: http://www.ema.europa.eu/docs/en_GB/docu ment_library/Scientific_guideline/2009/09/WC500003515.pdf

European Monitoring Centre for Drugs and Drug Addiction. 2012. Available from: http://www. ofdt.fr/BDD/publications/docs/OEDT121031siGEF.pdf

Finnegan LP, Kron RE, Connaugthon JF, Emich JP. A scoring system for evaluation and treatment of the neonatal abstinence syndrome: A clinical and research tool. In: Morselli PL, Garattini S, Sereni F, editors. Basic and therapeutic aspects of perinatal pharmacology. New York, NY: Raven; 1975. p. 139–53.

Finnegan L. Clinical effects of pharmacologic agents on pregnancy, the fetus, and the neonate. Ann N Y Acad Sci. 1976;281:74–89.

Finnegan LP. Pulmonary problems encountered by the infant of the drug-dependent mother. Clin Chest Med. 1980;1(3):311–25.

Finnegan LP. Neonatal abstinence syndrome: assessment and pharmacotherapy. In: Rubaltelli B, Granati B, editors. Neonatal therapy: an update. New York, NY: Excerpta Medica; 1986. p. 122–46.

Finnegan LP. Treatment issues for opioid-dependent women during the perinatal period. J Psychoactive Drugs. 1991;23(2):191–201.

Finnegan LP, Kandall SR. Perinatal substance Use. In: Galanter M, Kleber H, editors. Textbook of substance abuse treatment. Arlington, VA: American Psychiatric Publishing; 2004.

Finnegan LP, Kandall SR. Maternal and neonatal effects of alcohol and drugs. In: Lowinson JH, Ruiz P, Langrod J, editors. Substance abuse: a comprehensive textbook. Baltimore, MD: Lippincot Williams and Wilson; 2005.

Finnegan LP, Kandall SR. Perintal substance use, drug dependence, motherhood, and the newborn. In: Galanter M, Kleber H, editors. Textbook of substance abuse treatment. Arlington, VA: American Psychiatric Publishing; 2008.

Fischer G. Review of the literature on pregnancy and psychosocially assisted pharmacotherapy of opioid dependence (including withdrawal management, agonist and antagonist maintenance therapy and adjuvant pharmacotherapy). 1–39 Geneva, Switzerland; 2007.

Fitzsimons HE, Tuten M, Vaidya V, Jones HE. Mood disorders affect drug treatment success of drug-dependent pregnant women. J Subst Abuse Treat. 2007;32(1):19–25.

Franck L, Vilardi J. Assessment and management of opioid withdrawal in ill neonates. Neonatal Netw. 1995;14(2):39–48.

Glass L, Rajegowda BK, Kahn EJ, Floyd MV. Effect of heroin withdrawal on respiratory rate and acid-base status in the newborn. N Engl J Med. 1972;286(14):746–8.

Goel N, Beasley D, Rajkumar V, Banerjee S. Perinatal outcome of illicit substance use in pregnancy–comparative and contemporary socio-clinical profile in the UK. Eur J Pediatr. 2011;170(2):199–205.

Goldenberg RL, Culhane JF, Iams JD, Romero R. Epidemiology and causes of preterm birth. Lancet. 2008;371(9606):75–84.

Green M, Suffet F. The Neonatal Narcotic Withdrawal Index: a device for the improvement of care in the abstinence syndrome. Am J Drug Alcohol Abuse. 1981;8(2):203–13.

Greenfield SF, Back SE, Lawson K, Brady KT. Substance abuse in women. Psychiatr Clin North Am. 2010;33(2):339–55.

Gyarmathy VA, Giraudon I, Hedrich D, Montanari L, Guarita B, et al. Drug use and pregnancy - challenges for public health. Euro Surveill. 2009;14(9):33–6.

Gynecologists ACoOa. Committee on Health Care for underserved Women and the American Society of Addicition Medicine "Opioid Abuse, Dependence, and Addicition in Pregnancy". Obstetrics & Gynecology, Commitee Opinion. 2012; p. 524

Haasen C, Prinzleve M, Zurhold H, Rehm J, Guttinger F, et al. Cocaine use in Europe - a multi-centre study. Methodology and prevalence estimates. Eur Addict Res. 2004;10(4):139–46.

Haddad PM, Pal BR, Clarke P, Wieck A, Sridhiran S. Neonatal symptoms following maternal paroxetine treatment: serotonin toxicity or paroxetine discontinuation syndrome? J Psychopharmacol. 2005;19(5):554–7.

Havens JR, Cornelius LJ, Ricketts EP, Latkin CA, Bishai D, et al. The effect of a case management intervention on drug treatment entry among treatment-seeking injection drug users with and without comorbid antisocial personality disorder. J Urban Health. 2007;84(2):267–71.

Havens JR, Simmons LA, Shannon LM, Hansen WF. Factors associated with substance use during pregnancy: results from a national sample. Drug Alcohol Depend. 2009;99(1–3):89–95.

Headley J, Northstone K, Simmons H, Golding J. Medication use during pregnancy: data from the Avon Longitudinal Study of Parents and Children. Eur J Clin Pharmacol. 2004;60(5):355–61.

Heberlein A, Leggio L, Stichtenoth D, Hillemacher T. The treatment of alcohol and opioid dependence in pregnant women. Curr Opin Psychiatry. 2012;25(6):559–64.

Heil SH, Jones HE, Arria A, Kaltenbach K, Coyle M, et al. Unintended pregnancy in opioid-abusing women. J Subst Abuse Treat. 2011;40(2):199–202.

Henry A, Crowther C. Patterns of medication use during and prior to pregnancy: the MAP study. Aust N Z J Obstet Gynaecol. 2000;40(2):165–72.

Herzlinger RA, Kandall SR, Vaughan Jr HG. Neonatal seizures associated with narcotic withdrawal. J Pediatr. 1977;91(4):638–41.

Higgins ST, Washio Y, Heil SH, Solomon LJ, Gaalema DE, et al. Financial incentives for smoking cessation among pregnant and newly postpartum women. Prev Med. 2012;55(Suppl):S33–40.

Hodgson ZG, Abrahams RR. A rooming-in program to mitigate the need to treat for opiate withdrawal in the newborn. J Obstet Gynaecol Can. 2012;34(5):475–81.

Holbrook A, Kaltenbach K. Co-occurring psychiatric symptoms in opioid-dependent women: the prevalence of antenatal and postnatal depression. Am J Drug Alcohol Abuse. 2012;38(6):575–9.

Hudak ML, Tan RC, Committee on Drugs, Committee on Fetus and Newborn, American Academy of Pediatrics. Neonatal drug withdrawal. Pediatrics. 2012;129(2):e540–60.

Johnson RE, Jones HE, Jasinski DR, Svikis DS, Haug NA, et al. Buprenorphine treatment of pregnant opioid–dependent women: maternal and neonatal outcomes. Drug Alcohol Depend. 2001;63(1):97–103.

Jones HE, Burns L, Gourarier L, Peles E, Springer-Kremser M, et al. A multi-national pre-consensus survey: the principles of treatment of substance Use disorders during pregnancy. Drug Alcohol Depend. 2010a;70(3):327–30.

Jones HE, Kaltenbach K, Heil SH, Stine SM, Coyle MG, et al. Neonatal abstinence syndrome after methadone or buprenorphine exposure. N Engl J Med. 2010b;363(24):2320–31.

Jones TB, Bailey BA, Sokol RJ. Alcohol use in pregnancy: insights in screening and intervention for the clinician. Clin Obstet Gynecol. 2013;56(1):114–23.

Kaltenbach K, Holbrook AM, Coyle MG, Heil SH, Salisbury AL, et al. Predicting treatment for neonatal abstinence syndrome in infants born to women maintained on opioid agonist medication. Addiction. 2012;107 Suppl 1:45–52.

Kandel DB, Huang FY, Davies M. Comorbidity between patterns of substance use dependence and psychiatric syndromes. Drug Alcohol Depend. 2001;64(2):233–41.

Kennare R, Heard A, Chan A. Substance use during pregnancy: risk factors and obstetric and perinatal outcomes in South Australia. Aust N Z J Obstet Gynaecol. 2005;45(3):220–5.

Kessler RC, McGonagle KA, Zhao S, Nelson CB, Hughes M, et al. Lifetime and 12-month prevalence of DSM-III-R psychiatric disorders in the United States. Results from the National Comorbidity Survey. Arch Gen Psychiatry. 1994;51(1):8–19.

Kessler RC. The epidemiology of dual diagnosis. Biol Psychiatry. 2004;56(10):730–7.

Klug MG, Burd L. Fetal alcohol syndrome prevention: annual and cumulative cost savings. Neurotoxicol Teratol. 2003;25(6):763–5.

Kraft WK, Dysart K, Greenspan JS, Gibson E, Kaltenbach K, et al. Revised dose schema of sublingual buprenorphine in the treatment of the neonatal opioid abstinence syndrome. Addiction. 2011;106(3):574–80.

Kraigher D, Schindler S, Ortner R, Fischer G. Pregnancy and substance dependency. Gesundheitswesen. 2001;63 Suppl 2:S101–5.

Law KL, Stroud LR, LaGasse LL, Niaura R, Liu J, et al. Smoking during pregnancy and newborn neurobehavior. Pediatrics. 2003;111(6 Pt 1):1318–23.

Lim S, Prasad MR, Samuels P, Gardner DK, Cordero L. High-dose methadone in pregnant women and its effect on duration of neonatal abstinence syndrome. Am J Obstet Gynecol. 2009;200(1): 70e1–70.e5.

Lipsitz PJ. A proposed narcotic withdrawal score for use with newborn infants. A pragmatic evaluation of its efficacy. Clin Pediatr. 1975;14(6):592–4.

Lumley J, Chamberlain C, Dowswell T, Oliver S, Oakley L, Watson L. Interventions for promoting smoking cessation during pregnancy. Cochrane Database Syst Rev. 2009 (3):CD001055.

Lund N, Pedersen LH, Henriksen TB. Selective serotonin reuptake inhibitor exposure in utero and pregnancy outcomes. Arch Pediatr Adolesc Med. 2009;163(10):949–54. Erratum in: Arch Pediatr Adolesc Med. 2009 Dec;163(12):1143.

Madden JD, Chappel JN, Zuspan F, Gumpel J, Mejia A, et al. Observation and treatment of neonatal narcotic withdrawal. Am J Obstet Gynecol. 1977;127(2):199–201.

Mangham LJ, Petrou S, Doyle LW, Draper ES, Marlow N. The cost of preterm birth throughout childhood in England and Wales. Pediatrics. 2009;123(2):e312–27.

Martin PR, Arria AM, Fischer G, Kaltenbach K, Heil SH, et al. Psychopharmacologic management of opioid-dependent women during pregnancy. Am J Addict. 2009;18(2):148–56.

Martin JA, Hamilton BE, Ventura SJ, Osterman MJ, Kirmeyer S, et al. Births: final data for 2009. Natl Vital Stat Rep. 2011;60(1):1–70.

McCarthy JJ, Posey BL. Methadone levels in human milk. J Hum Lact. 2000;16(2):115–20.

Metz V, Jagsch R, Ebner N, Wurzl J, Pribasnig A, et al. Impact of treatment approach on maternal and neonatal outcome in pregnant opioid-maintained women. Hum Psychopharmacol. 2011; 26(6):412–21.

Metz V, Kochl B, Fischer G. Should pregnant women with substance use disorders be managed differently? Neuropsychiatry. 2012;2(1):29–41.

Moore BC, Easton CJ, McMahon TJ. Drug abuse and intimate partner violence: a comparative study of opioid-dependent fathers. Am J Orthopsychiatry. 2011;81(2):218–27.

Najavits LM, Gastfriend DR, Nakayama EY, Barber JP, Blaine J, Frank A, et al. A measure of readiness for substance abuse treatment. Psychometric properties of the RAATE-R interview. Am J Addict. 1997;6(1):74–82.

National Drug Strategy Household Survey Report. 2011. Available from: http://www.fare.org.au/wp-content/uploads/2011/07/Alcohol-Consumption-During-Pregnancy-Final.pdf

National Survey on Drug Use and Health. 2007. Available from: http://www.samhsa.gov/data/2k7/pregCigs/pregCigs.pdf

National Survey on Drug Use and Health 2012. Available from: http://www.samhsa.gov/data/NSDUH/2012SummNatFindDetTables/NationalFindings/NSDUHresults2012.htm-ch2.6.

National Survey on Drug Use and Health. 2013. Available from: http://www.samhsa.gov/data/ NSDUH/2012SummNatFindDetTables/NationalFindings/NSDUHresults2012.htm#ch2.6

Nature Editorial. Putting gender on the agenda. 2010;465(7299):665.

Newman RG, Gevertz SG. Efficacy versus effectiveness of buprenorphine and methadone maintenance in pregnancy. J Addict Dis. 2011;30(4):318–22.

O'Donnell M, Nassar N, Leonard H, Hagan R, Mathews R, et al. Increasing prevalence of neonatal withdrawal syndrome: population study of maternal factors and child protection involvement. Pediatrics. 2009;123(4):e614–21.

Olesen J, Gustavsson A, Svensson M, Wittchen HU, Jonsson B. The economic cost of brain disorders in Europe. Eur J Neurol. 2012;19(1):155–62.

Osborn DA, Jeffery HE, Cole MJ. Opiate treatment for opiate withdrawal in newborn infants. Cochrane Database Syst Rev. 2010 (10):CD002059.

Pajulo M, Savonlahti E, Sourander A, Helenius H, Piha J. Antenatal depression, substance dependency and social support. J Affect Disord. 2001;65(1):9–17.

Patrick SW, Schumacher RE, Benneyworth BD, Krans EE, McAllister JM, et al. Neonatal abstinence syndrome and associated health care expenditures: United States, 2000-2009. JAMA. 2012;307(18):1934–40.

Pediatrics AAo. Policy statement: breastfeeding and the use of human milk; 2005.

Pichini S, Puig C, Zuccaro P, Marchei E, Pellegrini M, et al. Assessment of exposure to opiates and cocaine during pregnancy in a Mediterranean city: preliminary results of the "Meconium Project". Forensic Sci Int. 2005;153(1):59–65.

Regier DA, Narrow WE, Rae DS, Manderscheid RW, Locke BZ, et al. The de facto US mental and addictive disorders service system. Epidemiologic catchment area prospective 1-year prevalence rates of disorders and services. Arch Gen Psychiatry. 1993;50(2):85–94.

Rogers CE, Kidokoro H, Wallendorf M, Inder TE. Identifying mothers of very preterm infants at-risk for postpartum depression and anxiety before discharge. J Perinatol. 2013;33(3):171–6.

Rosen TS, Pippenger CE. Pharmacologic observations on the neonatal withdrawal syndrome. J Pediatr. 1976;88(6):1044–8.

Seligman NS, Salva N, Hayes EJ, Dysart KC, Pequignot EC, et al. Predicting length of treatment for neonatal abstinence syndrome in methadone-exposed neonates. Am J Obstet Gynecol. 2008;199(4):396.

Stene LE, Dyb G, Jacobsen GW, Schei B. Psychotropic drug use among women exposed to intimate partner violence: A population-based study. Scand J Public Health. 2010;38(5 Suppl): 88–95.

Trull TJ, Sher KJ, Minks-Brown C, Durbin J, Burr R. Borderline personality disorder and substance use disorders: a review and integration. Clin Psychol Rev. 2000;20(2):235–53.

Unger A, Jung E, Winklbaur B, Fischer G. Gender issues in the pharmacotherapy of opioid-addicted women: buprenorphine. J Addict Dis. 2010;29(2):217–30.

Unger A, Jagsch R, Jones H, Arria A, Leitich H, et al. Randomized controlled trials in pregnancy: scientific and ethical aspects. Exposure to different opioid medications during pregnancy in an intra-individual comparison. Addiction. 2011;106(7):1355–62.

Unger A, Fischer G, Finnegan LP. Drug dependence during pregnancy and the postpartum period. In: Wenzel A, Stuart S, editors. Oxford handbook of perinatal psychology. New York, NY: Oxford University Press; 2013.

United Nations Office on Drug and Crime. World Drug Report 2013 United Nations Publications; 2013.

US National Institutes of Health. NIDA Survey Provides First National Data on Drug Use During Pregnancy. National Pregnancy and Health Survey; 1992.

Velez M, Jansson LM. The opioid dependent mother and newborn dyad: nonpharmacologic care. J Addict Med. 2008;2(3):113–20.

Wachman EM, Hayes MJ, Brown MS, Paul J, Harvey-Wilkes K, et al. Association of OPRM1 and COMT single-nucleotide polymorphisms with hospital length of stay and treatment of neonatal abstinence syndrome. JAMA. 2013;309(17):1821–7.

Weinberger SM, Kandall SR, Doberczak TM, Thornton JC, Bernstein J. Early weight-change patterns in neonatal abstinence. Am J Dis Child. 1986;140(8):829–32.

Weiner SM, Finnegan LP. Drug withdrawal in the neonate. In: Gardner SL, Carter BS, Enzman-Hines M, Hernandez JA, editors. Merenstein and Gardner's handbook of neonatal intensive care. 7th ed. St. Louis: Mosby Elsevier; 2011. p. 201–22.

Werler MM, Bower C, Payne J, Serna P. Findings on potential teratogens from a case-control study in Western Australia. Aust N Z J Obstet Gynaecol. 2003;43(6):443–7.

Windsor RA, Boyd NR, Orleans CT. A meta-evaluation of smoking cessation intervention research among pregnant women: improving the science and art. Health Educ Res. 1998; 13(3):419–38.

Winklbaur B, Baewert A, Jagsch R, Rohrmeister K, Metz V, et al. Association between prenatal tobacco exposure and outcome of neonates born to opioid-maintained mothers. Implications for treatment. Eur Addict Res. 2009;15(3):150–6.

Winklbaur-Hausknost B, Jagsch R, Graf-Rohrmeister K, Unger A, Baewert A, et al. Lessons learned from a comparison of evidence-based research in pregnant opioid-dependent women. Hum Psychopharmacol. 2013;28(1):15–24.

Wojnar-Horton RE, Kristensen JH, Yapp P, Ilett KF, Dusci LJ, et al. Methadone distribution and excretion into breast milk of clients in a methadone maintenance programme. Br J Clin Pharmacol. 1997;44(6):543–7.

Wouldes TA, Woodward LJ. Maternal methadone dose during pregnancy and infant clinical outcome. Neurotoxicol Teratol. 2010;32(3):406–13.

Zahorodny W, Rom C, Whitney W, Giddens S, Samuel M, et al. The neonatal withdrawal inventory: a simplified score of newborn withdrawal. J Dev Behav Pediatr. 1998;19(2):89–93.

Complements and Alternatives to Psychopharmacology During Pregnancy

13

Kelly Brogan

Abstract

A discussion of pharmacologic and non-pharmacologic management of mental disorders in the pregnant woman is presented, with a focus on alternative health approaches and putative environmental/lifestyle contributors to depression and anxiety. The chapter explores some considerations of "modifiable risk factors" thought to play a role in epigenetic manifestations of infant and child illness. Several case examples illustrate the potential for integrative medicine in patients of reproductive age. Non-pharmacologic treatments reviewed include Bright Light Therapy, S-adenosylmethionine (SAMe), Cranial Electrical Stimulator, Essential Fatty Acids, Folate/L-methylfolate, Vitamin D, Diet, Exercise, Mindfulness.

Keywords

Alternative medicine • Integrative psychiatry • Fish oil • B vitamins • Bright light therapy • Diet • Exercise • Meditation

Women of reproductive age represent a population whose treatment demands expert consideration of a complex web of risks and benefits. Between 10 and 18 % of women suffer from depression and anxiety at a time in their lives when expectations are high for stability and wellness (Heron et al. 2004). A comprehensive approach to patient care endeavors to identify root causes of illness (digestive, nutrient, hormonal, and fatty acid imbalances) and to provide patients with tools for self-care that extend beyond compliance with a prescription and for alternatives to medication when that preference is expressed.

Kate: Discontinuation of medication

Board certified in Psychiatry, Psychosomatic Medicine, and Integrative and Holistic Medicine

K. Brogan (✉)
Faculty Member NYU/Bellevue Hospital Center, New York, NY 10016, USA
e-mail: drbrogan@kellybroganmd.com

M. Galbally et al. (eds.), *Psychopharmacology and Pregnancy*,
DOI 10.1007/978-3-642-54562-7_13, © Springer-Verlag Berlin Heidelberg 2014

Kate is a 32-year-old woman with a history of dysthymia and one depressive episode in college following a romantic disappointment. Her doctor has treated her since with sertraline. She married and seeks a consultation regarding discontinuation of her medication prior to attempting conception.

This patient represents an ideal candidate for a trial off medication and consideration of alternatives that may be more consistent with her preferences. During or after a taper of medication, risks and benefits of treatment with bright light therapy, S-adenosylmethionine (SAMe), and cranial electrical stimulation (CES) can be explored.

13.1 Bright Light Therapy

Often viewed as an evidence-based intervention for seasonal depression, bright light therapy continues to accrue data for treatment in the pregnant patient. In an open study on antenatal Major Depression, 60 min daily at 10,000 lux for 3 weeks resulted in a 49 % improvement as measured by the Hamilton Rating Scale for Depression (HAM-D) (Oren et al. 2002), and a 10-week, double-blind, randomized, placebo-controlled trial of 7,000 versus 500 lux demonstrated an effect size of 0.43 for the 7,000 lux group after 5 weeks, which could be considered comparable to antidepressant treatment (Epperson et al. 2004). In a study of patients with antepartum Major Depressive Disorder treated with 7,000 lux light therapy, there was an 81 % response rate with 69 % achieving remission (Wirz-Justice et al. 2011). A typical recommendation is for patients to get 30 min of morning exposure to a UV-filtered, 10,000 lux lamp, at the appropriate distance, with the lamp shining down on the face. Risk considerations include headache and activation in patients with a history of Bipolar Disorder.

13.2 SAMe

SAMe is a naturally occurring methyl donor in the human body that participates in a variety of synthetic reactions, including the formation of neurochemicals, methylation of phospholipids, glutathione synthesis, myelination, coenzyme q10, carnitine, creatine synthesis, and DNA transcription. To date, 48 clinical trials have been completed including head-to-head studies with traditional medications and randomized, placebo-controlled trials (Brown et al. 2002).

In a population of postpartum patients with subjective reports of depressive symptoms, doses of SAMe up to 1,600 mg achieved a 75 % reduction of symptoms in 30 days (50 % in 10 days) relative to placebo (Cerutti et al. 1993). There are eight studies (n = ~150) looking at the use of SAMe in the pregnant population for the treatment of cholestasis, which support its safety (Hardy et al 2003). SAMe is generally well tolerated with potential side effects including insomnia, anxiety, and gastrointestinal upset. Dosing is typically 400–2,400 mg depending on severity and tolerance.

13.3 Cranial Electrical Stimulation

Cranial electrical stimulators are FDA-approved patient-administered devices. They are indicated for the treatment of anxiety, depression, and insomnia. A low-intensity alternating current is transmitted across the skull for 20 min once-twice daily to promote alpha wave activity and to modulate neurotransmitters, endorphins, and cortisol (Gunther and Phillips 2010).

The five meta-analyses include 67 human studies ($n = 2,910$) and demonstrate the efficacy of the devices without report of adverse events (Smith 2008). There are no perinatal studies of the device; however, given the relative safety of electroconvulsive treatments in the pregnant population, adverse effects are unlikely. This device may represent a first-line option for women given that is it noninvasive with a low-side-effect profile.

Kate's therapy

After serial introduction of both light box therapy for 30 minutes in the morning, and cranial electrical stimulation for 20 minutes twice daily, Kate was successfully tapered off of her SSRI and went on to conceive 4 months later. She maintained this treatment throughout her pregnancy.

Tasha: Polypharmacy to monotherapy

Tasha is a 30-year-old woman with a history of recurrent depression, panic disorder, and generalized anxiety, currently treated with citalopram and prn lorazepam. She has been hospitalized twice for passive suicidality. She is at 8 weeks gestation and is not in a supportive relationship. She follows a vegan diet and exercises several times a week.

The goal in this patient is to optimize medication treatment towards monotherapy, as there is sparse evidence supporting the safety of polypharmacy. Augmenting or complementing her treatment with low risk, potentially high yield, choices might be a consideration. Essential fatty acids, vitamin D, L-methylfolate, and mindfulness meditation/breathing exercises would all be considerations.

13.4 Essential Fatty Acids

Phospholipids, free fatty acids, and triglycerides provide sources of energy and storage, structural support for membrane receptors, peptides, channels, and nuanced signaling systems as eicosanoid precursors.

Omega-3 fatty acids come under the umbrella of essential polyunsaturated fatty acids, which refers to their dietary requirement, and to their carbon/hydrogen structure. The best-studied representatives are docosahexaenoic acid (DHA) and eicosapentaenoic acid (EPA). EPA is a relatively minor structural component of nerve cell membranes influencing fluidity, but a major prostaglandin precursor, and DHA is a primary component of brain gray matter. Humans are assumed to be relatively inefficient at converting essential linoleic acid and alpha-linolenic acid precursors into the highly unsaturated fats and eicosanoids such as the omega-6 fatty acids dihomogammalinolenic acid (DGLA) and arachidonic acid (AA) and the omega-3 fatty acid EPA derived primarily from fish and pastured meat. A high carbohydrate diet and associated elevation in insulin and glucose levels may upregulate phospholipase A2 that cleaves fatty acids from phospholipids, disturbing membrane structure. Given the prevalence of refined vegetable oils in the American diet, some researchers posit that omega 6 fatty acids dominate dietary sources of omega-3s (a point of question is whether these vegetable oils in commercial foods represent trans or distorted fats when incorporated into human phospholipids). The anti-inflammatory effect of omega-3 fatty acids may be related to their interference with key inflammatory cytokines and competitive inhibition of the cyclo-oxygenase pathway, but there may also be a role in neurotrophic growth, genetic expression, and neurotransmitter production and function.

Currently, the only means of assessing individual fatty acid needs is through erythrocyte analysis, and the optimal dietary ratio ranges from 4:1 to 1:1 omega 6:3 depending on the source consulted. Disparity in benefit with omega-3 supplementation may relate to a lack of individual assessment of need. There is a risk that chronic oversupplementation of omega-3 from flax and/or fish oil may impair the production of omega-6 highly unsaturated fatty acids such as gamma linolenic acid (GLA), DGLA, and AA (precursors to prostaglandin E1 and prostacyclin) and contribute to imbalance through competitive inhibition of desaturase enzymes (Niculescu et al. 2013). The effect of GLA administration can be simplistically attributed to structural membrane support and production of the eicosanoid DGLA that serves to regulate AA (promoting its retention in the membrane) through its conversion to PGE1. At least three randomized, placebo-controlled trials of evening primrose oil (0.5–2 mg) in premenstrual syndrome suggest that GLA is an effective intervention potentially related to its potentiation of PGE1 and attenuation of prolactin sensitivity at the receptor site in the membrane (Horrobin 1983). The importance of the individual biochemical profile is an essential consideration.

Epidemiologic data suggests that prevalence of perinatal depression is inversely associated with fish consumption (Hibbeln 2002) and breast milk levels of DHA (Golding et al. 2009). A prospective cohort study of 54,000 women found that the lowest fish intake during pregnancy raised the likelihood of treatment with an antidepressant for up to 1 year postpartum (Strøm et al. 2009). Since this data emerged, four placebo-controlled, double-blind interventional trials have been done to assess the link between omega-3 fatty acids and perinatal depression, one of which has shown an association between supplementation and decrease in depressive symptoms (Su et al. 2008; Freeman 2009; Mozurkewich et al. 2013). These studies were limited by short duration (6–8 weeks), inconsistency in assessment for indication of supplementation, timing of intervention, confirmation of serum fatty acid response, high placebo response, and small size. A recent randomized trial of EPA, DHA, or soy-oil placebo demonstrated an inverse relationship between DHA supplementation/serum levels and Beck Depression Inventory (BDI) score for at-risk women (based on history and initial BDI score) in the third trimester, but improvement did not reach significance (Mozurkewich et al. 2013). Recent meta-analyses support dosing of a 3:2 EPA:DHA, 1–3 g daily supplement relative to placebo (Sublette et al. 2011). Given data that supports mitigation of risk for preterm birth, preeclampsia, and even behavioral development, supplementation is thought to represent a low risk, high yield option. It may be advisable to balance such supplementation with GLA from evening primrose given the limited duration of these studies and the aforementioned impact on omega-3 and omega-6 metabolism with omega-3 supplementation.

In the postpartum period, there is concern for the maternal reservoir of essential nutrients having been largely depleted by the needs of the growing fetus. Without appropriate repletion, these deficits may represent an underlying etiology of postpartum depression and anxiety. Immediately following delivery, omega-3 fatty acids are lower and omega 6:3 ratios higher in women who develop depressive symptoms at 6–10 months postpartum (De Vriese et al. 2003). One study demonstrated that recovery of maternal DHA levels at 32 weeks postpartum was slower in women with postpartum depressive symptoms (Otto et al. 2003), potentially reflecting reduced membrane fluidity. A prospective cohort study demonstrated that women with dietary ratios of omega-6 to omega-3 fats greater than 9:1 (unclear if adequate control for trans fat intake) had a higher incidence of postpartum depression as assessed by the Edinburgh Postnatal Depression Scale (EPDS). Given concerns over pollutants and mercury contamination of marine sources, many patients may benefit from considering a molecularly distilled, third party checked supplement.

13.5   Folate/Folic Acid/L-methylfolate

Folate (B9) is found in leafy greens, lentils, broccoli, and sunflower seeds and is an important cofactor in the synthesis of monoamines, reduction of homocysteine, and slowing brain breakdown of tryptophan. The relationship between folate and depression has been explored in studies linking low serum levels to poor treatment response, elevated homocysteine, to depression incidence (Folstein et al. 2007), and augmentation to increased likelihood of remission (Coppen and Bailey 2000). There are four transformation steps required to render folic acid a biologically available form of folate that can cross the blood–brain barrier to participate in the production of neurochemicals. One of these metabolites, 5-MTHF or L-methylfolate, is required for the production of biopterin, a cofactor for neurotransmitter production, and of methionine/SAMe from homocysteine (with B12 as a cofactor), influencing the production and function of neurotransmitters, DNA, and enzymes. Recent literature has focused on the role of genetic polymorphism for MTHFR in the metabolism of folate and associations with depressive illness (Gilbody et al. 2007).

For individuals with variants in one of two known genes C677T and 1298C, efficiency of conversion of folate or folic acid to L-methylfolate is compromised to varying extents. Bioavailability of folate and its metabolites can theoretically impact homocysteine and neurotransmitter levels as well as global DNA methylation, including placental methylation. Maternal MTHFR polymorphisms are associated with antenatal depression and may influence the fetal programming of serotonin transporter methylation and future functioning (Devlin et al. 2010). A recent study in the postpartum population demonstrated benefit with regard to EPDS scores at 21 months postpartum for women with C677TT polymorphism who supplemented with folic acid during pregnancy (Lewis et al. 2012). Bypassing this enzymatic conversion with supplementation of bioactive folate appears to be a potentially important treatment option. Thus, it is important to assess individual risk factors in terms of dietary/supplement intake in the first trimester and biomarkers for methylation.

13.6 Vitamin D

Our growing insight into the myriad of immune modulating, bone supporting, and mood modifying actions of vitamin D, a steroid hormone, has served to reveal its complexity. Several studies have suggested a relationship between low serum vitamin D (25OH) levels and depression, particularly in women, and in premenstrual dysphoria and seasonal depression. A recent study of 178 pregnant African-American women demonstrated a relationship between low first trimester 25-hydroxyvitamin D serum levels and second trimester antenatal depression diagnosed by the CES-D (Cassidy-Bushrow et al. 2012). Optimizing levels during pregnancy and postpartum likely represents a high yield intervention given the limitations of its endogenous production. While small amounts of vitamin D may be obtained through fish, eggs, and cod liver oil, sunlight has historically been the primary source. Monitoring levels with consideration of higher dosing ranges may be a reasonable approach; particularly given data suggests that doses of 4,000 IU in the second and third trimester may minimize risk of pregnancy complications such as gestational diabetes and preeclampsia. Supplementation to achieve a serum level above 40 ng/ml, which has been found to be the lower threshold required to optimize 1,25(OH)2D levels, often requires more than the recommended 400 IU daily, even up to 4,000 IU daily (Wagner et al. 2012). An Amsterdam birth cohort demonstrated that deficiency/insufficiency of vitamin D, as demonstrated by serum levels at 13 weeks gestation, was associated with significant depressive symptoms at 16 weeks of gestation (Brandenbarg et al. 2012). Postpartum serum levels less than 32 ng/ml have been correlated with increased incidence of depressive symptoms as quantified by the EPDS (Murphy et al. 2010).

Tasha's therapy

After an assessment of her vitamin D status, homocysteine, and MTHFR genetic profile, Tasha decided to focus on dietary changes including incorporating wild salmon and sardines twice a week, sunflower seeds, walnuts, pumpkin seeds, and pastured eggs and poultry. She obtained daily sun exposure of approximately 20 minutes from the hours of 10 to 2. These efforts, along with an established breathing practice helped to eliminate her need for additional benzodiazepine throughout her pregnancy.

Maggie: Postpartum mood disorder

> Maggie is a 34-year-old woman with a history of treatment with venlafaxine in the past and several failed trials of SSRIs. She is now 4 months postpartum with tearfulness, forgetfulness, weight gain, amotivation, fatigue, and mood flatness. She describes a diet consisting primarily of refined carbohydrates and sweet snacks.

Consideration of medication treatment in a breastfeeding mother is one that relies on technical case report/series data about maternal/fetal serum levels of drugs, protein binding, and peaks and troughs. Based on the work of lactation specialists and pharmacologists such as Thomas Hale, a collective assumption is made among providers that an infant serum level of less than 10 % of the maternal dose is considered a clinically insignificant exposure.

Prior to the consideration of medication treatment for new-onset postpartum depression, anxiety, and/or often comorbid obsessive/compulsive symptoms, a thorough evaluation for root cause etiology must be performed. The experience of pregnancy is one that draws heavily on a woman's native nutrient stores, and involves fluctuations in hormone levels and immunologic parameters. The anabolic state of pregnancy demands a synergy of nutrients not only to nourish the growing fetus, but also to support the tissues of reproduction (mammary, placental). Some theorize that the relative deficiencies of certain critical nutrients may make some women more vulnerable to postpartum psychiatric symptoms. A study of pregnant American women found that the majority were consuming below recommended amounts of iron, zinc, calcium, magnesium, folate, and vitamins D and E (Giddens et al. 2000) and that selenium supplementation may protect against the development of postpartum depression (Mokhber et al. 2011). Screening for serum levels of B12/methylmalonic acid, copper, chromium, magnesium, and zinc is indicated.

Immune modulation in the postpartum contributes to conservative estimates of a 10 % incidence of postpartum thyroiditis. Up to one-third of women experience thyroiditis with insomnia, anxiety, palpitations, irritability, and weight loss occurring 1–4 months postpartum, followed by hypothyroidism which may present 4–8 months postpartum and continue for 9–12 months. These symptoms may include weight fluctuations, constipation, hair and skin changes, depression, psychomotor slowing, and fatigue. While many cases spontaneously resolve within 1 year from onset, treatment is often indicated. Of 31 inpatient women with a diagnosis of postpartum psychosis, 19 % had detectable thyroid autoantibodies and 67 % of these women developed thyroid dysfunction by 6 months as compared to 20 % in the controls (Bergink et al. 2011). TSH at delivery has been shown to be a predictor of postpartum depression at 6 months postpartum (Sylvén et al. 2013). Screening for thyroid autoantibodies, levels of free hormone (T3 & T4), and TSH is the appropriate method of assessment.

For women with diagnosed hypothyroidism on T4 monotherapy, T3 may represent an appealing option for augmentation prior to consideration of antidepressant treatment (Nygaard et al. 2009). Given an established history in psychiatry of T3 augmentation, the support of active thyroid hormone is likely to improve mood and wellness parameters based on limited central nervous system conversion of T4 to T3, a nutrient-dependent process impeded by elevated cortisol (Cooke et al. 1992).

Maggie's Therapy

After serum screening, it was noted that Maggie had values consistent with B12 deficiency and hypothyroidism. Her symptoms resolved after 3 weeks on replacement therapy.

13.7 Oxidative Stress

Oxidative stress refers to an imbalance between the oxidant substances produced by mitochondrial metabolism and antioxidant neutralization through superoxide dismutase and glutathione peroxidase, vitamin E, flavonoids, copper, vitamin C, zinc, and selenium. Reactive oxygen species or free radicals that are not neutralized may then compromise the mitochondrial machinery, DNA, and the delicate polyunsaturated fats in cell membranes, rendering the cell unstable.

Specific inflammatory cytokines such as IL1B have been identified as potential early warning indicators of postpartum depression developing at 1 month (Corwin et al. 2008). Biochemical individuality, in concert with limited access to nutrient-dense foods and the metabolic demands placed on us by our chemical exposures, leads to a vulnerability that can be mitigated with some attention to these areas.

Studies are being published, demonstrating that whole food diets exert a protective effect with regard to depressive incidence and diets consisting of commercial and processed foods confer a dose-dependent risk (Sánchez-Villegas et al. 2012). Sugar and trans fats (hydrogenated and heated/processed vegetable oils) are implicated as an element of the modern diet that spurs pro-inflammatory cytokines and oxidative stress. One of the biomarkers of this biochemical stress is elevated homocysteine; another is preferential formation of quinolinic acid which 'steals' tryptophan from serotonin formation thought to occur in pro-inflammatory states associated with postpartum depression (Maes et al. 2002). Some experts theorize that processing of foods has rendered certain molecules inflammatory/neuroactive when undigested and absorbed through the gut wall. Two studies have raised questions about the role of foods such as gluten and dairy in the development of postpartum depression and psychosis, finding that plasma/cerebrospinal fluid morphine-like fragments derived from casein and gluten may have an association with maternal psychopathology (Lindström et al. 1984) and potentially mental illness in the child.

Generationally transferred alterations in microbial flora resultant from surgical birth, formula feeding (Song et al. 2013), antibiotics, medications such as proton pump inhibitors, and dietary exposures may account for intestinal dysbiosis and attendant psychiatric and immunologic sequelae. Preliminary investigation into the anxiolytic properties of probiotics is based on the bidirectional communication between the enteric and central nervous system through the vagus nerve (Messaoudi et al. 2011). With altered flora comes poor enterocyte health, poor micronutrient production by native bacteria, poor absorption and digestion (particularly of peptides) with zonulin-mediated intestinal permeability (Fasano 2012), and production by pathogenic bacteria and fungi of inflammatory cytokines (Campbell-McBride 2010). Congenital heart defects, preterm birth, and psychiatric pathology in the offspring are all outcomes that have been examined in the study of the impact of antenatal depression and antidepressant treatment in pregnancy. We may mitigate a third path of influence by promoting a diet devoid of trans fat, refined carbohydrates, and minimized in inflammatory sugars and associated advanced glycation end products.

Other sources of oxidative stress include environmental exposures to chemicals that place a metabolic burden on the system. With 80,000 registered agents in the Toxic Substances Inventory, a mere 200 have been studied for human safety parameters. An important case series supported by the Environmental Working Group and the Red Cross examined umbilical cords, identifying 287 toxic chemicals, 217 of which are known neurotoxins. Polybrominated diphenyl ethers (PDBE) flame retardants, pthalates, and bisphenol A (BPA) have been associated with adverse cognitive, endocrine, and motor outcomes in children (Jurewicz and Hanke 2011), and while environmentally ubiquitous, represent a modifiable exposure in our immediate environment.

Treatment between 1948 and 1971 of pregnant women with a synthetic estrogen, diethylstilbestrol, demonstrated epigenetically driven reproductive effects two generations later, leading to its subsequent ban. Intergenerational epigenetic changes may also be influencing the pregnancies we are working so hard to take into treatment consideration. Examination of germ cell inheritance of chronic disease phenotypes (tumors, kidney disease, immune dysfunction) in fourth-generation rats born of pesticide exposed ancestors has demonstrated, once again, that these non-DNA-sequence-related phenotypes could be passed down (Anway and Skinner 2006). This research serves to sound the alarm on understudied environmental toxins and their role in consideration of pregnancy exposures.

Given the myriad of epigenetic variables that are just now being explored in the literature, the most prudent approach appears to be one that advocates for an organic, whole foods, low-glycemic diet, awareness of environmental chemical exposures, focus on stress management behaviors and techniques, and a personally tailored treatment plan that reflects patient preference for evidence-based alternatives to medication and/or medications with a history of treatment benefit in the patient.

Conclusion

When a woman is planning a pregnancy, is pregnant, or postpartum, she may reach out to a mental health provider for expertise in this developing field of study. Each patient's history and current symptoms will inform the risk/benefit analysis around medication treatment during this sensitive period. After an informed consent and review of current psychotropic literature, the patient's preferences should play an integral role in the treatment plan. Complementary and alternative medicine offers an improved capacity to individualize treatment rather than providing a "yes" or "no" to a given prescription. Whether optimizing underlying nutritional factors associated with depression such as folate, essential fatty acids, and vitamin D or using targeted therapies such as

SAMe, cranial electrical stimulation, and bright light therapy, options for intervention multiply. Consideration of health and wellness parameters such as education around a whole food diet and minimization of environmental toxic exposures will also support a healthy pregnancy and postpartum experience for mother and baby.

References

Anway MD, Skinner MK. Epigenetic transgenerational actions of endocrine disruptors. Endocrinology. 2006;147(6 Suppl):S43–9.

Bergink V, Kushner SA, Pop V, Kuijpens H, Lambregtse-van den Berg MP, Drexhage RC, et al. Prevalence of autoimmune thyroid dysfunction in postpartum psychosis. Br J Psychiatry. 2011;198(4):264–8.

Brandenbarg J, Vrijkotte TGM, Goedhart G, Van Eijsden M. Maternal early-pregnancy vitamin D status is associated with maternal depressive symptoms in the Amsterdam born children and their development cohort. Psychosom Med. 2012;74(7):751–7.

Brown RP, Gerbarg P, Bottiglieri T. Adenosylmethionine (SAMe) for depression: biochemical and clinical evidence. Psychiatr Ann. 2002;32(1):29–44.

Campbell-McBride N. Gut and psychology syndrome. Cambridge: Medinform Publishing; 2010.

Cassidy-Bushrow AE, Peters RM, Johnson DA, Li J, Rao DS. Vitamin D nutritional status and antenatal depressive symptoms in African American women. J Women's Health. 2012;21 (11):1189–95.

Cerutti R, Sichel MP, Perin M, Grussu P, Zulian O. Psychological distress during puerperium: a novel therapeutic approach using S-adenosylmethionine. Curr Ther Res. 1993;53(6):707–16.

Cooke RG, Joffe RT, Levitt A. T3 augmentation of antidepressant treatment in T4-replaced thyroid patients. J Clin Psychiatry. 1992;53(1):16–8.

Coppen A, Bailey J. Enhancement of the antidepressant action of fluoxetine by folic acid: a randomised, placebo controlled trial. J Affect Disord. 2000;60(2):121–30.

Corwin EJ, Johnston N, Pugh L. Symptoms of postpartum depression associated with elevated levels of interleukin-1 beta during the first month postpartum. Biol Res Nurs. 2008;10 (2):128–33.

De Vriese SR, Christophe AB, Maes M. Lowered serum n-3 polyunsaturated fatty acid (PUFA) levels predict the occurrence of postpartum depression: Further evidence that lowered n-PUFAs are related to major depression. Life Sci. 2003;73(25):3181–7.

Devlin AM, Brain U, Austin J, Oberlander TF. Prenatal exposure to maternal depressed mood and the MTHFR C677T variant affect SLC6A4 methylation in infants at birth. PLoS One. 2010;16 (8):e12201.

Epperson CN, Terman M, Terman JS, Hanusa BH, Oren DA, Peindl KS, et al. Randomized clinical trial of bright light therapy for antepartum depression: preliminary findings. J Clin Psychiatry. 2004;65(3):421–5.

Fasano A. Leaky gut and autoimmune diseases. Clin Rev Allergy Immunol. 2012;42(1):71–8.

Folstein M, Liu T, Peter I, Buell J, Arsenault L, Scott T, et al. The homocysteine hypothesis of depression. Am J Psychiatry. 2007;164(6):861–7.

Freeman MP. Complementary and alternative medicine for perinatal depression. J Affect Disord. 2009;112(1–3):1–10.

Giddens JB, Krug SK, Tsang RS, Guo S. Pregnant adolescent and adult women have similarly low intakes of selected nutrients. J Am Diet Assoc. 2000;100(11):1334–40.

Gilbody S, Lewis S, Lightfoot T. Methylenetetrahydrofolate reductase (MTHFR) genetic polymorphisms and psychiatric disorders: a HuGE review. Am J Epidemiol. 2007;165 (1):1–13.

Golding J, Steer C, Emmett P, Davis JM, Hibbeln JR. High levels of depressive symptoms in pregnancy with low omega-3 fatty acid intake from fish. Epidemiology. 2009;20(4):598–603.

Gunther M, Phillips K. Cranial electrotherapy stimulation for the treatment of depression. J Psychosoc Nurs Ment Health Serv. 2010;48(11):37–42.

Hardy ML, Coulter I, Morton SC, Favreau J, Venuturupalli S, Chiappelli F, Rossi F, Orshansky G, Jungvig LK, Roth EA, Suttorp MJ, and Shekelle P. S-Adenosyl-L-Methionine for Treatment of Depression, Osteoarthritis, and Liver Disease. Evidence Report/Technology Assessment (Summary). 2003 Aug;(64):1–3.

Heron J, O'Connor TG, Evans J, Golding J, Glover V. The course of anxiety and depression through pregnancy and the postpartum in a community sample. J Affect Disord. 2004;80 (1):65–73.

Hibbeln JR. Seafood consumption, the DHA content of mothers' milk and prevalence rates of postpartum depression: a cross-national, ecological analysis. J Affect Disord. 2002;69 (1–3):15–29.

Horrobin D. The role of essential fatty acids and prostaglandins in the premenstrual syndrome. J Reprod Med. 1983;28(7):465–8.

Jurewicz J, Hanke W. Exposure to phthalates: reproductive outcome and children health. A review of epidemiological studies. Int J Occup Med Environ Health. 2011;24(2):115–41.

Lewis SJ, Araya R, Leary S, Smith GD, Ness A. Folic acid supplementation during pregnancy may protect against depression 21 months after pregnancy, an effect modified by MTHFR C677T genotype. Eur J Clin Nutr. 2012;66(1):97–103.

Lindström L, Nyberg F, Terenius L. CSF and plasma beta-casomorphin-like opioid peptides in postpartum psychosis. Am J Psychiatry. 1984;141(9):1059–66.

Maes M, Verkerk R, Bonaccorso S, Ombelet W, Bosmans E, Scharpé S. Depressive and anxiety symptoms in the early puerperium are related to increased degradation of tryptophan into kynurenine, a phenomenon which is related to immune activation. Life Sci. 2002;71 (16):1837–48.

Messaoudi M, Lalonde R, Violle N, Javelot H, Desor D, Nejdi A, et al. Assessment of psychotropic-like properties of a probiotic formulation (Lactobacillus helveticus R0052 and Bifidobacterium longum R0175) in rats and human subjects. Br J Nutr. 2011;105(5):755–64.

Mokhber N, Namjoo M, Tara F, Boskabadi H, Rayman MP, Ghayour-Mobarhan M, et al. Effect of supplementation with selenium on postpartum depression: a randomized double-blind placebo-controlled trial. J Matern Fetal Neonatal Med. 2011;24(1):104–8.

Mozurkewich EL, Clinton CM, Chilimigras JL, Hamilton SE, Allbaugh LJ, Berman DR, et al. The mothers, omega-3, and mental health study: a double-blind, randomized controlled trial. Am J Obstet Gynecol. 2013;208(4):313.e1-9.

Murphy PK, Mueller M, Hulsey TC, Ebeling MD, Wagner CL. An exploratory study of postpartum depression and vitamin D. J Am Psychiatr Nurses Assoc. 2010;16(3):170–7.

Niculescu MD, Lupu DS, Craciunescu CN. Perinatal manipulation of α-linolenic acid intake induces epigenetic changes in maternal and offspring livers. FASEB J. 2013;27(1):350–8.

Nygaard B, Jensen EW, Kvetny J, Jarløv A, Faber J. Effect of combination therapy with thyroxine (T4) and 3,5,3'-triiodothyronine versus T4 monotherapy in patients with hypothyroidism, a double-blind, randomised cross-over study. Eur J Endocrinol. 2009;161(6):895–902.

Oren DA, Wisner KL, Spinelli M, Epperson CN, Peindl KS, Terman JS, et al. An open trial of morning light therapy for treatment of antepartum depression. Am J Psychiatry. 2002;159 (4):666–9.

Otto S, De Groot RH, Hornstra G. Increased risk of postpartum depressive symptoms is associated with slower normalization after pregnancy of the functional docosahexaenoic acid status. Prostaglandins Leukot Essent Fatty Acids. 2003;69(4):237–43.

Sánchez-Villegas A, Toledo E, de Irala J, Ruiz-Canela M, Pla-Vidal J, Martínez-González MA. -Fast-food and commercial baked goods consumption and the risk of depression. Public Health Nutr. 2012;15(3):424–32.

Smith R. Cranial electrotherapy stimulation: Its first fifty years, plus three: a monograph. Tate Publishing & Enterprises: Oklahoma; 2008.

Song SJ, Dominguez-Bello MG, Knight R. How delivery mode and feeding can shape the bacterial community in the infant gut. Can Med Assoc J. 2013;185(5):373–4.

Strøm M, Mortensen EL, Halldorsson TI, Thorsdottir I, Olsen SF. Fish and long-chain n-3 polyunsaturated fatty acid intakes during pregnancy and risk of postpartum depression: a prospective study based on a large national birth cohort. Am J Clin Nutr. 2009;90(1):149–55.

Su KP, Huang SY, Chiu TH, Huang KC, Huang CL, Chang HC, et al. Omega-3 fatty acids for major depressive disorder during pregnancy: results from a randomized, double-blind, placebo-controlled trial. J Clin Psychiatry. 2008;69(4):644–51.

Sublette ME, Ellis SP, Geant AL, Mann JJ. Meta-analysis of the effects of eicosapentaenoic acid (EPA) in clinical trials in depression. J Clin Psychiatry. 2011;72(12):1577–84.

Sylvén SM, Elenis E, Michelakos T, Larsson A, Olovsson M, Poromaa IS, et al. Thyroid function tests at delivery and risk for postpartum depressive symptoms. Psychoneuroendocrinology. 2013;38(7):1007–13.

Wagner CL, Taylor SN, Johnson DD, Hollis BW. The role of vitamin D in pregnancy and lactation: emerging concepts. Womens Health. 2012;8(3):323–40.

Wirz-Justice A, Bader A, Frisch U, Stieglitz R-D, Alder J, Bitzer J, et al. A randomized, double-blind, placebo-controlled study of light therapy for antepartum depression. J Clin Psychiatry. 2011;72(7):986–93.

Electroconvulsive Therapy in Pregnancy

14

Raju Lakshmana, Richard Hiscock, Megan Galbally, Alison Fung, Susan Walker, Gaynor Blankley, and Anne Buist

Abstract

Modified Electroconvulsive Therapy (ECT) is a highly effective treatment in psychiatry despite variable community views. It is considered a first-line treatment option for severe depression (associated with high suicide risk, catatonic signs, and/or psychotic symptoms), functional catatonia, and severe psychotic agitation (acute mania or psychosis). It is also an effective treatment option for depression that is unresponsive to multiple trials of antidepressant medications with response rates close to 70 % in some studies. The current evidence suggests that pregnant women who present with the above indications for ECT should not per se be excluded from accessing ECT. There are specific considerations associated with ECT use in pregnancy and this chapter will summarize the principles of safety and effective use of ECT in pregnant patients to optimize perinatal outcomes. The chapter will not go into details of ECT electrophysiology and techniques that can be accessed from other texts and guidelines.

Keywords

Electroconvulsive therapy (ECT) • Pregnancy

R. Lakshmana (✉)
University of Melbourne, Melbourne, Australia

Northpark Private Hospital, Cnr Plenty and Greenhills Roads, Bundoora, Victoria 3083, Australia
e-mail: rraju@unimelb.edu.au

R. Hiscock • S. Walker
University of Melbourne, Melbourne, Australia

Mercy Hospital for Women, 163 Studley Rd Heidelberg, VIC 3084, Australia

M. Galbally • A. Fung • G. Blankley
Mercy Hospital for Women, 163 Studley Rd Heidelberg, VIC 3084, Australia

A. Buist
University of Melbourne, Melbourne, Australia

14.1   Introduction

Electroconvulsive Therapy (ECT) is an effective treatment for severe depression, with both rapid onset of action and high response rates compared to available pharmacological treatments (Pagnin et al. 2004). However, the evidence for safety and efficacy of ECT specifically in pregnancy is limited. There are no randomized controlled trials and the literature tends to be limited to case reports, case series, and review articles.

The stigma and concerns that limit the use of ECT in the general adult population also limit the numbers of pregnant patients receiving ECT, making it a relatively rare treatment. The infrequency with which it occurs necessitates that all possible precautions should be undertaken and that ideally women who require ECT in pregnancy should be managed in a setting that has adequate experience and resources to ensure safety for both the pregnant woman and the fetus.

There are specific concerns associated with the use of ECT in pregnant patients and these relate to the effects of general anesthesia and electrical induction of seizure on maternal, fetal, and obstetric outcomes. Clinicians undertaking ECT in pregnant women should also be cognizant of potential medico-legal issues.

This chapter will cover the key areas for administration of ECT in pregnancy, namely indications, barriers, and risks of ECT in pregnancy including longer term outcomes in children born to women who have received ECT during pregnancy. It will conclude with a discussion of guiding principles and specific recommendations for safe administration of ECT in pregnancy

14.2   Indications and Barriers for ECT in Pregnancy

14.2.1 Indications

Indications for ECT in pregnancy are similar to those in non-pregnant adult patients (Table 14.1). There is good evidence to support the consideration of ECT treatment in severe depression, particularly where there has been a failure to respond to medication (Prudic et al. 1990, 1996), or when the risks associated with the illness require a quicker treatment response than that usually occurs with pharmacological treatment (Pagnin et al. 2004). ECT is also one of the most effective treatment options for puerperal psychosis (Reed et al. 1999). When considering the place of ECT as a treatment for severely unwell pregnant women it must be compared to both pharmacological treatments that also carry a significant risk–benefit profile (see Chap. 6 for further discussion) and the risks of not treating the patient (Fig. 14.1). Three reviews (Saatcioglu and Tomruk 2011; Anderson and Reti 2009; Miller 1994) and a recent retrospective case series (Bulut et al. 2013) all conclude that ECT is relatively safe and effective as a treatment in pregnancy.

Anderson and Reti reviewed all published literature relating to ECT in pregnancy (2009). They described a total of 339 women receiving ECT during pregnancy; 25 adverse fetal effects were reported of which 11 were deaths. However,

Table 14.1 Indications for ECT in pregnancy

Moderate to severe Major Depression (unipolar or bipolar):
- Where there has been a failure of antidepressant medication or
- If the severity of symptoms and the risk to life is such that there is a need for rapid improvement
  - Suicidal
  - Inadequate oral intake and is at risk of malnutrition or dehydration
  - Severe psychotic features
  - Agitation
  - Catatonia

Catatonic states associated with any psychiatric condition

Mania

Mixed Affective states

Schizophrenia with prominent affective symptoms

Schizoaffective disorders

Puerperal Psychosis

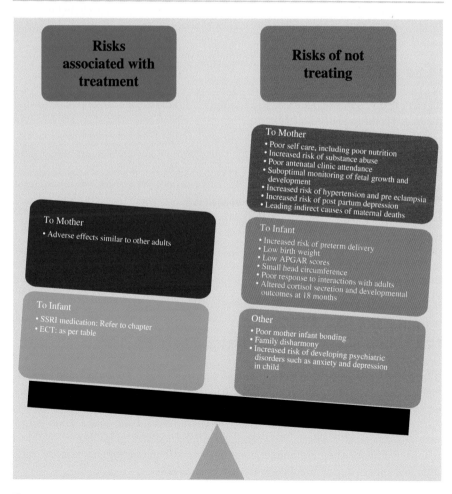

Fig. 14.1 Balancing risks of treating depression in pregnancy

only one death seemed to be related to ECT (Anderson and Reti 2009) [see Sect. 14.3.1, point (4)]. In another review of all reported cases of ECT in pregnancy between 1942 and 1991, adverse events or complications were reported in 28 cases (9.3 %)—miscarriage was reported in 5 cases (1.6 %) which is comparable to the general population, and neonatal death or still birth was noted in 3 cases; however, factors other than ECT were considered responsible in these cases (Miller 1994). Another case report of miscarriage following ECT in the first trimester was published in 1998 (Echevarria Moreno et al. 1998): the patient developed profuse vaginal bleeding after the third ECT session and lost the fetus at 8 weeks gestation.

Collectively theses studies suggest an incidence of adverse events close to 10 %. With limited evidence to support biological plausibility and the virtual impossibility of demonstrating association by clinical studies, one has to exercise caution in utilizing ECT during all trimesters of pregnancy (Richards 2007). These clinical concerns over potential risks, as well as women's treatment preferences, make this a rarely used treatment. Interestingly, Wheeldon et al. (1999) found over 80 % of patients receiving ECT were 'satisfied' with their treatment experience; however, these findings were not supported by a later systematic review (Rose et al. 2003).

14.2.2 Barriers

Barriers to ECT in pregnancy are not simply attitudinal, but also involve having adequate facilities and sufficiently experienced staff to ensure that it is carried out in a safe manner for the pregnant woman and fetus. This includes psychiatrists experienced in having administered ECT in pregnancy, obstetric and midwifery staff with mental health competencies and willingness to attend the ECT suite if required, access to fetal monitoring equipment and anesthetic staff who are familiar with protocols around administering anesthesia to pregnant women and for ECT. This inherently limits ECT to centers where maternity care and psychiatric care coincide. The geographical barriers and costs associated with this level of care may be prohibitive for both individuals and services. In some regions, there are legislative barriers for ECT treatment such as the requirement for clearance from a legislative body if the patient is unable to provide informed consent to the proposed treatment (e.g., Mental Health Act).

14.2.3 Risks of Untreated Psychiatric Illness (Fig. 14.1)

All treatments in pregnancy carry potential risks, not just for the expectant mother, but also for the fetus. Studies in the area of psychotropic medication exposure suggest that examination of risks should not just focus on those apparent at delivery, such as malformations, prematurity, and impaired fetal growth, but also on longer term outcomes for children. However, potential concerns must also be weighed against the increasing literature about risks to offspring born to women with untreated illness during pregnancy (Deave et al. 2008).

Adverse outcomes for the women with untreated mental illness during pregnancy include poor self-care and poor nutrition (Zuckerman et al. 1989), increased risk of substance abuse, poor antenatal clinic attendance, suboptimal monitoring of fetal growth and development (Leigh and Milgrom 2008; Bonari et al. 2004; Bansil et al. 2010), increased risk of hypertension and pre-eclampsia (Kurki et al. 2000), and increased risk of postpartum depression (Evans et al. 2001). Also, maternal mental illness has been one of the leading indirect causes of maternal deaths in the UK and Australia (Oates 2003). Adverse outcomes for the infants born to women with untreated mental illness during pregnancy include increased risk of preterm delivery (Wisner et al. 2009; Alder et al. 2007), low birth weight (Diego et al. 2009; Field et al. 2004, 2006), low APGAR scores (Alder et al. 2007), small head circumference (Lusskin et al. 2007), poor response to interactions with adults (Field et al. 2006), altered cortisol secretion and altered developmental outcomes at 18 months (Deave et al. 2008). In addition, prenatal depression has been associated with poor mother–infant bonding (Lusskin et al. 2007), family disharmony (Burke 2003), and long-term effects on offspring, with adolescents at increased risk of developing psychiatric disorders such as anxiety and depression (Halligan et al. 2009; Pawlby et al. 2009).

ECT is a faster and more effective treatment for severe depression than the available pharmacological treatments (Pagnin et al. 2004). These benefits need to be balanced against the potential maternal and fetal risks of ECT during pregnancy, these issues are discussed below.

14.3 Risks Associated with ECT in Pregnancy

14.3.1 Risks Related to Electrical Stimulus and Seizure During ECT

1. **Premature Labor**: Induction of premature labor appears to be the most frequent adverse maternal event in ECT. Preterm labor and/or increased uterine activity were reported in 3.5 % of 339 cases reviewed (Anderson and Reti 2009). Given that the electroconvulsive current does not pass through the uterus, other physiologic and pathophysiologic factors must be considered. After electroconvulsive stimulation, levels of several hormones change—oxytocin rises and reaches a peak a few minutes post seizure and may induce labor by stimulating uterine contractions (Griffiths et al. 1989). In addition, infection, dehydration, and hypoxia are all risk factors for premature labor. Tocodynamometry during ECT administration can be used to monitor uterine activity. In the event of uterine contractions, tocolysis with beta 2-adrenergic agonists, such as terbutaline, can be administered (UK ECT Review Group 2003).

2. **Issues Related to Seizure Activity**: Expectant mother's motor activity during ECT is not detrimental to the fetus; however, physical injury to the expectant mother or resultant hypoxia in the expectant mother could be harmful to the fetus. This can be prevented by both pre-oxygenation and monitoring for hypoxemia using pulse-oximetry, adequate muscle relaxation, and taking prompt steps to limit prolonged seizures (>120 s) or delayed seizures. There

has been one case report of fetal demise linked to status epilepticus in an expectant mother following an ECT session where the mother had a prolonged seizure for 200 s (Balki et al. 2006). There is no harmful impact of the charge delivered on the fetus as the current does not pass through the uterus. Similarly, procedures such as cardioversion, which utilize electrical charges similar to ECT, are not associated with any specific fetal adverse effects (Lam and Chow 2003).

3. **Placental Abruption**: There is a profound sympathetic discharge associated with the tonic-clonic phase of a seizure that can lead to significant utero-placental vasoconstriction, severe maternal hypertension, and fluctuations in blood pressure—all of these can theoretically cause fetal distress. Transient hypertension may also increase the risk of placental abruption (Sherer et al. 1991).

4. **Neonatal Mortality**: There is one report of multiple deep interhemispheric cerebral infarcts in a baby born to a mother who received multiple ECT treatments during pregnancy; her last ECT treatment was 2 weeks prior to birth of the baby whose delivery was induced due to pre-eclampsia. The authors discuss that a cause and effect relationship cannot be established, but highlight the need for vigilance and monitoring in view of the temporal correlation of the adverse event to ECT (Pinette et al. 2007; Richards 2007).

5. **Non-Pregnancy-Related Complications**: As with non-pregnant patients, con-fusion, memory loss, muscle soreness, and headache can occur post-ECT (Smith 1956).

14.3.2 Risks Associated with Anesthesia for ECT in Pregnancy and Strategies to Minimize them

The general principles of anesthesia for ECT in the non-pregnant patient apply in the pregnant woman. If the gestation is less than 14–16 weeks, these techniques can be safely used without modification. After this gestation, the physiological and anatomical changes associated with pregnancy require additional measures to maximize the safety of both mother and fetus.

1. **Fetal Arrhythmias**: Fetal bradyarrhythmias are common, they occurred at a rate of 2.7 % in cases reviewed by Anderson and Reti (2009), and these are mostly transient and are most likely secondary to fetal hypoxia experienced during the procedure. Adequate pre-oxygenation is essential, but hyperventilation should be avoided as respiratory alkalosis can hinder transfer of oxygen to fetal hemoglobin from the maternal circulation (Miller 1994). Maintenance of adequate oxygenation during the apneic period is also critical. The combination of both increased oxygen consumption and ventilation perfusion mismatch predisposes to hypoxemia. Pre-oxygenation with 100 % oxygen, for at least 3 min, delivered at high flow via an anesthetic circuit using a well-applied anesthetic facemask is recommended.

2. **Aspiration Pneumonitis**: Progesterone-related relaxation of the lower esopha-geal sphincter and a rise in intra-gastric pressure (secondary to the gravid uterus) lead to an increased risk of gastric reflux. Furthermore, pregnancy-related gastric

hyperacidity increases the risk of acid aspiration syndrome should substantial reflux occur. All pregnant women should receive pre-induction antacid prophylaxis. This may be achieved using a once-daily oral dose of a proton pump inhibitor over the duration of ECT therapy (Yau et al. 1992). Protected rapid sequence intubation using both cricoid pressure and tracheal intubation with a cuff endotracheal tube is required for airway protection. Estuation should only be performed when the patient is awake with intact airway reflexes.

3. **Risks Associated with Induction Agents**: Methohexitone or propofol alone is commonly used for ECT anesthesia in the adult non-pregnant patient. Currently these, and many other anesthetic agents, are under investigation for an association with neuronal cell injury in the fetal and early neonatal period (Davidson 2011); therefore it is prudent to minimize the dose of these agents. Combining them with a short acting (alfentanil) or ultrashort acting (remifentanil) narcotic substantially reduces the dose required, thereby reducing fetal drug exposure. The duration of effect is suitable for ECT treatment and assists with both stability of cardiovascular parameters and achieving a therapeutic seizure of adequate duration. These narcotic agents are considered safe in pregnancy (Smith et al. 2003; Nguyen et al. 1997). Methohexitone and propofol have a long history of safe use as the induction agents in women having cesarean section under general anesthesia and neither drug is associated with teratogenicity, and the doses required for ECT are expected to be similar to that required for the non-pregnant patient (Mongardon et al. 2009; Gin et al. 1997).

4. **Risks Associated with Muscle Relaxants**: The duration of action of suxamethonium increases after 30 weeks gestation secondary to fall in plasma pseudocholine esterase activity. Consideration should be given to substituting suxamethonium with the non-depolarizing muscle relaxant rocuronium which can then be rapidly (in less than 2 min) and completely reversed using sugammadex (Kadoi et al. 2011). The dose of sugammadex is based upon the dose of rocuronium administered and the interval between administration and reversal—requires a dose of 8–16 mg/kg in this setting (de Boer et al. 2007).

   Dosage of either agent should be chosen to achieve rapid neuromuscular blockade (suxamethonium 1–1.5 mg/kg, rocuronium 1.2 mg/kg), these being substantially larger than usually administered for ECT. Thus increased duration of suxamethonium action will require a longer time until extubation and therefore may require additional doses of induction agents to prevent awareness in the partially paralyzed patient.

   Suxamethonium and rocuronium in these doses do not cross the placenta in detectable amounts (Moya and Kvisselgaard 1961; Pacifici and Nottoli 1995).

5. **Aortocaval Compression and the Supine Hypotension Syndrome**: After 18–20 weeks gestation, when supine, the uterus falls posteriorly compressing the inferior vena cava and to a lesser extent the aorta. When combined with venodilatation and reduced sympathetic outflow secondary to anesthetic induction agents, marked falls in mean arterial pressure with reduced uterine perfusion can occur (Eckstein and Marx 1974; Kinsella and Lohmann 1994). From this period of gestation onwards all women should be positioned in a 10–15° left lateral tilt,

Table 14.2 Summary of risks

	Anesthesia		Electrical stimulus/ induced seizure	Other factors related to anesthesia
	Inducing Agent (propofol/ methohexitone)	Muscle relaxant (succinyl choline)		
Mother	No significant issues	Duration of action increases after 30 weeks of gestation	Status Epilepticus	Aspiration
Fetus	Potential neuronal cell injury (under investigation). Neither drug is associated with teratogenicity.	Passes placental barrier in negligible quantities	Fetal distress from fluctuations in maternal blood pressure and uterine hypo-perfusion	Bradyarrythmia due to hypoxemia during apnoeic phase
Pregnancy	Long history of use of propofol and methoxitone in pregnancy for caesarian section		Induction of premature contractions or labor; abdominal pain; placental abruption	Aortocaval compression and the supine hypotension syndrome after 18 weeks gestation

prior to induction, and this position should be maintained until the patient is awake and normotensive.

6. **Other Considerations**: Severe pre-eclampsia is associated with significant hypertension (systolic BP > 160 mmHg) and (often) upper airway edema. If any of these features are present, induction of anesthesia and the cardiovascular changes associated with ECT place the mother at high risk of complication beyond those already outlined. Consideration should be given to the timely delivery of the baby with ECT postponed until resolution of pre-eclampsia related changes in the early postpartum period. Table 14.2 summarizes the risks associated with ECT to mother, fetus and pregnancy.

14.3.3 Longer Term Effects in Children of Mothers Who Were Exposed to ECT During Pregnancy

Follow-up of children (up to 6 years after birth) born to women who received ECT during pregnancy did not show any significant abnormalities in children (Forssman 1955; Smith 1956). Impastato et al. (1964) in their follow-up of 79 children described two as "mentally deficient"; however, they conclude that these abnormalities are unlikely due to ECT and recommend ECT as a treatment of choice in psychotic unmanageable women (Impastato et al. 1964). None of these studies used any standardized tools to screen for developmental issues and relied only on clinical impression.

14.3.4 Guiding Principles and Specific Recommendations for ECT in Pregnancy (Fig. 14.2)

Principles to Guide Clinicians Prescribing and Providing ECT to Pregnant Women

Pre-ECT
1. A thorough and collaborative assessment is required before a decision to prescribe ECT for a pregnant woman is made:
   (a) Clarifying clear indication for ECT: a second opinion from a perinatal psychiatrist is recommended in all cases to ensure that all other treatment options have been considered. It may be important to define symptoms that ECT is anticipated to relieve and these symptoms (e.g., suicidal thoughts) monitored using a validated scale.
   (b) Informed and collaborative decision making: a decision to prescribe ECT must involve obtaining informed consent from the patient and their significant carer/s where possible. Involving carers and families is critical in situations where the patient is clinically unable to provide informed consent due to their psychiatric condition. This decision must weigh up risks associated with ECT, the risks of not undertaking ECT and maintaining status quo (with possibility of deterioration in mental state), and risks of alternative treatments for their condition on expectant mother, fetus, and the pregnancy. This process needs to be documented as per informed consent guidelines of the hospital/health service.
   (c) Discussion with the patient's obstetric team: the decision to proceed with antenatal ECT treatment, rather than expedite delivery and treat postnatally, will be informed by the presence of concurrent obstetric morbidities (such as pre-eclampsia), fetal well-being, and gestational age.
   (d) Medico-legal issues: the decision to prescribe ECT or process of consenting a patient for ECT is determined by legislation in most places and this may vary from state to state within the same country (Harris 2006; Loo et al. 2010), and all practitioners must familiarize themselves with legislative requirements in their jurisdiction.
2. Clear communication and robust consultation: there should be adequate and documented consultation with an Obstetrician, Anesthetist (with experience in obstetrics), and Pediatrician (or Neonatologist) to assess suitability of the patient for general anesthesia and ECT. It is strongly recommended to convene a conference with all specialists and formulate a documented plan for the patient whilst receiving ECT.
3. Rationalization of pharmacotherapy to minimize effect on seizure threshold: all medications with potential anticonvulsant action should be ceased a few days prior to ECT, especially benzodiazepines and anticonvulsant mood stabilizers.

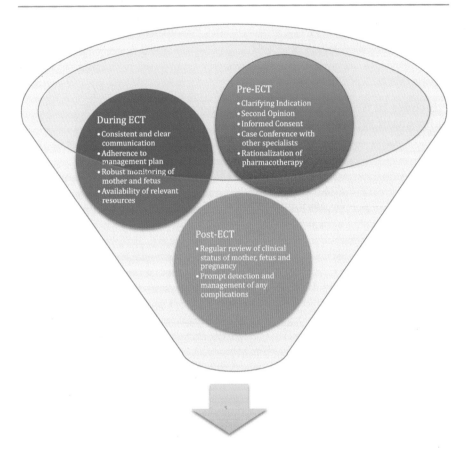

Critical Success Factors

Fig. 14.2 Principles guiding ECT in pregnancy

This will decrease the electrical dose required to induce a seizure and is likely to decrease the incidence of prolonged seizures or post-ictal confusion, both of which are common adverse effects when patients receive ECT whilst on such medication.

4. Careful evaluation of the need for concurrent treatment with other medications (e.g., antidepressants or antipsychotics): this needs to be undertaken utilizing a risk–benefit analysis framework in collaboration with the patient and their carer/s. ECT is effective in ameliorating acute symptoms, but has a limited role as continuation or maintenance therapy in pregnancy; however, the treatments may be spaced out prior to cessation of the acute course to assess stability of response. However, there are a few case reports of continuation ECT in pregnancy

(O'Reardon et al. 2011; Bozkurt et al. 2007) and they indicate no adverse events, but we are wary of recommending continuation or maintenance ECT during pregnancy.

During ECT

5. Consistency of adhering to a management plan during ECT: this is critical to ensuring adequate monitoring and preventing negative outcomes for patients and practitioners. Most ECT is provided by specialists and clinicians who are not necessarily part of the primary treatment team and are on a roster; therefore adherence to a management plan and clear communication between the ECT teams and the treating team is of paramount importance.
6. It is advisable that the patient spends the least amount of time under general anesthesia. The use of lower doses of anesthetic agents and ECT techniques that limit the time needed under anesthesia is recommended. Consideration may be given to bilateral ECT (bitemporal placement of electrodes), given its superiority in the rate of symptom reduction (Kellner et al. 2010a) and speed of onset of antidepressant effect (Kellner et al. 2010b) when compared to other commonly used electrode placements.
7. Adequate monitoring of potential risks should be undertaken and both documented and reviewed.

Post-ECT

8. Clinical review and monitoring of the patient, the fetus, and the gestation-appropriate pregnancy-related issues should occur on a daily basis. ECT may be discontinued or withheld in case of any doubt till the patient is reassessed and it is safe to continue with ECT.
9. Regular ongoing fetal surveillance with ultrasound and/or cardiotocography (CTG) is recommended for women undergoing ECT to evaluate serial fetal growth and well-being. CTG and biophysical profiles may be difficult to interpret in the setting of sedation and other medications; therefore, feto-placental Doppler may be a useful adjunct to assess placental sufficiency and fetal well-being.
10. Prompt detection and management of any complications related to the procedure.
11. ECT course should cease once the target symptoms improve in response to ECT.

Recommended Practice (Table 14.3)

- Specialized anesthetic requirements in patients after 14 weeks gestation include:
  1. Maintenance of uterine perfusion (IV crystalloid fluid preloading, left lateral or pelvic wedge tilt, and maternal blood pressure control).
  2. Avoidance of maternal hypoxemia (pre-oxygenation with 100 % FiO2 for 3 min).

Table 14.3 Recommended practice whilst performing ECT during pregnancy

Anesthetic	Obstetric	Psychiatric
Maintenance of uterine perfusion Avoidance of maternal hypoxaemia Maternal airway protection Minimal effective dosing of anesthetic agents Monitoring of vital signs until patient is stable.	If gestational age is 14–25 weeks, monitor the fetal heart rate via handheld Doppler If gestational age is 26+ weeks, an obstetrician or senior obstetric trainee to be present (where possible) to continuously monitor the fetus using CTG before, during and post-ECT until the trace returns to normal	Monitor and prevent prolonged seizure Avoid hyperventilation to lower seizure threshold Recommend bilateral ECT, avoids multiple stimulations Close monitoring of mental state to assess response to ECT

3. Maternal airway protection (usually rapid sequence endotracheal intubation with cricoid pressure).
4. Minimal effective dosing of induction agent/s.
5. Maximal muscle relaxation to achieve a well-modified seizure with ECT.
6. Close monitoring of vital signs and maintenance of adequate oxygenation and maternal blood pressure.

- Obstetric monitoring:
  1. A baseline assessment of fetal growth and well-being, including relevant feto-placental Doppler examination, is recommended, given the potential for placental insufficiency and provoking fetal compromise in patients undergoing ECT.
  2. If gestational age is 14–25 weeks, an appropriately trained clinician (e.g., Midwife) should be present in the ECT suite to monitor the fetal heart rate pre- and post-ECT via handheld Doppler.
  3. If gestational age is 26+ weeks, an obstetrician or senior obstetric trainee should be present in ECT suite, where possible, to continuously monitor the fetus using CTG before, during, and post-ECT to ensure fetal well-being. The complex clinical setting of anesthesia and induced seizure due to ECT in women who may be receiving multiple or high-dose psychiatric medications may affect CTG interpretation, but the presence of a prolonged bradycardia should prompt intervention with standard intrauterine resuscitative measures including control of blood pressure, left lateral tilt, fluid resuscitation, and tocolysis in the event of significant uterine activity.

- Psychiatric aspects:
  1. ECT dosing and administration can proceed as normal. However, it is important to avoid a prolonged seizure and the seizure must be terminated promptly if it is prolonged (longer than 120 s).
  2. It is preferable to use techniques that both minimize the time under anesthesia and are likely to produce an effective treatment (supra-threshold seizure). We would recommend utilization of bilateral placement of electrodes as this technique has quick onset of action, requires less elaborate titration, and has

been in use for the longest period (Kellner et al. 2010a, b). However, the technique and dosing strategies may be tailored according to patient preferences and outcomes (especially cognitive) after discussion with the patient and consultation with a peer who is experienced in ECT.

3. The mental state of the patient needs to be closely monitored so that the course of ECT can be completed as soon as the target symptoms (e.g., suicidality, catatonia) improve.

Conclusion

Pregnancy is a time of increased risk of depressive symptoms and these symptoms can range in severity. Untreated depression in pregnancy has been associated with perinatal and neonatal complications and may even have longer term implications on infant development. Maternal mental illness has been one of the leading indirect causes of maternal deaths in both the UK and Australia. While many women are successfully managed with either psychological and pharmacological treatments or both, for a small minority the severity of symptoms and the risks to mother and baby may require consideration of ECT as a treatment option. ECT can be safely utilized in pregnancy provided careful consideration is given to potential ethical, medico-legal, and clinical risk issues.

References

Alder J, Fink N, Bitzer J, Hösli I, Holzgreve W. Depression and anxiety during pregnancy: a risk factor for obstetric, fetal and neonatal outcome? A critical review of the literature. J Matern Fetal Neonatal Med. 2007;20(3):189–209.

Anderson EL, Reti IM. ECT in pregnancy: a review of the literature from 1941 to 2007. Psychosom Med. 2009;71(2):235–42. doi:10.1097/PSY.0b013e318190d7ca.

Balki M, Castro C, Ananthanarayan C. Status epilepticus after electroconvulsive therapy in a pregnant patient. Int J Obstet Anesth. 2006;15(4):325–8. doi:10.1016/j.ijoa.2006.01.005.

Bansil P, Kuklina EV, Meikle SF, Posner SF, Kourtis AP, Ellington SR, et al. Maternal and fetal outcomes among women with depression. J Womens Health (Larchmt). 2010;19(2):329–34. doi:10.1089/jwh.2009.1387.

Bonari L, Pinto N, Ahn E, Einarson A, Steiner M, Koren G. Perinatal risks of untreated depression during pregnancy. Can J Psychiatry. 2004;49(11):726–35.

Bozkurt A, Karlidere T, Isintas M, Ozmenler NK, Ozsahin A, Yanarates O. Acute and maintenance electroconvulsive therapy for treatment of psychotic depression in a pregnant patient. J ECT. 2007;23(3):185–7. doi:10.1097/YCT.0b013e31806db4dd.

Bulut M, Bez Y, Kaya MC, Copoglu US, Bulbul F, Savas HA. Electroconvulsive therapy for mood disorders in pregnancy. J ECT. 2013;29(2):e19–20. doi:10.1097/YCT.0b013e318277cce2.

Burke L. The impact of maternal depression on familial relationships. Int Rev Psychiatry. 2003; 15(3):243–55.

Davidson AJ. Anesthesia and neurotoxicity to the developing brain: the clinical relevance. Paediatr Anaesth. 2011;21(7):716–21. doi:10.1111/j.1460-9592.2010.03506.x.

de Boer H, Driessen J, Marcus M, Kerkkamp H, Heeringa M, Klimek M. Reversal of rocuronium-induced (1.2 mg/kg) profound neuromuscular block by sugammadex. Anesthesiology. 2007; 107(2):239–44.

Deave T, Heron J, Evans J, Emond A. The impact of maternal depression in pregnancy on early child development. BJOG. 2008;115(8):1043–51.

Diego MA, Field T, Hernandez-Reif M, Schanberg S, Kuhn C, Gonzalez-Quintero VH. Prenatal depression restricts fetal growth. Early Hum Dev. 2009;85(1):65–70.

Echevarria Moreno M, Martin Munoz J, Sanchez Valderrabanos J, Vazquez GT. Electroconvulsive therapy in the first trimester of pregnancy. J ECT. 1998;14(4):251–4.

Eckstein KL, Marx GF. Aortocaval compression and uterine displacement. Anesthesiology. 1974; 40(1):92–6.

Evans J, Heron J, Francomb H, Oke S, Golding J. Cohort study of depressed mood during pregnancy and after childbirth. BMJ. 2001;323(7307):257–60.

Field T, Diego M, Dieter J, Hernandez-Reif M, Schanberg S, Kuhn C et al. Prenatal depression effects on the fetus and the newborn. Infant Behav Dev 2004; 27 SRC - GoogleScholar: 216–29.

Field T, Diego M, Hernandez-Reif M. Prenatal depression effects on the fetus and newborn: a review. Infant Behav Dev. 2006;29(3):445–55.

Forssman H. Follow-up study of sixteen children whose mothers were given electric convulsive therapy during gestation. Acta Psychiatrica et Neurologica Scandinavica. 1955;30(3):437–41.

Gin T, Mainland P, Chan M. Decreased thiopental requirements in early pregnancy. Anesthesiology. 1997;1997(86):73–8.

Griffiths EJ, Lorenz RP, Baxter S, Talon NS. Acute neurohumoral response to electroconvulsive therapy during pregnancy. A case report. J Reprod Med. 1989;34(11):907–11.

Halligan SL, Murray L, Martins C, Cooper PJ. Maternal depression and psychiatric outcomes in adolescent offspring: a 13-year longitudinal study. J Affect Disord. 2009;97:145–54.

Harris V. Electroconvulsive therapy: administrative codes, legislation, and professional recommendations. J Am Acad Psychiatry Law. 2006;34(3):406–11.

Impastato DJ, Gabriel AR, Lardaro HH. Electric and insulin shock therapy during pregnancy. Dis Nerv Syst. 1964;25:542–6.

Kadoi Y, Hoshi H, Nishida A, Saito S. Comparison of recovery times from rocuronium-induced muscle relaxation after reversal with three different doses of sugammadex and succinylcholine during electroconvulsive therapy. J Anesth. 2011;25(6):855–9.

Kellner CH, Knapp R, Husain MM, Rasmussen K, Sampson S, Cullum M, et al. Bifrontal, bitemporal and right unilateral electrode placement in ECT: randomised trial. Br J Psychiatry. 2010a;196(3):226–34. doi:10.1192/bjp.bp.109.066183.

Kellner CH, Tobias KG, Wiegand J. Electrode placement in electroconvulsive therapy (ECT): a review of the literature. J ECT. 2010b;26(3):175–80. doi:10.1097/YCT.0b013e3181e48154.

Kinsella SM, Lohmann G. Supine hypotensive syndrome. Obstet Gynecol. 1994;83(5 Pt 1):774–88.

Kurki T, Hiilesmaa V, Raitasalo R, Mattila H, Ylikorkala O. Depression and anxiety in early pregnancy and risk for preeclampsia. Obstet Gynecol. 2000;95(4):487–90.

Lam CM, Chow KM. Electric shock during pregnancy. Can Fam Physician. 2003;49:737.

Leigh B, Milgrom J. Risk factors for antenatal depression, postnatal depression and parenting stress. BMC Psychiatry. 2008;8:24.

Loo C, Trollor J, Alonzo A, Rendina N, Kavess R. Mental health legislation and psychiatric treatments in NSW: electroconvulsive therapy and deep brain stimulation. Australas Psychiatry. 2010;18(5):417–25. doi:10.3109/10398562.2010.508125.

Lusskin SI, Pundiak TM, Habib SM. Perinatal depression: hiding in plain sight. Can J Psychiatry. 2007;52(8):479–88.

Miller LJ. Use of electroconvulsive therapy during pregnancy. Hosp Community Psychiatry. 1994;45(5):444–50.

Mongardon N, Servin F, Perrin M, Bedairia E, Retout S, Yazbeck C. Predicted propofol effect-site concentration for induction and emergence of anesthesia during early pregnancy. Anesth Analg. 2009;109(1):90–5.

Moya F, Kvisselgaard N. The placental transmission of succinylcholine. Anesthesiology. 1961;22: 1–6.

Nguyen T, Chibber A, Lustik S, Kolano J, Dillon P, Guttmacher L. Effect of methohexitone and propofol with or without alfentanil on seizure duration and recovery in electroconvulsive therapy. Br J Anaesth. 1997;79(6):801–3.

Oates M. Suicide: the leading cause of maternal death. Br J Psychiatry. 2003;183:279–81.

O'Reardon JP, Cristancho MA, von Andreae CV, Cristancho P, Weiss D. Acute and maintenance electroconvulsive therapy for treatment of severe major depression during the second and third trimesters of pregnancy with infant follow-up to 18 months: case report and review of the literature. J ECT. 2011;27(1):e23–6. doi:10.1097/YCT.0b013e3181e63160.

Pacifici GM, Nottoli R. Placental transfer of drugs administered to the mother. Clin Pharmacokinet. 1995;28(3):235–69.

Pagnin D, de Queiroz V, Pini S, Cassano GB. Efficacy of ECT in depression: a meta-analytic review. J ECT. 2004;20(1):13–20.

Pawlby S, Hay DF, Sharp D, Waters CS, O'Keane V. Antenatal depression predicts depression in adolescent offspring: prospective longitudinal community-based study. J Affect Disord. 2009; 113(3):236–43.

Pinette MG, Santarpio C, Wax JR, Blackstone J. Electroconvulsive therapy in pregnancy. Obstet Gynecol. 2007;110(2 Pt 2):465–6. doi:10.1097/01.AOG.0000265588.79929.98.

Prudic J, Sackeim HA, Devanand DP. Medication resistance and clinical response to electroconvulsive therapy. Psychiatry Res. 1990;31(3):287–96.

Prudic J, Haskett RF, Mulsant B, Malone KM, Pettinati HM, Stephens S, et al. Resistance to antidepressant medications and short-term clinical response to ECT. Am J Psychiatry. 1996; 153(8):985–92.

Reed P, Sermin N, Appleby L, Faragher B. A comparison of clinical response to electroconvulsive therapy in puerperal and non-puerperal psychoses. J Affect Disord. 1999;54(3):255–60.

Richards DS. Is electroconvulsive therapy in pregnancy safe? Obstet Gynecol. 2007;110(2 Pt 2): 451–2. doi:10.1097/01.AOG.0000277540.63064.d3.

Rose D, Fleischmann P, Wykes T, Leese M, Bindman J. Patients' perspectives on electroconvulsive therapy: systematic review. BMJ. 2003;326(7403):1363. doi:10.1136/bmj.326.7403.1363.

Saatcioglu O, Tomruk NB. The use of electroconvulsive therapy in pregnancy: a review. Isr J Psychiatry Relat Sci. 2011;48(1):6–11.

Sherer DM, D'Amico ML, Warshal DP, Stern RA, Grunert HF, Abramowicz JS. Recurrent mild abruptio placentae occurring immediately after repeated electroconvulsive therapy in pregnancy. Am J Obstet Gynecol. 1991;165(3):652–3.

Smith S. The use of electroplexy (E.C.T.) in psychiatric syndromes complicating pregnancy. J Ment Sci. 1956;102(429):796–800.

Smith D, Angst M, Brock-Unte J, DeBattista C. Seizure duration with remifentanil/methohexital vs. methohexital alone in middle -aged patients undergoing electroconvulsive therapy. Acta Anaesthesiol Scand. 2003;47(9):1064–6.

UK ECT Review Group. Efficacy and safety of electroconvulsive therapy in depressive disorders: a systematic review and meta-analysis. Lancet. 2003;361(9360):799–808. doi:10.1016/S0140-6736(03)12705-5.

Wheeldon TJ, Robertson C, Eagles JM, Reid IC. The views and outcomes of consenting and non-consenting patients receiving ECT. Psychol Med. 1999;29(1):221–3.

Wisner KL, Sit DKY, Hanusa BH, Moses-Kolko EL, Bogen DL, Hunker DF, et al. Major depression and antidepressant treatment: impact on pregnancy and neonatal outcomes. Am J Psychiatry. 2009;166(5):557–66.

Yau G, Kan AF, Gin T, Oh TE. A comparison of omeprazole and ranitidine for prophylaxis against aspiration pneumonitis in emergency caesarean section. Anaesthesia. 1992;47(2):101–4.

Zuckerman B, Amaro H, Bauchner H, Cabral H. Depressive symptoms during pregnancy: relationship to poor health behaviors. Am J Obstet Gynecol. 1989;160(5 Pt 1):1107–11.

Index

M. Galbally et al. (eds.), *Psychopharmacology and Pregnancy*,
DOI 10.1007/978-3-642-54562-7, © Springer-Verlag Berlin Heidelberg 2014